COMPARISON OF TYPE I AND TYPE II DIABETES

Similarities and Dissimilarities in Etiology, Pathogenesis, and Complications

ADVANCES IN EXPERIMENTAL MEDICINE AND BIOLOGY

Recent Volumes in this Series

A Continuation Order Plan is available for this series. A continuation order will bring delivery of each new volume immediately upon publication. Volumes are billed only upon actual shipment. For further information please contact the publisher.

COMPARISON OF TYPE I AND TYPE II DIABETES

Similarities and Dissimilarities in Etiology, Pathogenesis, and Complications

Edited by

Mladen Vranic

Departments of Physiology and Medicine
and Banting and Best Diabetes Centre
University of Toronto
Toronto, Canada

Charles H. Hollenberg

Department of Medicine and
Banting and Best Diabetes Centre
University of Toronto
Toronto, Canada

and

George Steiner

Departments of Medicine and Physiology
and Banting and Best Diabetes Centre
University of Toronto and
Division of Endocrinology and Metabolism
Toronto General Hospital
Toronto, Canada

SPRINGER SCIENCE+BUSINESS MEDIA, LLC

Library of Congress Cataloging in Publication Data

Main entry under title:

Comparison of type I and type II diabetes.

(Advances in experimental medicine and biology; v. 189)
"Proceedings of a satellite symposium of the VIIth International Congresses of Endo-
crinology . . . held June 28–29, 1984, in Toronto, Canada" — T.p. verso.
Includes bibliographies and index.
1. Diabetes — Congresses. 2. Non-insulin-dependent diabetes — Congresses. I. Vranic,
Mladen. II. Hollenberg, Charles H., 1930–   . III. Steiner, George. IV. International
Congresses of Endocrinology (7th: 1984: Québec, Québec) V. Title: Comparison of
type one and type two diabetes. VI. Title: Comparison of type 1 and type 2 diabetes.
VII. Series. [DNLM: 1. Diabetes Mellitus, Insulin-Dependent — congresses. 2. Diabetes
Mellitus, Non-Insulin-Dependent — congresses. W1 AD559 v.189/WK 810C737 1984]
RC660.A15C66   1985   616.4′62   85-12159
ISBN 978-1-4757-1852-2   ISBN 978-1-4757-1850-8 (eBook)
DOI 10.1007/978-1-4757-1850-8

Proceedings of a satellite symposium of the VIIth International Congress
of Endocrinology entitled Comparison of Type I and Type II Diabetes:
Similarities and Dissimilarities in Etiology, Pathogenesis, and Complications,
held June 28–29, 1984, in Toronto, Canada

©1985 Springer Science+Business Media New York
Originally published by Plenum Press, New York in 1985

PREFACE

　　Five years ago, a new system of classification of the various types of diabetes was proposed. This publication provides an integrated picture of the latest information on the similarities and dissimilarites of two types of diabetes. It contains contributions from morphologists, physiologists, biochemists, immunologists, pathologists, geneticists, clinicians and epidemiologists. In the first section, the basis for the present classification and its limitations are discussed. In addition, there is a discussion of gestational diabetes and heterogeneity of some sub-classes of diabetes. The next section deals with genetics and immunology. The third section discusses abnormalities of insulin secretion and action on both the receptor and post-receptor levels. The role of gastrointestinal peptides in Type I and Type II diabetes is also considered. In the last section, both types of diabetes are compared with respect to diabetic complications. The closing section summarizes the present status and offers a stimulating view of future development. We hope that this book will be a useful source of information for both researchers and practicing clinicians.

M. Vranic
G. Steiner
C.H. Hollenberg

ACKNOWLEDGEMENTS

The Symposium from which this volume arose (June 28-29, 1984) was organized by the Banting and Best Diabetes Centre, University of Toronto. We would like to express our appreciation to the following sponsors: Ames Educational Institute, Ayerst Laboratories, Becton Dickinson Canada Inc., Canadian Soft Drink Association, Connaught Laboratories Limited, Connaught Novo Ltd., Eli Lilly Canada Inc., Hoechst Canada Inc., The Hospital for Sick Children Foundation, Nordisk, Nova Research Institute, Ross Laboratories, Sandoz Inc., Ault Dairies (Division of Ault Foods Ltd.), The Upjohn Company of Canada, Air Canada. The Symposium was part of the Ontario Bicentennial celebrations.

Special thanks is due to Dr. A.K. Hanna, Co-chairman of the organizing committee, Drs. A. Angel, J. Dupre, R.M. Ehrlich, E.A. Sellers, B. Zinman and especially to Mrs. Norah Rankin for their contribution to the organization of the Symposium.

ACKNOWLEDGMENTS

CONTENTS

ix

CONTENTS

COMPLICATIONS

CONCLUSIONS

CONTENTS

IDENTIFICATION OF SOME ISSUES AND QUESTIONS TO BE ANSWERED IN COMPARING TYPE I AND TYPE II DIABETES

Mladen Vranic

Department of Physiology & Medicine
University of Toronto
Toronto, Ontario

This chapter will attempt to identify some of the issues and questions arising from the present classification of and comparisons between Type I and Type II diabetes. Because these issues will also be dealt with in other chapters of this book in depth, it was not considered necessary to include herein a complete list of references.

It was felt that it was timely to review the present classification. About five years ago the National Diabetes Data Group proposed a new system for classification and diagnosis of diabetes mellitus and other categories of glucose intolerance.[1] This nomenclature has also been accepted by the World Health Organization's Expert Committee on Diabetes. Many questions and some controversies arose from this endeavour. At that time, the hope was expressed that this plan would stimulate further research so that some of the queries could be clarified in the ensuing years. The most pertinent conclusion of the classification system was that there is a clear distinction between Type I and Type II diabetes. A third subclass deals with diabetes caused by other conditions, while gestational diabetes is also identified as a separate entity. The nomenclature also identifies impaired glucose tolerance, previous abnormality of glucose tolerance and potential abnormality of glucose tolerance. In addition, criteria for diagnosis of diabetes have been standardized.

The following definitions are summarized from some of the conclusions of the National Diabetes Data Group entitled: "Classification and Diagnosis of Diabetes Mellitus and Other Categories of Glucose Intolerance".[1] It is proposed that this classification be used as a uniform framework in which to conduct clinical and epidemiological research so that more meaningful and

1

comparative data will be obtained on the scope and impact of the various forms of diabetes and other classes of glucose intolerance.

1. Insulin-dependent, ketosis-prone type of diabetes, which is associated with increased or decreased frequency of certain histocompatibility antigens (HLA) on chromosome 6 and with islet cell antibodies, be considered A DISTINCT SUBCLASS OF DIABETES (IDDM).

2. The noninsulin-dependent, nonketosis-prone types of diabetes, which are not secondary to other diseases be considered a SECOND DISTINCT SUBCLASS OF DIABETES (NIDDM). This subclass has been divided according to whether or not obesity is present and is further characterized by the type of treatment the patients receive or by other characteristics. It is believed that further heterogeneity within NIDDM and IDDM will be demonstrated.

3. Types of diabetes CAUSED BY OTHER CONDITIONS be considered A THIRD SUBCLASS OF DIABETES MELLITUS.

4. GESTATIONAL DIABETES be restricted to women in whom glucose intolerance develops or is discovered during pregnancy.

5. Individuals with plasma glucose levels between those considered normal and those considered diabetic be termed to have IMPAIRED GLUCOSE TOLERANCE.

6. Individuals with normal glucose tolerance who have experienced transient hyperglycemia be classed as PREVIOUS ABNORMALITY OF GLUCOSE TOLERANCE.

The suggestion that there are at least two subclasses of diabetes is not a new one. It has been put forward that dietary and exercise prescriptions contained in the book "Chikits Sthana"[2], written by the Indian physician Sushruta as early as 600 B.C. might have referred to Type I and Type II diabetics, one lean and emaciated, the other obese. In textbooks of diabetes one will find detailed descriptions of these types of diabetes and very often the focus is on the difference between them. We felt that insufficient emphasis has been placed on comparing the two diseases with respect to genetics, pathophysiology, metabolic abnormalities and complications. As it is necessary to review both similarities and dissimilarities, ideally each item under discussion should go through the process of comparing as well as contrasting. The impact of discovery of insulin on the well-being of Type I diabetes is well documented. However, throughout the world most diabetics can be classified as Type II. Moreover, it is only in a very small part of the world that Type I diabetes has such a prevalence that it affects up to 10% of the total diabetic population. Therefore, the importance of insulin discovery has not had such a dramatic impact in those ethnic groups where Type I diabetes is unknown or very rare. As indicated by Zimmet[3] and other epidemiologists, these groups include Japanese, Indians, Chinese, Phillipinos, American Indians, Eskimos, Maltese, Sri Lankans, South African Negroes, Polynesians, Micronesians and Melanesians. The impact of the discovery of insulin on Type II diabetes has not as yet been fully documented. The National Diabetes Data Group pointed out that in Type II diabetes, insulin treatment is needed only when other treatment modalities fail to maintain glucose values within acceptable limits. Since Type II diabetes is accompanied by insulin resistance, the indications of insulin treatment need to be more precisely outlined because excess insulin could further increase insulin resistance.

It is particularly important to evaluate at the present time the progress achieved with respect to the three aims for the new classification as identified by the National Data Group.

1. To serve as A UNIFORM BASIS on which to plan and conduct clinical research in diabetes, including its causes, treatment, development of complications, and prevention.

2. To serve as A FRAMEWORK for the collection of epidemiologic data on the etiology, natural history, and impact of diabetes and its complications in diverse populations throughout the world.

3. To aid the clinician in categorizing patients who have GLUCOSE INTOLERANCE or are at INCREASED RISK of developing diabetes.

The question which is germane to all topics covered in this book is whether or not the classification has indeed provided a uniform basis on which to plan and conduct clinical research in diabetes.

IS THE PRESENT CLASSIFICATION VALID AND SUFFICIENT?

The chapters of Drs. Bennett and Keen provide information as to whether a framework has indeed been provided for collection of epidemiological data. It is also of specific interest to find out more about epidemiology of patients with glucose intolerance who may be at increased risk of developing diabetes. Dr. Bennett[4] feels that the current system has at last begun to bring about some degree of standardization in relation to diabetes and that there is wider acceptance of the current criteria than had ever previously been achieved. However, the classification focuses on the phenotypic expressions of the disease with the hope that this could be adopted to incorporate new future findings in etiopathology. Some confusion still persists between the use of etiological and clinical parameters in differentiating diabetic types. The classification still omits the condition referred to as tropical diabetes, Type J or

malnutrition diabetes. Dr. Keen[5] feels that the greatest problem
is to determine where normality ends and the disease begins and that
is particularly dramatic with respect to impaired glucose tolerance,
where there is still discrepancy between the present nomenclature
and the WHO criteria. Due to inadequacies to defining impaired
glucose tolerance, the present ability to identify those at risk for
increased cardiovascular morbidity and mortality, or for development
of frank diabetes is limited. The definitions of Type I and Type II
diabetes are not perfect synonyms fo IDDM and NIDDM because epidemiologists do not as yet have precise measures for susceptibility
and environmental determinants.

Criteria for diagnosis of gestational diabetes had not been
fully developed 5 years ago. Drs. Freinkel and Metzger[6] described
how normal pregnancy alters every aspect of maternal fuel metabolism. A fraction of pregnant women (2.4%) is unable to cope with
those changes leading to glucose intolerance and gestational
diabetes which can be associated with increased perinatal complications and an increased risk of progression of frank diabetes.
Absolute insulinopenia is the most striking characteristic of
gestational diabetes. A longitudinal study is underway with the aim
of establishing abnormalities in the mother, which persist after
delivery. They feel that gestational diabetes with its effects on
the mother and child is one of the major public health frontiers in
diabetes.

It is further stipulated that the requirements of the classification are that THE CLASSES SHOULD BE MUTUALLY EXCLUSIVE, AND BE AS
HOMOGENEOUS AS POSSIBLE, AND THE PHENOTYPIC EXPRESSION OF THE
ABNORMALITY SHOULD BE WELL DEFINED. Yet, there is considerable
heterogeneity in both the Type I and Type II diabetes. Dr. Fajans[7]
describes in great detail a special form of diabetes which was
defined as maturity-onset diabetes in the young (MODY). It is a
non- or slowly-progressive diabetes in children, adolescents and
young adults with a strong familial association of diabetes. He
feels that both NIDDM and MODY exhibit a slow progression of glucose
intolerance while in Type I diabetes the development of this
decompensation is much faster. Sulfonylurea treatment of MODY
patients show clear extrapancreatic effects and an enhanced insulin
secretory response can persist over many years. Also, in contrast
to NIDDM, there is frequently normal sensitivity to exogenous
insulin. Therefore, it is important that MODY are not misdiagnosed
as Type I diabetics.

GENETICS AND IMMUNOLOGY

The observations which are crucial in the understanding of
differences between different types of diabetes relate to genetics.
Dr. Permutt indicates that concordance of diabetes in monozygotic

twins is more than 90% for NIDDM, but only 50% for IDDM. Genetic
studies indicate that most of the genetic liability for susceptibility to IDDM resides within the HLA gene locus alone located on
the short arm of chromosome 6. These studies became possible with
development of DNA recombinant technology. It is particularly
important that, as it appears, there is no HLA association with
NIDDM. Heterogeneity of the disease, and importance of many
environmental factors make it difficult to delineate genetics of
this disease more precisely at the present time. The main question
asked is whether regulatory and/or structural gene mutations are
contributing to NIDDM. Dr. Lernmark[9] indicates that in IDDM there
may be a defective immune response which leads to damage of
pancreatic beta cells. Indeed, inflammatory cells were found in the
pancreas of some patients. Many such patients have islet cell
surface antibodies specific for beta cells: 60% at diagnosis, but
only 25% after two years. It also appears that these patients may
exhibit cellular hypersensitivity to pancreatic extracts, indicating
an auto-antigen.

PATHOPHYSIOLOGY AND METABOLIC ABNORMALITIES

    The requirements further stipulate that THE CLASSIFICATION
SHOULD REQUIRE ONLY SIMPLE CLINICAL MEASUREMENTS. The
classification is, therefore, mainly based on measurements of plasma
glucose, be it in the fasting state or following a glucose
challenge. Yet, diabetes is characterized by abnormalities in
carbohydrate, lipid and protein metabolism and in electrolyte
fluxes. These abnormalities can reside at pre-receptor, receptor
and post-receptor levels. The classification system deals only with
glucose concentration measurements and does not take into account
abnormalities in fluxes of metabolites and electrolytes, and all the
parameters which are considered are static and not dynamic. Yet,
abnormalities in fluxes could precede the abnormalities identified
on the basis of concentration measurements. The question arises
whether such a classification does not lead to oversimplifications
which could distort events which occur at a level of higher
complexity. The question, therefore, arises whether the present
classification is sufficiently flexible to incorporate new research
findings with respect to the large variety of metabolic abnormalities. In both types of diabetes there is an abnormality in both
insulin secretion and tissue sensitivity to insulin. The question
arose which of these abnormalities is primary in diabetes. The
answer depends on available methology to accurately measure in man
and in animal models of diabetes, insulin secretion and sensitivity
of peripheral tissues and the liver to the action of insulin.

    Insulin resistance has been studied using a variety of steady
state techniques based on glucose clamp and insulin suppression

tests, and furthermore, from the dose-response curves it was possible to indicate whether the abnormality of insulin sensitivity is at the receptor and/or post-receptor level.[9,10,11,12,13,14] In order to study insulin release and insulin sensitivity in type 2 diabetics, a glucose infusion test (GIT) was designed which led to development of a mathematical model which made it possible to make quantitative measurements in a large population of diabetics.[15,16] It was suggested that impaired insulin release might represent a primary defect.[17] In addition, it appears that in normal populations, individuals can be classified as low or high insulin responders with respect to a glucose challenge. It could be that low insulin responders are at higher risk of developing glucose intolerance or diabetes.[10,15] The present classification, however, does not consider whether responsivenes of beta cells may be in any way related to the risk for development of diabetes.

More recently, a new mathematical approach based on minimal modelling has been proposed. This latter approach allows for estimation of the insulin sensitivity index from the dynamic responses of plasma glucose and insulin to a glucose injection. By the use of computer modelling it was possible to sever the feedback loop between plasma insulin and glucose.[18,19] The modelling approaches[15,17,18,19] require only simple experimental designs and therefore can be used for wide epidemiological studies to define more precisely the abnormalities of insulin secretion and sensitivity.

The use of radioactive glucose tracers made it possible to assess insulin resistance with respect to liver glucose production and overall glucose uptake, and this methodology[20] was validated both in and out of steady state.[21,22] As tracer methodology developed, a more refined approach to abnormalities in metabolism became possible.

Dr. Reaven[23] compared insulin resistance in Type I and Type II diabetes using both the older technique of insulin suppression and the newer technique of insulin clamp. He demonstrated insulin resistance in both types of diabetes. However, in Type I, it is only present under conditions of poor metabolic control and therefore it seems to be a secondary phenomenon. Insulin resistance was related to degree of control and could be overcome by improved control. He suggested that insulin resistance is much greater in Type II than in Type I. He feels that in Type II, insulin resistance is a primary defect, less related to the degree of control and with good control unable to return insulin action to normal. Diabetes caused by pancreatitis is different than NIDDM as insulin resistance could not be demonstrated. Porte et al.[24] reviewed the differences in abnormalities in insulin secretion between the two types of diabetes. Their approach was to consider the feedback loop system for regulation of plasma glucose. In IDDM, there is a considerable loss of this regulation system, due to an almost complete loss of islet function. This leads to decompensated hyperglycemia and a need for insulin treatment. In constrast, in NIDDM there is a steady state reregulation of plasma glucose at an elevated level. Hyperglycemia compensates for the partial loss of islet function leading to restoration of glucose uptake in the periphery and to partial suppression of hepatic glucose production. The cost of this compensation is persistant hyperglycemia.

The abnormalities of insulin action can occur at different levels of subcellular structures. The signalling starts when insulin binds to receptor, but interestingly this is followed by internalization of the insulin receptor complex. Posner et al.[25] reviewed their work demonstrating that insulin receptors are located not only on the cell surface but also intracellularly. The insulin-receptor complex is internalized into a vesicular structure called the endosome. Insulin is metabolized and receptor recycled back to the cell surface. The endosomal insulin receptors seem to be active since they contain a protein kinase activity. The question is whether degradation products of insulin may play some role in insulin action and whether the complex in the endosome exhibits a biological activity within the cells. These new methodologies will perhaps be important to explain in part, some defects of insulin action occurring in the different classes of diabetes.

Olefsky et al.[26] reviewed the methodology whereby dose response curves (insulin vs glucose utilization) are used to outline whether the defect in glucose utilization resides in receptor and/or post-receptor levels in the different classes and subclasses of diabetes. This methodology offers important opportunities for researchers to outline metabolic heterogeneities of diabetes and perhaps to search for the different subcellular locations where the lesion may reside. Thus, insulin resistance in impaired glucose tolerance is due to decreased insulin receptors, while in NIDDM, there is a combination of receptor and postreceptor defects. With increased severity of diabetes, postreceptor defect predominates and one acquired postreceptor abnormality is a decrease in the rate of glucose transport. Consistent with this is the observation that postreceptor defect is partially reversible with insulin therapy. Insulin resistance was only detected in poorly controlled IDDM patients and can be completely reversed by intensive insulin therapy.

As indicated earlier, the use of radioactive glucose tracers made it possible to assess insulin resistance with respect to glucose production in the liver and overall glucose utlization both in and out of steady state. As described in another chapter of this book[27] we have used a method of graded glucagon to assess insulin resistance in obesity[28] and in lean hypertriglyceridemic patients[29] by measuring nonsteady glucose kinetics. This tracer method assesses only changes in the overall glucose utilization, but cannot differentiate between abnormalities in peripheral and liver glucose utilization. Glucose uptake in the liver in man is diffi- cult to assess because the first-pass glucose uptake by the liver is much smaller than was previously thought to be the case.[30] With the error contained in the double tracer method used to assess glucose uptake in the liver, it may not be possible to detect differences which may exist between a normal population and differ- ent classes of diabetics. If, however, a given metabolic event is characteristic of only one organ, metabolic abnormalities specific for that organ can be detected in vivo in man and in animals without using invasive surgical methodology.

A novel possibility to assess the possible role of the liver in overall insulin resistance emerged when liver futile cycles were measured in lean and obese mild type II diabetics.[31,32] Since glucose futile cycle occurs essentially only in the liver, it is possible to sequester a liver defect from the overall defect in glucose utilization. This study was designed to assess the relative contributions of the liver and the periphery to excessive hyper- glycemia during glucose infusions in the diabetic. In lean, normal man with the present methodology we could not detect the futile cycling. However, in mild type II diabetics both in basal state and particularly during glucose challenge futile cycling became an important feature of glucose metabolism in the liver. We concluded that glucose intolerance in mild type II diabetics[31,32,33] is not only due to a decreased peripheral glucose phosphorylation but also to a defect in the liver. As a result of this, a significant part of glucose phosphorylated in the liver cannot be further utilized, since it is dephosphorylated through a glucose cycle. In addition, glucose production in the liver is inadequately suppressed by hyper- glycemia. We speculated that contributions of liver and periphery to glucose intolerance in those diabetics could be of similar magni- tude. This methodology could thus be useful in comparing some post-receptor abnormalities in the liver in different classes of diabetes.

New developments of tracer methodology offer also new possi- bilities to measure gluconeogenesis in vivo quantitatively, taking into account the loss of labelled precursors which occurs in some common pools in the liver.[34]

Regulation of insulin secretion is very complex. Normal pancreatic beta cell responds to a variety of metabolic neural and hormonal signals. Dupre et al.[35] reviewed the importance of signals generated by gastrointestinal peptides. A number of new peptides which respond to a food challenge have been identified and in addition to insulin mediated effects, these peptides may also act directly on metabolism. In type I diabetes, abnormalities of secretion of gastrointestinal peptides are likely a consequence of insulin deficiency. Since insulin is not administered through its physiological-portal route, such abnormalities may persist even in well treated patients. In type II diabetes, abnormalities of secretion of gastrointestinal peptides may at least in some cases represent a primary metabolic disorder.

New methodology to measure secretion and metablolism of insulin in vivo was reviewed by Radziuk et al.[36] This methodology combines measurements of C-peptide, which is not metabolized in the liver with an infusion of tritiated insulin to assess rate of insulin appearance in the posthepatic circulation. This methodology involves computer modelling and can measure insulin secretion and metabolism both in steady and nonsteady states. Measurements of insulin concentrations do not always reflect its rate of secretion because it is possible that in insulin resistant states, not only glucose uptake is impaired, but also insulin metabolism may be decreased, since binding of insulin to its receptors is impaired. It seems that tritiated insulin is the only insulin tracer whose kinetics are identical to those of native insulin.[37]

In addition to abnormalities in insulin secretion, the release of counterregulatory hormones (glucagon, catecholamines, cortisol) is also abnormal in diabetes. The question of how heterogeneous these abnormalities are in various classes in diabetes is an important one, and represents a task for further research. It is well known that in uncontrolled diabetes, there is an exaggerated counterregulatory response to stress and exercise. In stress, exaggerated release of these hormones, and particularly glucagon contribute to hyperglycemia.[38,39,40] The onset of diabetes often coincides with an episode of stress. The deterioration of metabolic control of diabetes, which can lead to ketoacidosis, not only in type I but also in type II diabetics, is also associated with severe stress. Yet, it is unknown whether there are abnormalities in the secretion of counterregulatory hormones which could precede the onset of diabetes. Do the responses of counterregulatory hormones to stress differ in various subclasses of diabetes or are they related to metabolic control or to complications of diabetes? Recently, many laboratories have outlined the fact that, in chronic diabetes, the glucagon response to hypoglycemia and later that of the catecholamines, becomes deficient.[41,42,43,44,45] The cause of this is not known but it could be related, at least in part, to diabetic neuropathy. This is why the risk of hypoglycemic reactions due to insulin treatment and often associated with exercise increases with duration of diabetes. Very little is known about potential abnormalities of counterregulatory responses in type II diabetics who are either insulin treated or are not exposed to insulin therapy.

In addition to hyperglucagonemia which has been implied to play a diabetogenic role in both types of diabetes,[46] it appears that the release of the other pancreatic peptide, somatostatin, may also be impaired.[47] Whether these impairments are primary or secondary and how they present in the two types of diabetes still remains to be determined. At least one recent report has demonstrated an impaired response of somatostatn to an oral glucose challenge in type II diabetes.[48] It was also demonstrated that release of endogenous opiates is involved in the complex counterregulatory responses to a variety of stress stimuli. It is indicated that one such endogenous opiate, beta-endorphin, not only affects the endocrine pancreatic function[49] but can also interfere with the effects of epinephrine.[50] Interestingly, blockade of opiate receptors affects counterregulatory responses to insulin induced hypoglycemia[51] in normal dogs. The intriguing question to be explained is how these complexities of counterregulatory cascades are involved in the two types of diabetes, and whether some of the impairments could represent a primary defect in some cases.

In comparing type I and type II diabetics with respect to metabolic challenges, one important area is the metabolic effect of exercise. It has become apparent that the decrease of plasma glucose during exercise in type I diabetics is related to insulin treatment.[52,53,54] In normal post absorptive man or animals, glucose production and utilization increase during exercise concurrently and therefore normoglycemia is maintained. Suppression of insulin secretion during exercise facilitates mobilization of glucose by the liver so that the increased energy needs of the working muscle can be met. When insulin is injected subcutaneously, there is increased mobilization of insulin from the subcutaneous depots, and depending on timing of exercise hyperinsulinemia is frequently encountered even before initiation of exercise. Hyper-insulinemia interferes with adequate glucose mobilization by the liver and since muscle glucose utilization is increased plasma glucose decreases. When, however, insulin is infused at basal and a constant rate in type I diabetics glucose homeostasis is maintained as in normal subjects. Interestingly, exercise induces a decrease in plasma glucose also in the postabsorptive type II diabetics.[55] This is again related to inadequate mobilization of glucose by the liver. Due to insulin resistance there is basal hyperinsulinemia in these patients, and insulin secretion is not suppressed during exercise, perhaps due to neuropathy of nerves supplying the endocrine pancreas. It is also surprising that despite marked insulin resistance during exercise, the increase in peripheral glucose utilization is not less than in normal subjects. The question of how acute exercise affects insulin resistance in type II diabetes needs to be further explored. The effect of training on natural history of human type I and type II diabetes has been extensively explored.[38,39] When exercise is associated with proper diets there is improvement in insulin sensitivity and in lipoprotein profiles. This effect, however, seems to cease when the training programme is discontinued. It requires a heavy training programme, and seems to be more beneficial in type II than in type I diabetes.

COMPLICATIONS

     The least understood aspects of diabetes are its complica-
tions. It is well known that despite reasonable treatment which
results in acceptable metabolic control, diabetic complications
develop, sometimes rapidly, sometimes slowly, and in some cases are
virtually absent. From the point of view of prognosis it would be
crucial to find markers which could predict the prevalence and the
incidence of these complications in various subclasses of diabetes.
One could envisage a totally different basis of classification which
would be based not on glucose profiles, but on the history of the
development of diabetic complications. At the present time, due to
the lack of availability of such markers, no attempts have been made
to take such an approach. The marked heterogeneity in developments
of complications raises the question of the underlying genetic basis
which could delay or accelerate the development of these complications. Some degenerative changes characteristic of diabetic complications are also seen in non-diabetic populations and are related to
the aging process. In the aging process, as well as in diabetes,
heterogeneity is also apparent. This raises the question of whether
these genetic factors which facilitate the development of some
diabetic complications are evenly distributed in diabetic and non-
diabetic populations or the genetic predisposition for diabetes and
for diabetic complications are linked together.

     Interestingly, it seems that all diabetic complications develop
both in type I and in type II diabetes, but precise data on the
prevalence and incidence of these complications in each type of
diabetes are still lacking. An important question to be answered is
whether or not type I diabetes is associated with higher prevalence
of complications. The high rate of complications in type II
diabetes is surprising because the metabolic abnormalities in this
disease are usually milder than in type I. This is attributed to
the fact that the diagnosis of type II diabetes is delayed, and
therefore the duration of diabetes before the onset of complications
is difficult to ascertain. The underlying metabolic cause of
diabetic complications seems to be assoicated with either an
increased glycosylation of a variety of proteins or an increased
flux of sorbitol in some tissues.

     Dr. Steiner[56] reviewed the field of diabetes and athero-
sclerosis and indicated that there is an increased risk of coronary
heart disease, cerebrovascular accidents and peripheral vascular
disease, particularly in women. Comparison between type I and type
II diabetes is difficult because of such complicating factors as
patient's age, onset and duration of diabetes and other risk factors. He indicated that hyperinsulinemia may represent an increased
risk for coronary artery disease independent of other factors.
Insulin could act on artery wall or promote specific vascular
elements. It is also possible that an increase in turnover of

triglyceride rich particles in association with hyperinsulinemia could generate atherogenic intermediate-density lipoproteins.

Dr. Maurer[57] indicates that diabetes is the most important cause of end-stage renal disease (ESRD) in the western world. While both types of diabetes contribute to ESRD, the prevalence of ESRD is higher in type I. The question whether precise regulation of plasma glucose can prevent nephropathy in diabetes is still unanswered. Dick et al.[58] indicate that the main questions to be answered are whether peripheral neuropathy is more frequent in type I than in type II diabetes, and whether complications of neuropathy are related to severity and duration of hyperglycemia. There are three primary classes of neuropathy, namely, disfunction of motor neurons, of sensory nerves and of autonomic neurons. Neuropathy is hetero-geneous, but it seems that both small blood vessels and nerve conduction involvement are important. Very often in the same patients one observes all three complications, namely neuropathy, nephropathy and retinopathy.

Davis et al.[59] outlined that it appears that proliferative diabetic retinopathy is the major problem in type I diabetics, whereas macular edema in the eye is the more prevalent condition in type II diabetes. Some of these conclusions were derived from a large epidemiological study of diabetic retinopathy conducted at the University of Wisconsin. It is apparent that the study of diabetic complications in various classes of diabetes is a major frontier in diabetes research today.

This book concludes with the challenging remarks of Dr. Chaill,[60] with the aim of integrating the most important new data generated in recent years.

REFERENCES

1.   National Diabetes Data Group. Classification and diagnosis of diabetes mellitus and other categories of glucose intolerance, Diabetes 28, 1039-1057 (1979).
2.   S.C. Sushruta, "Vaidya Jadavaji Trikamji Acharia," Nirnyar Sasar Press, Bombay (1938) (The original book was published in 500 B.C).
3.   P. Zimmet, Epidemiology of diabetes mellitus, in: "Diabetes Mellitus - Theory and Practice," M. Ellenberg and H. Rifkin, eds., Medical Examination Pub. Co. Inc., New York (1983).
4.   P. Bennett, Basis of the present classification of diabetes, in: "Comparison of Type I and Type II Diabetes" (1985).
5.   H. Keen, Limitations of the present classification of diabetes from an epidemiological point of view, Ibid (1985).

6. N. Freinkel and B.E. Metzger, Gestational diabetes: Problems in classification and implications for long range prognosis, Ibid (1985).

7. S.S. Fajans, Heterogeneity within type II and MODY diabetes, Ibid (1985).

8. M.A. Permutt, Genetics of type I and type II diabetes. Analysis by recombinant DNA methods, Ibid (1985).

9. A. Lernmark, Immunological aspects of etiology and pathogenesis of type I and type II diabetes, Ibid. (1985).

10. S. Efendic, R. Luft and A. Wajngot, Endocrine Reviews 5:95–410 (1984).

11. S.W. Shen, G.M. Reaven, and J.W. Farquhar, J. Clin. Invest. 49:2151 (1970).

12. R.A. DeFronzo, J.D. Tobin, and R. Andres, Am. J. Physiol. 237:E214 (1979).

13. O.G. Kolterman, L.J. Insel, M. Sackow, and J.M. Olefsky, J. Clin. Invst. 65:1272 (1980).

14. C.R. Kahn, "Metabolism," 27:1893 (1978).

15. E. Cerasi, and R. Luft, Acta Endocriol (Copenh) 55:278:304 (1967).

16. E. Cerasi, Acta Endocrinol (Copenh) 55:163 (1967).

17. E. Cerasi, R. Luft, Diabetes 16:615:627 (1967).

18. R.N. Bergman, Y.Z. Ider, C.R. Bowden, and C. Cobelli, Am. J. Physiol. 236:E667 (1979).

19. D.T. Finegood, G. Pacini, and R.N. Bergman, Diabetes 33:362 (1984).

20. R.C. De Bodo, R. Steele, N. Altszuler, A. Dunn, and J.S. Bishop, Recent Prog. Horm. Res. 19:445–488 (1963).

21. J.S. Cowan and G. Hetenyi, Metabolism 20:360–373 (1971).

22. J. Radziuk, K.H. Norwich, and M. Vranic, Am. J. Physiol. 234: E84–93 (1978).

23. G. Reaven, Insulin stimulated glucose disposal in patients with type I (IDDM) and type II (NIDDM) diabetes mellitus, in: "Comparison of Type I and Type II Diabetes," Plenum Press (1985).

24. W.K. Ward, J.C. Beard, J.B. Halter, and D. Porte, Pathophysiology in insulin secretion in diabetes mellitus, Ibid. (1985).

25. B. Posner, M.N. Kahn, and J.J.M. Bergeron, Internalization of insulin structure involved and their significance, Ibid (1985).

26. J.M. Olefsky, R.R. Revers, M. Prince, R. Henry, W.T. Garvey, J.A. Scarlett, and O.G. Kolterman, Insulin resistance in non insulin dependent (type II) and insulin dependent (type I) diabetes mellitus, Ibid (1985).

27. M. Vranic, A. Wajngot, and S. Efendic, New probes to study insulin resistance in men: futile cycle and glucose turnover, Ibid. (1985).

28. M. Vranic, S. Morita, and G. Steiner, Diabetes 29:169–176 (1980).

29. G. Steiner, S. Morita, and M. Vranic, Diabetes 29:889-905 (1980).

30. J. Radziuk, T.J. McDonald, D. Rubenstein, and J. Dupre, Metabolism 28:300-307 (1979).

31. S. Efendic, A. Wajngot, and M. Vranic, Proc. Natl. Acad. Sci. U.S.A. (1985, in press).

32. S. Karlander, A. Roovete, A. Vajngot, M. Vranic, and S. Efendic, Diabetologia 27:294A. Abstract 260 (1984).

33. A. Wajngot, A. Roovete, M. Vranic, R. Luft, and S. Efendic, Proc. Natl. Acad. Sci, USA 79:4432-4436 (1982).

34. G. Hetenyi Jr., Can. J. Physiol, Pharmacol 57:767-770 (1979).

35. J. Dupre, A. Baer, M. Lee, J.T. McDonald, J. Radziuk, N.W. Rodger, and S. Sullivan, Insulin mediated and non-insulin mediated effects of gastroentoeropancreatic peptides in type I and type II diabetes, in: "Comparison of Type I and Type II Diabetes," Plenum Press (1985).

36. J. Radziuk, and T. Morishima, New methods for the analysis of insulin kinetics in vivo, Ibid (1985).

37. M. Berger, P.A. Halban, W.A. Muller, R.E. Offord, A.E. Renold and M. Vranic, Diabetologia 15:133-140 (1978).

38. M. Vranic, F.W. Kemmer, P. Berchtold, and M. Berger, Hormonal intereactions in control of metabolism during exercise in physiology and diabetes, in: "Diabetes Mellitis - Theory and Practice," M. Ellenberg, and H. Rifkin, eds., Medical Examination Pub. Co. Inc., New York (1983).

39. M. Vranic, and L. Lickley, Exercise and stress in Diabetes Mellitus, in: "Clinical Diabetes Mellitus," J.K. Davidson, ed., Thieme-Stratton Inc. (In press) Ch. 15. (1985).

40. G. Perez, F.W. Kemmer, H.L.A. Lickley, and M. Vranic, Am. J. Physiol 241:E328-335 (1981).

41. J.E. Gerich, V. Schneider, S.E. Dippe, M. Longlois, C. Nuacco, J.H. Karam and P.H. Forsham, Science 182:171-173 (1973).

42. T.D. Maher, R.J. Tannenberg, B.Z. Greenberg, J.E. Hoffman, R.P. Doe, and F.C. Goetz, J. Clin. Endocrionol. Metab. 44:459-464 (1977).

43. J. Hilsted, S. Marsbad, T. Krazup, L. Sestoft, N.J. Christensen, B. Tronier, and H. Galbo, Diabetes 30:626-632 (1983).

44. G. Bolli, P. DeFeo, P. Compagnucci, M. Castechini, G. Angeletti, F. Santeusanio, P. Brunetti, and J.E. Gerich, Diabetes 32:134-141 (1983).

45. P.E. Cryer, and J.G. Gerich, Diabetes Care 6:95-99 (1983).

46. R.H. Unger, and L. Orci, "Glucagon Physiology, Pathophysiology and Morphology of the Pancreatic A Cell," Esevier, New York (1981).

47. V. Schusdziarra, D. Rouiller, V. Harris, J.M. Coulon, and R.H. Unger, Endocrinology 103:2264 (1978).

48. V. Grill, M. Gutniak, A. Roovete, and S. Efendic, J. Clin. Endocrinol. (In press) (1984).

49. E. Ipp, R.E. Dobbs, and R.H. Unger, Nature 276:190-191 (1981).

50. K. El Tayebn, P. Brubaker, L. Lickley, and M. Vranic, The International Congress of Endocrinology, Excerpta Medica International Congress Series 652:477, Abstract #434 (1984).
51. K. El Tayeb, P. Brubaker, L. Lickley, and M. Vranic, Diabetes 33, Suppl. 1, 51a. Abstract #202 (1984).
52. M. Vranic, R. Kawamori, S. Pek, N. Kovacevic, and G.A. Wrenshall, J. Clin. Invest. 57:245-255 (1975).
53. R. Kawamori, and M. Vranic, J. Clin. Invest. 59:331-337 (1977).
54. B. Zinman, F.T. Murray, M. Vranic, A.M. Albisser, B.S. Leibel, P.A. McClean, and E. Marliss, J. Clin. Endocrinol. Metab. 45:641-652 (1977).
55. H.L. Minuk, M. Vranic, E.B. Marliss, A.K. Hanna, A.M. Albisser and B. Zinman, Am. J. Physiol. 240:E458-464 (1981).
56. G. Steiner, Atherosclerosis, the major complication of diabetes, in: "Comparison of Type I and Type II Diabetes," Plenum Press (1985).
57. S.M. Mauer, B.M. Chavers, A comparison of kidney disease in type I and type II diabetes, Ibid (1985).
58. J. Dick, A. Windebank, H. Yasuda, J. Service, R. Rizza, and B. Zimmerman, Functional and pathological alterations in human diabetic nephropathy, Ibid. (1985).
59. R. Klein, M.D. Davis, S.E. Moss, E.K.B. Klein, and D.L. de Mets, The Wisconsin Epidemiological study of diabetic neuropathy, Ibid. (1985).
60. G. Cahill, Some summarizing thoughts. Ibid. (1985).

BASIS OF THE PRESENT CLASSIFICATION OF DIABETES

Peter H. Bennett

Epidemiology and Field Studies Branch
NIADOK, NIH
Phoenix, Arizona, U.S.A.

ABSTRACT

The present classification of diabetes most widely used is that recommended by the National Diabetes Data Group and subsequently endorsed by the World Health Organization. This classification is primarily a clinical classification of diabetes because in most instances the etiology is unknown. The need for a standardized classification arose out of the recognition that diabetes was a syndrome rather than a single disease and the different terminologies which emerged. While certain types of diabetes can be classified according to specific etiology or associations with specific syndromes, the vast majority cannot. Insulin-dependent and noninsulin-dependent diabetes usually represent syndromes whose etiopathology is believed to differ and their clinical characteristics are usually distinctive. As evidence of etiological heterogeneity has increased there has been a tendency to adopt the terms Type I and Type II diabetes to indicate different etiologies, although the original usage of these terms was as a clinical classification to differentiate between insulin dependent and non-insulin-dependent disease. At present the use of the four terms to describe the common types of diabetes leads to confusion, which could readily be resolved by arriving at agreed definitions for each of these terms. While the NDDG-WHO classification has served to standardize terminology and stimulate research into the different causes of diabetes, some further refinement of the classification, together with some additional definition of terms, should be considered.

The classification of diabetes most widely used at the present time is that suggested by the National Diabetes Data Group (NDDG) in the United States in 1979,[15] which was subsequently recommended by the World Health Organization (WHO) Expert Committee on Diabetes Mellitus in 1980.[20] It should be stressed that this classification was intended to be a uniform framework for clinical and epidemiological research, and that the classification would almost certainly have to be modified on the basis of new knowledge in the future.

HISTORICAL BACKGROUND

History undoubtedly plays an important part in shaping current concepts and this has certainly been true in arriving at the current classification of diabetes. There would probably be little reason for discussion of the subject today if the etiology of all that is now considered to be diabetes were established. Unfortunately, this is not the case. Consequently, we are presently torn between a classification scheme which incorporates what we do know about etiology; descriptions of what we recognize on clinical grounds as being related, but which is of uncertain or unknown etiology and which may be heterogeneous; and the extent to which we believe we can safely venture in classifying individual subjects into the categories which we define.

Although diabetes has been recognized for over 2000 years and in spite of the fact that it has emerged as one of the most common chronic diseases, it is in only a minority of cases in which the etiology is sufficiently clear that the cause can reasonably be stated as known. In the vast majority the common feature is chronic hyperglycemia of unknown or uncertain etiology.

DIABETES AS A SYNDROME

The recognition of diabetes as more than a single disease goes back for more than a century. Bouchardat, in 1875,[3] proposed a classification of diabète maigre and diabète gras to distinguish between two syndromes which he recognized as having a different prognosis and in which different forms of clinical management were indicated. This distinction appears to have been lost in the early part of the present century where the tendency was to consider "mild" and "severe" forms of the disease. This concept was followed by attempts to explain the differences in terms of the numbers of diabetes genes inherited, or in terms of the age of onset of the condition. These concepts in turn led to the introduction of terms such as "brittle" and "stable" diabetes and "juvenile" and "maturity onset" diabetes, but the idea that these subgroups represented a spectrum of one and the same disease pervaded. During the 1930's, however, the concept of Secondary diabetes to describe diabetes associated with hemachromatosis, acromegaly, chronic pancreatitis, etc., gained acceptance. The term Secondary diabetes was used in contradistinction to Primary, Idiopathic or Hereditary diabetes. There were then many attempts to stage primary or idiopathic diabetes according to its natural history, leading to a host of terms including potential diabetes, prediabetes, latent diabetes, asymptomatic diabetes, chemical diabetes, subclinical diabetes, and overt diabetes. Further confusion arose when these terms were used in different ways by different authors in different countries.

Exceptions to the viewpoint that the commonly encountered forms of diabetes were variations of a single disease then started to appear. Sir Harold Himsworth, for example, in 1949, stated clearly that diabetes mellitus is not one disease entity, but a syndrome which includes a group of disorders differing in their clinical features, biochemistry and causes.[4] Himsworth recognized that the syndrome could frequently be characterized as "insulin sensitive" or "insulin resistant".[10] Following this, R.D. Lawrence in his presidential address to the Section of Endocrinology of the Royal Society of Medicine in 1950[14] proposed a classification scheme which included diabetes due to primary pancreatic destruction; due to a primary disturbance of other endocrines, e.g. pituitary, adrenal disease and pheochromocytoma; due to disturbances of fat storage, in particular lipoatrophic diabetes and the most common form of diabetes – lipoplethoric diabetes – associated with obesity and without ketosis; and insulin deficient diabetes, characterized by ketosis which in the absence of insulin treatment leads to coma. He also pointed out that the analysis of over 1000 cases performed by Harris in 1950[9] suggested that the insulin deficient type and the lipoplethoric type tended to run separately in families and may be due to separate genetic influences. Lawrence[14] summarized his presentation by saying human diabetics are divided clinically into two main types 1) those who are probably not insulin deficient and 2) those who certainly are.

In 1955 Hugh-Jones[12] appears to have introduced the terminology, Type 1 and 2, as a clinical classification. He characterized Type 1 diabetes as "starting in young people who are often underweight; it is severe in that the patient depends on the administration of insulin to prevent ketosis". Type 2 diabetes is mild and characteristically arises in middle age patients who are often obese (lipoplethoric diabetes of Lawrence) and seldom requires insulin except during added infection. Hugh-Jones then went on to describe a third type of diabetes, found in Jamaica, Type J, which he characterized as "occurring in young adults and even in children who persistently require large doses of insulin to control glycosuria and maintain their weight, and who are relatively sensitive to infection, and show little or no ketosis if insulin is withheld." The terminology, Type 1 and 2, then appeared to lie dormant until rediscovered or revived in 1976 by the late Dr. Andrew Cudworth, who subsequently popularized its use.

Cudworth[4] introduced his classification (Table 1) by stating that "diabetes in a clinically heterogeneous disorder and that any investigation into the etiology of diabetes should first take into consideration the role of genetic determination." He continued, "there are obvious dangers in taking differences in phenotype as a basis for investigating basic heterogeneity," but "despite these notes of caution it seems reasonable to assume there are two aetiologically distinct forms of the disease determined by differences in age of onset, relative abruptness of onset, tendency to ketoacidosis and dependence on insulin."

He then argued that "in primary diabetes the terms 'juvenile onset' and 'maturity onset' are too rigid and should perhaps be discarded in favor of Type 1 and Type 2 diabetes, respectively. While well-recognized by clinicians that Type 1 diabetes presents mainly in childhood and adolescence, it can also occur in the insulin dependent syndrome of typically abrupt onset at all ages including the elderly. It is conceivable that in these late onset insulin-dependent cases the same pathogenic factors are operating as those that trigger the disease seen predominantly in the young." The question of maturity onset diabetes of the young (MODY) is then discussed, and Cudworth concluded, "but whether this is a different disease to Type 2 diabetes observed predominantly in older age groups remains speculative."

Cudworth then went on to justify the classification of Type I

Table 1: Clinical and Aetiological Classification of
          Diabetes

Primary Diabetes

          type 1 - juvenile onset or insulin-dependent
          type 2 - maturity onset or noninsulin-dependent

Secondary Diabetes

          pancreatic disease
          liver disease
          hormone induced (endogenous or exogenous)
          obesity
          drugs

(From Cudworth A.G. Br. J. Hosp. Med. 16:207-216 (1976)

---

as a separate entity by pointing out the then recently established HLA associations, the excess of diabetes in HLA and haplo-identical siblings and the association with the presence of islet cell anti-bodies. In subsequent paper[5] he reviewed the evidence that Type I diabetes was more common in the siblings and parents of insulin-dependent diabetics even when the probands had an onset of 20 years of age and over, as compared to the excess of Type II diabetes in relatives when the proband was insulin independent.

In 1977, Irvine[13] wrote in a paper on the Classification of Idiopathic Diabetes that "Type 1 includes classic insulin dependent juvenile onset diabetes, insulin-dependent diabetes presenting in later life, and diabetes initially adequately controlled for at least 3 months on oral hypoglycemic agents, but with islet cell antibody in the serum. Type 11 includes classical maturity onset insulin-dependent diabetes and the rarer insulin independent diabetes presenting at a younger age in patients whose serum is negative for islet cell antibodies at the time of diagnosis." He then subdivided Type 1 diabetes into three subtypes according to whether the main factor is a genetically determined diathesis towards autoimmunity (Type 1a); islet damage by appropriate viral infection or other agent in the absence of islet cell autoimmunity (Type 1c); or a combination of the two diatheses (Type 1b). He also points out that his classification was similar to that utilized a year earlier by Bottazzo and Doniach,[6] except that the Irvine Type 1a more closely corresponded to the Bottazzo and Doniach Type 1b. Interestingly, Bottazzo and Doniach[6] while espousing the Type 1 classification of Cudworth,[4] point out that insulin requirement is sometimes delayed in individuals who are islet cell antibody positive, and Type 1 diabetes is not necessarily insulin-dependent at the time of diagnosis though it usually becomes so later.

The move towards a numerical classification of diabetes was clearly driven by the desire to arrive at an etiological classi-fication, incorporating the concept of the heterogeneity of diabetes mellitus, that had reemerged over the previous decade, and to supplant the terms "juvenile onset" diabetes and "maturity onset," which had come into wide usage, but were now recognized as inadequate.

THE PRESENT CLASSIFICATION

In April 1978, a workgroup under the sponsorship of the National Diabetes Data Group was convened to discuss and make recommendations about terminology and arrive at a working classi-fication that reflects the current knowledge about the disease.[15] Their deliberations were subsequently circulated widely to the diabetes community prior to publication. They were subsequently adopted by the WHO Expert Committee on Diabetes Mellitus and hence, became the internationally recognized classification of diabetes.[20]

The main aims of the classification of the National Diabetes Data Group were (1) to serve as a uniform basis for the conduct of clinical research in diabetes, (2) to serve as a framework for the collection of data on the etiology, natural history and impact of diabetes, and (3) to aid the clinician in categorizing patients with varying degrees of glucose tolerance. The terminology and classification were designed so that (1) the classes were mutually exclusive and that an individual at a given point in time could be placed only in one class, although this could subsequently change, (2) the classification should require only simple clinical or descriptive observations, (3) the classes should be as precise and well-defined as current knowledge of the etiopathology of diabetes permits, (4) the terminology would describe the phenotypic expression of the abnormality, and (5) the classification should be able to incorporate new findings on the etiopathology of diabetes.

THE CURRENT NDDG AND WHO CLASSIFICATION

The NDDG presented three clinical classes of diabetes mellitus (Table 2). Each class was described in terms of its clinical characteristics and they stated that multiple etiologies are probably present in all.

The first class, Insulin-dependent diabetes (IDDM) – Type 1, contains persons who are dependent on injected insulin to prevent ketosis and to preserve life. The description states that the onset, while generally in youth, may occur at any age, and that there may be noninsulin-dependent phases in the natural history of the disease. The presence of associations with certain HLA types and abnormal immune responses is acknowledged and it is stated that islet cell antibodies are frequently present at diagnosis.

The second class, Noninsulin-dependent diabetes mellitus (NIDDM) – Type 2, contains persons who are not insulin-dependent or ketosis prone, although they may use insulin for the correction of symptomatic or persistent hyperglycemia and can develop ketosis under special circumstances such as during episodes of infection or stress. While the onset of the disease is most often after the age of 40 and most are obese at the time of onset, the classification also clearly recognized Maturity Onset Diabetes of the Young (MODY) as belonging to this class, and that hyperinsulinemia and insulin resistance characterize some patients in the class. NDDG recommended subdivision into two subtypes – nonobese and obese NIDDM.

The third class is Other types of diabetes, including diabetes associated with pancreatic disease, hormonal abnormalities, drug or chemical induced diabetes, insulin receptor abnormalities and

certain specified genetic syndromes. This class contains subjects
in whom the etiology of the diabetes is established or those which
show an intimate relationship with some other well-defined genetic
syndrome such as Type 1 glycogen storage disease, ataxic telangiec-
tasia, Werner's syndrome, etc., in which the etiologies of the
diabetes are likely to be different from those of the commonly
encountered forms, and where the distinctive features can be recognized because of the association with other findings. Conceptually,
if the etiology of all types of diabetes were established, all cases

Table 2   Classification of Diabetes Mellitus and Other Categories
           of Glucose Intolerance

Clinical classes

    Diabetes mellitus (DM)

        Insulin-dependent type (IDDM): Type 1
        Noninsulin-dependent type (NIDDM): Type 11

            Nonobese
            Obese

        Other types (includes diabetes mellitus associated with
        certain conditions and syndromes)

            Pancreatic disease
            Disease of hormonal etiology
            Drug- or chemical-induced condition
            Insulin receptor abnormalities
            Certain genetic syndromes
            Miscellaneous

    Impaired glucose tolerance (IGT)

            Nonobese
            Obese
            Impaired glucose tolerance associated with certain
            conditions and syndromes

    Gestational diabetes (GDM)

Statistical risk classes (subjects with normal glucose tolerance but
substantially increased risk of developing diabetes)

    Previous abnormality of glucose tolerance
    Potential abnormality of glucose tolerance

---

of diabetes would be classified specifically and appear in this
category.

The NDDG also defined two other clinical classes. The first,
Impaired glucose tolerance (IGT), contains persons with a degree of
glucose intolerance intermediate between that of normal and
diabetic. It was recognized that assignment to this class could
only be made on the basis of a glucose tolerance test and that this
abnormality may be attributable to normal variation in glucose
tolerance, or may represent a stage in the development of NIDDM, or
IDDM, or Other types of diabetes, even though many persons with IGT
will not develop either of these conditions. The reasons for recognizing this class separately were that some studies have shown an
increased prevalence of arterial disease, and that such subjects,
while at increased risk of developing IDDM or NIDDM do not yet have
definitive evidence of these diseases, and may never do so, and,
therefore, they should not be stigmatized by being labeled as such.

The final clinical class, Gestational diabetes (GDM), contains
pregnant women who have glucose intolerance which has its onset or
recognition during pregnancy (thus excluding diabetics who become
pregnant). While women with gestational diabetes have an increased
risk for progression to diabetes later, the classification demands
that the pregnant woman be reclassified after pregnancy is termi-
nated. (It should be noted that while the nomenclature is similar
for the NDDG and WHO classification, the diagnostic criteria for
gestational diabetes differ). The justification for this class is
that glucose intolerance during pregnancy carries an increased risk
of perinatal morbidity and mortality, some of which appears to be
preventable by careful management. While such women are at a higher
risk of developing diabetes in the future, the type of diabetes
which these women may subsequently develop cannot be predicted and
in any event their glucose tolerance often reverts to normal after
parturition.

To accommodate the classification of persons who have previously had an abnormality of glucose tolerance, such as those who
have had gestational diabetes and have now returned to normal, or
those whose glucose tolerance may have returned to normal after
weight loss, or who have exhibited glucose intolerance only at a
time of severe stress or injury, a statistical risk class of
Previous Abnormality of Glucose Tolerance (PrevAGT) was defined.
Furthermore, the NDDG suggested the term Potential Abnormality of
Glucose Tolerance (PotAGT) as a statistical risk class for those
who, while never yet exhibiting abnormal glucose tolerance, are at
substantially increased risk of developing diabetes. These subjects
include persons with normal glucose tolerance who have islet cell
antibodies or the nondiabetic monozygous twin of a diabetic, and an
HLA or haplo-identical sibling of a diabetic. Although proposed by
the NDDG and WHO these two statistical risk categories do not appear

to have been used very extensively.

Besides these clinical classifications and statistical risk classes the NDDG hinted at the need for a further subclassification for research purposes. The provisional classification proposed included dividing insulin dependent diabetes mellitus into sub-classes 1a, b and c depending upon the presence of organ specific autoimmune phenomena, and the presence and persistence or absence of islet cell antibodies. Noninsulin-dependent diabetes was subclassified according to the degree of obesity, but further subclassification of this entity was stated to be inappropriate at the time the recommendations were formulated.

PROBLEMS WITH THE PRESENT CLASSIFICATION SYSTEM

The present NDDG-WHO classification was designed to categorize patients on the basis of the clinical manifestations, or phenotypic expressions of diabetes at a given point in the course of the disease. While an etiological classification would have been desirable, it was believed at the time that knowledge of the etiology of the common forms of diabetes was sufficiently incomplete and uncertain that only a clinical categorization could be justified and widely accepted for the classification of the majority of diabetics.

DEFINITIONS OF TYPE 1 AND TYPE 2 DIABETES

A major problem has evolved for the usage of the terms Type I and Type II (or 1 and 2) diabetes. The NDDG and WHO classification, unfortunately perhaps, implied an equivalence of these terms, yet the authors who initially popularized their usage,[4,5,13] had justified and made the distinction on etiological grounds, rather than on the basis of clinical descriptors as used by the NDDG-WHO classification. On the other hand, the original usage of Type 1 and Type 2 had been simply a convenient way of labeling the clinical entities of insulin dependent and noninsulin-dependent diabetes, before any details of the differences in etiopathology were defined.[12] This situation has led to continued confusion in the literature. Some authors using Type I and II (or 1 and 2) to indicate forms of diabetes which are believed to have different etiologies, and others simply using the terms as clinical descriptors for insulin-dependent diabetes and noninsulin-dependent diabetes. The trend appears towards the use of Type I and Type II in relation to different etiologies, and to retain IDDM and NIDDM as a clinical classification. This matter is presently in urgent need of resolution.

There have been marked advances in the past six years in the understanding of one form of diabetes which often ends in the development of insulin-dependent diabetes. It is now recognized that the HLA and haplo-identical siblings of insulin-dependent diabetics are at increased risk of this form of diabetes[8] and that in the Caucasian population subjects with HLA-DR3/4 are also more likely to carry genetic susceptibility to this form of the disease than those with other HLA-DR types, especially HLA-DR2.[16] Persons with islet cell antibodies, particularly if these are present on several occasions and are of the complement fixing type, also carry an increased risk for developing this disease,[7] as do siblings of IDDM patients who have impaired glucose tolerance.[17] Subjects with this syndrome may also manifest diabetes which is not insulin-dependent and their glycemia may be controlled with oral hypoglycemic agents for a period of time before insulin dependency supervenes. The period between the development of islet cell anti-bodies and the appearance of insulin dependency has been shown to be at least several years in some instances.[7] Furthermore, after an acute episode of hyperglycemia, and sometimes ketoacidosis, the aggressive treatment with insulin is often followed by a period in which insulin therapy can be completely withdrawn and this period can perhaps be prolonged by immunosuppression.[18] Thus, at various stages according to the WHO-NDDG classification, the patient may have either a potential abnormality of glucose tolerance, IGT, a previous abnormality of glucose tolerance, NIDDM, or IDDM. Many authors have adopted the term Type 1 in describing this syndrome and, by implication, have introduced two dimensional classifica-tions, one based on a common etiopathology, and the other on clinical features of the syndrome. Thus, the various phases could be described as Type 1 IGT, Type 1 NIDDM, Type 1 IDDM, etc.

Such a scheme might have merit if there were agreement on the definition of the term Type 1. However, a number of problems remain. First, it is unclear what proportion of patients who ultimately develop IDDM share a common etiology. Secondly, the precipitating events which lead to islet cell destruction in this form of diabetes are unknown and while a case could be made for reclassifying this type of diabetes with Other types of diabetes due to specific causes, e.g. diabetes due to autoimmune destruction of the pancreas, it remains unclear whether this syndrome has the same etiology as that associated with the presence of other organ specific autoantibodies. Thirdly, the term Type 1 appears to imply to a single disease with a well-established single cause (cf. Type 1-glycogen storage disease) which is not yet the case. Fourthly, the use of a numeric term for an etiologic classification gives no indication of the cause of the disease, and other types of diabetes with defined causes are not numbered at this time.

The present definition of the term Type II appears to be arrived at by exclusion, i.e. diabetes that is not Type I, and that is not an Other type of diabetes due to specific causes. Further-more, it does not appear useful to use this term synonymously for

NIDDM since the extent to which the clinical entity has multiple causes is unknown. The use of this numeric descriptor, seems totally unjustified at present.

OTHER DEFINITIONAL PROBLEMS

There have also been other criticisms of the NDDG-WHO classification. Questions have arisen over the meaning insulin dependency and of the difficulty in defining proneness and resistance to ketosis. In particular, the classification of the older patient, who after some years of diabetes without dependency on insulin who then develops an infection or other stressful illness with an episode of ketosis and is then treated with insulin, or conversely, the young patient who develops severe hyperglycemia and who is treated promptly with insulin and who never develops an episode of ketoacidosis, both present the problem as to whether or not they are insulin dependent. Both are insulin treated, and may require insulin for glycemic control, but may or may not be prone to spontaneous ketosis. Such patients present classification dilemmas for those involved in clinical research and in epidemiological studies. Some distinction among insulin treated patients who are insulinopenic, and those who are not, may now be possible using serum or urinary C-peptide assays.[19,1]

DIFFERENCES IN NDDG AND WHO CRITERIA FOR CLASSIFICATION

The NDDG classification, because of the specifications for diagnostic criteria to be fulfilled to enter the classes, resulted in some glucose tolerance tests results being classified as "non-diagnostic." The classification, therefore, was not inclusive. On the other hand, WHO, recognizing this problem, modified the diagnostic criteria for IGT. WHO considered two-hour post-load venous plasma values below 140mg/dl as normal, those between 140-199/dl as IGT, whereas NDDG recommended, in addition, that an earlier value in the glucose tolerance test must exceed 200mg/dl to enter the IGT class. NDDG stated also that fasting venous plasma glucose levels of 115mg/dl and intermediate values of less than 200mg/dl were required to designate "normal glucose tolerance." Consequently the frequency of IGT by WHO criteria is appreciably greater, and the WHO IGT class includes a majority of the subjects who are categorized as "non-diagnostic" by NDDG criteria.[2]

IS IT TIME TO REVISE THE CLASSIFICATION?

In spite of these problems the NDDG-WHO classification has been broadly and widely embraced by the diabetes community. The adoption of the classification has led to a much wider awareness of the need for correct classification for clinical research, clinical manage-

ment and in epidemiological research, and appears to have served as
an impetus to search for the causes and etiologies of diabetes. A
primary reason for the present problems which are encountered in
applying the classification is the increased knowledge which has
come about, in part, as a result of the classification. Some of
these problems could readily be resolved by refining the definitions, and obtaining a wide concensus for their future usage. Other
features of the classification such as the confusion over the usage
of terms such as Type 11 and Type 1 could perhaps be eliminated by
agreement on an etiological classification of diabetes, and therefore, clearly separating the clinical classes (perhaps with some
redefinition) from the etiological categories in the future. In my
view the NDDG-WHO classification has been useful, and will continue
to be so if appropriate steps are taken to update the classification
to account for the recent advances in knowledge concerning the
etiology of diabetes, and eliminate some of the ambiguities in the
present definitions.

REFERENCES

1. J.P. Bantle, D.C. Laine, B.J. Hoogwerf, and F.C Goetz, The
    potential usefulnes of postprandial urine C-peptide measurement
    in classifying diabetic patients, Diabetes Care 7:202-203
    (1984).

2. P.H. Bennett, W.C. Knowler, D.J. Pettitt, and H.R. Baird,
    Differences in the National Diabetes Data Group (NDDG) and
    World Health Organization (WHO) criteria for diabetes (DM) and
    impaired glucose tolerance (IGT), Diabetes 32(Suppl. 1):110A
    (1983).

3. A. Bouchardat, De la glycosurie au diabète sucré: Son
    Traitment Hygiènique, Paris: Germer-Balliere, :180 (1875).

4. A.G. Cudworth, The aetiology of diabetes mellitus, Br. J. Hosp.
    Med. 16:207-216 (1976).

5. A.G. Cudworth, Type 1 diabetes mellitus, Diabetologia
    14:281-291 (1978).

6. G.F. Bottazzo, and D. Doniach, Pancreatic autoimmunity and HLA
    antigens, Lancet 2:800 (1976).

7. A.N. Gorsuch, K.M. Spencer, J. Lister, J.M. McNally, B.M. Dean,
    G.F. Bottazzo, and A.G. Cudworth, Evidence for a long
    prediabetic period in type 1 (insulin dependent) diabetes
    mellitus, Lancet 2:1363-1365 (1981).

8. A.N. Gorsuch, K.M. Spencer, J. Lister, E. Wolf, G.F. Bottazzo,
    and A.G. Cudworth, Can future Type 1 diabetes be predicted? A
    study of families of affected children, Diabetes 31:862-866
    (1982).

9. H. Harris, The familial distribution of diabetes mellitus: A
    study of the relatives of 1241 diabetic propositi, Ann. Eugen.
    15:95-119 (1950).

10. H.P. Himsworth, Diabetes mellitus: Its differentiation into insulin-sensitive and insulin-insensitive types, Lancet 1:117-120 (1936).
11. H.P. Himsworth, The syndrome of diabetes mellitus and its causes, Lancet 1:465-473 (1949).
12. P. Hugh-Jones, Diabetes in Jamaica, Lancet 2:891-897 (1955).
13. W.J. Irvine, Classification of idiopathic diabetes, Lancet 1: 638-642 (1977).
14. R.D. Lawrence, Types of human diabetes, Br. Med. J. 1: 373-375 (1951).
15. National Diabetes Data Group, Classification and diagnosis of diabetes mellitus and other categories of glucose intolerance, Diabetes 28:1039-1057 (1979).
16. J.Nerup, M. Christy, A. Green, M. Hauge, P. Platz, L.P. Ryder, A. Svejgaard, and M. Thompsen, HLA and insulin dependent diabetes - population studies, in: "The Genetics of Diabetes Mellitus," J. Kobberling and R. Tattersall, eds., Academic Press, London and New York, (1981), p.33-42.
17. A.L. Rosenbloom, S.S. Hunt, E.K. Rosenbloom, and N. Madaren, Ten-year prognosis of impaired glucose tolerance in siblings of patients with insulin-dependent diabetes, Diabetes 31:385-387 (1982).
18. C.R. Stiller, J. Dupre, M. Gent, M.R. Jenner, P.A. Keown, A. Laupacis, R. Martell, N.W. Rodger, B.V. Graffenried, and B.M.J. Wolfe, Effects of cyclosporine immunosuppression insulin-dependent diabetes mellitus of recent onset, Science 223: 1362-1367 (1984).
19. T.A. Welborn, P. Garcia-Webb, and A.M. Bousen, Basal C-peptide in the discrimination of type 1 from type 11 diabetes, Diabetes Care 4:616-619 (1981).
20. WHO Expert Committee on Diabetes Mellitus, in: "Second Report," World Health Organization Technical Report Series 646. Geneva: World Health Organization (1980).

LIMITATIONS AND PROBLEMS OF DIABETES CLASSIFICATION

FROM AN EPIDEMIOLOGICAL POINT OF VIEW

H. Keen

Guy's Hospital and Medical School
London, England

INTRODUCTION

Classifications of disease are man-made devices to assist in the ordering of thought or the organization of action. It follows that they depend upon the current state of knowledge and that as knowledge increases so classification may change. It also follows that the nature of the classification will depend upon the type of action to be organized. Thus a classification appropriate to a clinician whose concern is with diagnosis and treatment may well be inappropriate to a basic scientist whose concern is research strategy and experimental design. The public health agent will require a classification which assists in provision of health care resources and the planning of preventive approaches. Epidemiological needs will also make special demands of a classification, the main requirement being for clear, unambiguous definitions. The classification formulated by the US National Diabetes Data Group (NDDG)[1] and adopted in the Second Report of the World Health Organization Expert Committee on Diabetes Mellitus (WHO)[2] (see abbreviated version, Table 1) goes a long way to meet the varying needs of these different user groups but falls short of perfection as is inevitable in any attempt to meet them all. It is the residual problems, mainly those for the epidemiologist, that are dealt with here.

HISTORY

The contemporary format and shortcomings of the classification of diabetes can best be understood by viewing it in historical perspective.[3] The basic diagnostic concept of diabetes mellitus (DM), originated from purely clinical beginnings - from a striking syndrome identified in ancient writings and consisting of unassuag-

Table 1   Classification   of   Diabetes   Mellitus   and   Related
           Conditions [Abbreviated From (1)]

DIABETES MELLITUS (DM)

      I   INSULIN DEPENDENT DIABETES MELLITUS (IDDM)

      II   NON INSULIN DEPENDENT DIABETES MELLITUS (NIDDM)

          a) NON-OBESE   b) OBESE

          OTHER TYPES OF DIABETES MELLITUS (OTDM)

          i) PANCREATIC   ii) HORMONAL   iii) DRUG-INDUCED

          iv) INSULIN/RECEPTOR ABNORMALITIES v) GENETIC

          SYNDROMES vi) OTHER ASSOCIATION

      III   GESTATIONAL DIABETES MELLITUS (GDM)

IMPAIRED GLUCOSE TOLERANCE (IGT)

          a) NON OBESE   b) OBESE

STATISTICAL HIGH RISK CLASSES (NORMAL GTT)

      I   PREVIOUS ABNORMALITY OF GLUCOSE TOLERANCE (Prev. AGT)

      II   POTENTIAL ABNORMALITY OF GLUCOSE TOLERANCE (Pot AGT)

---

able thirst, profuse urination, rapid wasting and physical decline culminating 'in no long time' in drowsiness, hyperpnoeic coma and death.   Identification of urinary glucose as a diagnostic marker drew many more people into the class of DM and greatly changed its clearcut diagnostic image.   Unlike the youthful, wasted, grossly symptomatic prototypes these were usually older, often plumper, only mildly symptomatic people.   Their recruitment to the diagnostic class raised the apparent frequency of diabetes by an order of magnitude.   The further and most recent inflation of numbers of those diagnosed as diabetic followed upon the extension of automated

blood glucose screening to large, apparently normal populations
either in case-finding 'detection drives' or in epidemiological
investigations. Population screening led to the discovery of a high
proportion of people, ostensibly normal, but with blood glucose
concentrations (or glucose tolerance responses) which fell within,
often only just within, what had come to be the widely accepted
diagnostic glycaemic range for the disease. Inspecting these large
collections of data from typical mixed populations brought acutely
to attention the absence of any clear, natural division between the
normal and the diabetic in the frequency distribution of glucose
values. This led to great variation, even among 'experts'[4], in
the glycaemic values used for diagnostic criteria, generating the
potential for many fold variation in the apparent prevalence rates
for DM. The diagnostic distinction, and arbitrary cut-off, had to
be imposed upon what was, in essence, a variable, continuously
distributed and with positive skewing the degree of which increased
with advancing age. While the higher values in the distributions
were clearly 'diabetic', however this was defined, and while the
majority of the values falling in the main body of the distribution
were equally clearly normal, there was a substantial proportion of
intermediate, borderline values usually assigned to the diagnostic
category of diabetes. Their inclusion as diabetics greatly inflated
the apparent prevalence of DM so that, in large unselected
population groups, between 10 and 20% of those screened qualified
for the diagnosis. This final inflation as diabetes diagnosis
expanded from the classical, clinically defined syndrome to include
symptomless individuals defined entirely biochemically had several
consequences. Doubt about the significance and the treatment needs
of the many subjects with lesser degrees of glucose intolerance
brought large-scale, indiscriminate population screening virtually
to a stop. It was also the signal for organised epidemiological
validation of diagnostic criteria and classification against a
broader population background.

IMPAIRED GLUCOSE TOLERANCE (IGT)

It was to meet this proliferation of supposed 'early diabetes'
that the class of IGT was 'invented'. It described the metabolic
status of the large proportion of individuals with glycaemic
responses to a glucose load falling between those regarded by all
observers as unequivocally normal on the one hand, and those accepted by all as clearly diabetic on the other. By definition, an
individual can be assigned to this class of IGT only if blood
glucose responses fall within defined limits after a formal,
standardised test of oral glucose tolerance (OGTT).[1,2] The
possible significance of IGT to health and life has been the subject
of longterm epidemiological study in a number of populations. Does
it represent a period in the metabolic history of an individual
passing from the normal to the diabetic? Or is it an intermediate

metabolic track, followed by a person throughout life, neither reverting to normal nor deteriorating to diabetes? What underlying mechanism(s) is (are) responsible? What are its pathogenic implications? Is the development of IGT a 'normal' phenomenon of ageing? Should it be 'treated' and if so, how? Is it an homogeneous entity or is it, to use a currently much overused term, heterogeneous?

Follow-up studies[5,6,7,8,9] carried out in populations characterized initially by their glycaemic responses have contributed partial answers to some of these questions. Many individuals found on initial testing to show IGT revert, apparently spontaneously, to normal glucose tolerance, some of them no doubt illustrating the well-recognized statistical phenomenon of 'regression to the mean'. Others in this IGT group, perhaps 2 to 3% of them per annum, will show glycaemic deterioration to an unequivocally diabetic state. The rest will stay in the IGT zone. As a group, they are very unlikely to develop the so-called specific complications of DM (retinopathy, nephropathy, neuropathy). However, in some[10,11,12] but not all[13] large population follow-up studies, atherosclerotic disease occurs with significantly increased frequency in persons with IGT, at rates resembling those in the established diabetic. It is as yet uncertain what features predict ultimate deterioration of IGT to DM. There may be a delayed effect of obesity.[5,6] Those starting with the worse degrees of IGT are more likely to worsen to DM than those with lesser degrees. Though experience with the prospective Bedford study of newly detected IGT ('borderline diabetic') subjects did not suggest a predictive role for plasma insulin values, this was based upon the fasting and two hour concentrations, the only values measured. Similar conclusions were arrived at in studies of truly prediabetic Pima Indians.[14] In a recently published study on Japanese IGT subjects,[6] however, it was found that a low 30 min postload insulin response, particularly if associated with a high corresponding glucose concentration was a strong and independent predictor of worsening to diabetes.

It is not yet possible to offer a validated subclassification of IGT although, like DM, it is suggested that accompanying obesity (as defined) should be recorded as should any association with certain endocrine disorders, diabetogenic medications, genetic syndromes, etc. Clearly it would be valuable to distinguish those IGT individuals likely to revert to normal, those with persisting IGT and those liable to worsen to diabetes (bearing in mind that IGT may be the outward manifestation of more than one diabetogenic process). Other adverse outcomes which should be considered of importance in further classification of IGT are the increased susceptibility to arterial disease (coronary heart disease, stroke and peripheral vascular disease) and, possibly and contentiously[15,15a], the adverse outcome of pregnancy associated with IGT.

IGT, DM AND THE 'MID-TEST VALUE'

The value of replacing the older diabetic designation of glucose intolerance of lesser degree with the new category of IGT was recognised in the two major diagnostic reviews and recommendations of the early 1980s[1,2], and the social importance of not stigmatising such persons as diabetics has been widely accepted. However, the NDDG glycaemic definitions for DM and IGT differed in one (apparently) minor respect from those of the WHO Expert Committee on DM (Second Report). Both recommended the same fasting and 2 hour OGTT blood glucose values as diagnostic of IGT and DM but NDDG proposed that these should be accompanied by a mid-test (30, 60 or 90 minute) blood glucose concentration of 200 mg/dl (11.1mmol/1) or more (veinous plasma). WHO made no such mid-test value stipulation. Harris et al.[16] applied these two sets of glycaemic desiderata to 3701 OGTTs, assembled from a nationally based survey sample of American residents in the period 1976–1980. Of 191 responses qualifying for diagnosis of DM by WHO criteria, 12 failed to qualify by NDDG because of the mid-test value. Much more serious was the disagreement which occurred with the IGT category. Of the 532 tests so classified by WHO rules, 305 failed to do so by NDDG because of midtest values. Thus, this small difference in classificatory requirements has large effects in the numbers of individuals classified to IGT. One further drawback of the more demanding NDDG glycaemic requirement is the comparatively high proportion of tests that fall into the non-diagnostic or the unclassified group (538 of 3701 or 14.5%). The importance of this residual classificatory difference in epidemiological descriptions of populations is clearly demonstrated by the relatively high proportion of IGT subjects found in many population surveys (e.g. Bedford). In the American Second National Health and Nutrition Examination Survey (NHANES II) referred to above, 11.4% of the population aged between 20 and 74 years were classed as IGT by WHO criteria but only 4.8% were so classed by NDDG criteria. Taken along with the age standardised rate of 5.3% of known diabetics and 3.5% for newly found DM (WHO criteria, 3.3% NDDG criteria) in this population sample, the epidemiological scale of the overall metabolic problem becomes apparent as does the importance of using standardised methods and criteria for its ascertainment.

GLYCOSYLATED Hb AND CLASSIFICATION

On the face of it, the measurement of glycosylated Hb (GHb), as an integrated estimate of average glycaemia over the preceding month or two[17], would appear to be a useful diagnostic test, requiring no dietary and fasting preparation, no glucose loading, no timing of samples and measurable independently of time of day. However, as reviewed elsewhere[3] GHb, though of proven value in diabetes management and control, appears to lack sufficient discrimination to be used for diagnostic screening purposes. In particular, it fails to distinguish subjects with IGT from normals. This discriminatory failure may, in part, be due to the method of estimation employed. Methods vary considerably in which particular adducts are included as GHb and in whether only the stable ketoamine, or both this and unstable aldimine derivatives are included in the estimates. A recent paper[19] claims that, using an affinity chromatographic method, clear separation of GHb values from normal, impaired and diabetic responses in the OGTT can be achieved. This study included a very few IGT subjects and its findings were not upheld in a much larger population sample[19] of 2040 persons subjected to 100g glu- cose OGTT of whom 1058 also had measurement of GHb. This found extensive overlap of GHb values between different classes of glucose intolerance, even between normals and DM. It concluded that the 2 hour post glucose load value of blood glucose was a much more effec- tive single indicator of the diabetic state, and the one hour value, of overall glucose intolerance (IGT plus DM, NDDG criteria). One should just remain open to the possibility, however, that GHb repre- sents better the 'real-life' glycaemic milieu of the person's tissues than does the much more standardised - and perhaps much less repre- sentative-response to a large, unaccompanied glucose load.

CLASSES OF DIABETES MELLITUS

     The epidemiologist requires clear definitions before he can describe the distribution and associations of disease in populations. The major subclasses of the diabetic state were formulated in the NDDG classification and adopted (with some reservations) by the WHO Expert Committee, That classification represents a real advance on its predecessors but poses a number of problems for the epidemiologist.

     The two major subclasses recognised are insulin-dependent dia- betes mellitus (IDDM) and non insulin-dependent diabetes mellitus (NIDDM). It could be argued that all DM must be one or the other so that any further classification must be into subsets of these two major subclasses. However, the classification further recognizes 'other types of DM' (which may be insulin-dependent or not) and 'gestational DM' which is virtually, by definition, non insulin- dependent and which, to fulfill NDDG criteria, requires the application of quite different diagnostic methodologies and glycaemic criteria from diabetes diagnosis in the non-pregnant.[15] This for- mulation raises several theoretical and practical questions, one of the more troublesome being the definition of insulin dependency.

INSULIN DEPENDENCY

     As the term suggests, insulin dependency is essentially clini-

cally recognised. It describes a subclass readily recognizable in
its classical form (i.e. presenting in youth, with florid symptoms,
with ketosis and acidosis, lethal unless insulin is administered).
This last requirement, the ultimate proof of insulin dependency, can
now (since 1921) almost always be asserted only by inference; that
is to say that insulin dependent diabetes can be said to exist when,
in the judgement of the observer, death in ketoacidosis would follow
upon the withdrawal of insulin therapy. The 'honeymoon remission'
of ketoacidotic diabetes when insulin therapy may sometimes be completely withdrawn provides a classification problem but one that is
always only temporary. More troublesome is the young subject, perhaps related to a known insulin dependent diabetic, who is glucose
intolerant but not ketonuria, possibly already started on insulin
therapy in the expectation of deterioration but sometimes maintained
for many years on oral antidiabetic agents or even on diet alone.[20]
Is this 'preketotic' IDDM? A further classification problem is posed
by the lean, middle-aged patient, unremittingly hyperglycaemic from
diagnosis despite diet and oral agents, perhaps intermittently ketonuric, in whom insulin therapy is introduced to achieve glycaemic
control. What of the older patient, adequately maintained without
insulin for many years (and so unquestionably NIDDM) who then shows
progressive metabolic deterioration with progression to the ketosis-
prone state and in whom insulin therapy is judged to be mandatory
(now entirely acceptably IDDM)? And should one classify temporarily
as insulin-dependent the ordinarily adquately controlled NIDDM
patient who, under the stress of severe infection or a clinical event
such as myocardial infarction or physical trauma, for a period
requires insulin treatment to overcome a ketoacidotic response?

NDDG defined insulin dependency as a state 'characterized by an
abrupt onset of symptoms, insulinopenia, dependence on injected
insulin to sustain life, and proneness to ketosis. Classically this
type of diabetes occurs in juveniles... however, it can be recognized
and become symptomatic for the first time at any age ... in addition
to the ketosis prone stage it can also be recognised in a preketosis
stage'. While the clinician can cope with such a flexible definition, it may not be of great help to the epidemiologist confronted
with a large population of diabetic patients (or more likely their
clinical records) and called upon to separate the insulin-dependent
from the non insulin-dependent. In just such a position, Ng Tang
Fui et al.[21] used the following operational algorithm:

1. All diabetic patients not receiving insulin injections are
    NIDDM.

2. An unbroken (less than 1 month) record of daily insulin injec-
    tions from diagnosis defines IDDM.

3.   All others on insulin classified as NIDDM unless insulin was
     started during an episode of severe diabetic ketoacidosis and
     has been continued subsequently without interruption, which
     classifies to IDDM.

Of 800 randomly sampled diabetic outpatient records, only 4 could
not be classified using these rules.

Tattersall and colleagues[22] reviewed 100 consecutive new diabetic patients considered at diagnosis to require treatment with
insulin. As Table 2 shows, those diagnosed at age less than 20,
and those at age 21-40, conformed genetically closely to the 'classical' paradigm with over 90% of them HLA DR3, DR4 or DR3/4 hetero-
zygotes; however, in the subgroup aged 21-40 years only 42% had
demonstrable islet cell antibodies (ICA) compared with 88% with
earlier onset. Over age 40, these characteristics were much less
frequently present pointing to the possibility that more than one
pathogenic process may give rise to IDDM, especially when diagnosed
later in life.

Patients meeting the glycaemic requirements for DM and surviving
without insulin treatment are readily classified to NIDDM, though as
discussed above, their clinical evolution may later demand a change
of class. Although such changes of class are 'allowed for' in the
current classification they raise acutely the classificatory conflict
between clinical and pathogenic descriptors. The hope that the curi-
ous propensity of some NIDDM patients to flush when given a small
dose of alcohol (sherry) after pretreatment with the antidiabetic
agent chlorpropamide (chlorpropamide-alcohol flush, CPAF) might distinguish a genetically and clinically distinct subtype has not been
sustained.[21,23]

TYPE I AND TYPE II

Many people use the terms Type I and Type II diabetes interchangeably with IDDM and NIDDM respectively but that is unsatisfactory, both clinically and epidemiologically. Type I, as used, is
not so much of a description of a clinical state as of a presumed
pathogenic process. While this process may well be responsible for
many, probably most, cases of IDDM in peoples of European origin it
may also be responsible for a proportion of NIDDM patients[20] some
of whom go on to require insulin therapy. The Type I process may
also be associated with IGT and in some people with entirely normal
glucose tolerance (Figure 1). Furthermore, in some non-European
peoples (and perhaps in some Caucasoids as well - see above), IDDM
may result from other pathogenic processes. Thus, a single pathogenic process may manifest itself in a variety of clinical forms;
and a single clinical form of diabetes can result from a variety of
pathogenic processes. There is, of course, a broad parallelism

Table 2.   Analysis of 100 Patients Regarded as Insulin Requiring at
Diagnosis (Tattersall et al., 1984)

	AGE AT DIAGNOSIS			
	< 20	21 – 40	41 – 60	60+
Number	17	53	18	12
ISLET CELL Ab +ve(%)	88	42	22	17
HLA DR 3 or 4 (%)	94	93	61	59
KETONURIA > 2+ (%)	71	58	33	8
BODY MASS INDEX (Kg/m^2)	19	22	23	21
B GLUCOSE (mmol/L)	23.1	18.2	22.1	17.2
C PEPTIDE (nmol/L)	0.20	0.22	0.31	0.35
HbA (mean%)	16.3	15.2	15.0	14.9

100 consecutive patients presenting with what was clinically considered to be 'insulin requiring diabetes'* but not so severe as to
require admission to hospital. The group aged 40 years and under at
diagnosis are relatively homogeneous in respect of HLA types, GHb
and liability to ketonuria. Above that age, these associations are
all weaker.

*Two or more of: a) Ketonuria >++ b) abrupt symptomatic onset of <2
months duration c) severe symptoms of thirst of polyuria d) marked
weight loss e) first degree relative with insulin treated DM.

between pathogenic mechanism and clinical manifestation but the two
are not congruent; the attempt to make the one double for the other
in a classification generates anomalies and confusion. A more
logical classification might therefore, be based upon clinical
manifestation (e.g. IDDM, NIDDM) subdivided by pathogenic mechanism
(e.g. Type I, Type II, etc.) or vice versa.

    The problem of non-congruence of terms is further compounded by

difficulties in finding a definition for the term Type II. Probably
the best one can do is to define Type II as describing those
individuals qualifying for a diagnosis of DM who do not have Type I
(or gestational or 'other types' of diabetes). It is suggested,
therefore, that the term Type I should not be used to describe a
clinical form of diabetes but to denote, when sufficient information
is available to the classifier, a pathogenic process characterised
by certain immunological phenomena (as yet unstandardised in their
demonstration) occurring within individuals carrying the HLA
antigens DR3, DR4 or both (or some at present serologically
indistinguishable subtypes(s) of them). The Type I process may
manifest with a variety of presenting syndromes and evolving natural
histories; it may sometimes be associated with no demonstrable
clinical features at all. At present there is insufficient scientific evidence to talk in definable epidemiological terms about a
Type II process. Although there are indications that genetic
markers may be present near the insulin gene in some cases[24] it is
difficult to justify the use of the term Type II clinically or
scientifically. The application of these rather more rigorous
criteria to the use of terminology by editorial agencies of journals
and books would help to clear the ambiguities. Even the sponsors of
meetings and symposia may not be beyond criticism!

OTHER TYPES OF DM (OTDM)

      This broad category in the present classification accommodates
patients with a large number of known diabetogenic causal mechanism
and associations. Although the number of subgroups is very large
the category actually applies to a very small number of diabetic
patients. Individuals falling into these subgroups are of very
great scientific interest and importance but the epidemiologist,
concerned primarily with the recognition and enumeration of major
diabetes categories, could virtually ignore OTDM were it not for the
high prevalence of one particular subgroup, the so-called Tropical,
Pancreatic or Nutritional DM.[25] In global terms, this may well
exceed numerically the class of IDDM. This still incompletely
described and defined class appears to be restricted to the peoples
of developing tropical countries where malnutrition and infection
are rife. Occurring in youth, accompanied by severe cachexia,
without liability to keto-acidosis, intermittently insulin-dependent
and associated with a spectrum of pathological changes in the
pancreas ranging from diffuse fibrosis to gross intraductal
calcification, the syndrome deserves a much more prominent place in
the classification. An appeal that it should be called
Type III [26] has a more polemical than scientific basis, however.
As distinct causal mechanisms resulting in the diabetic state are
defined, increasing numbers of patients will be displaced from the
clinical 'parking' classes of IDDM and NIDDM into the process-
defined subclasses of OTDM, but that is some way off.

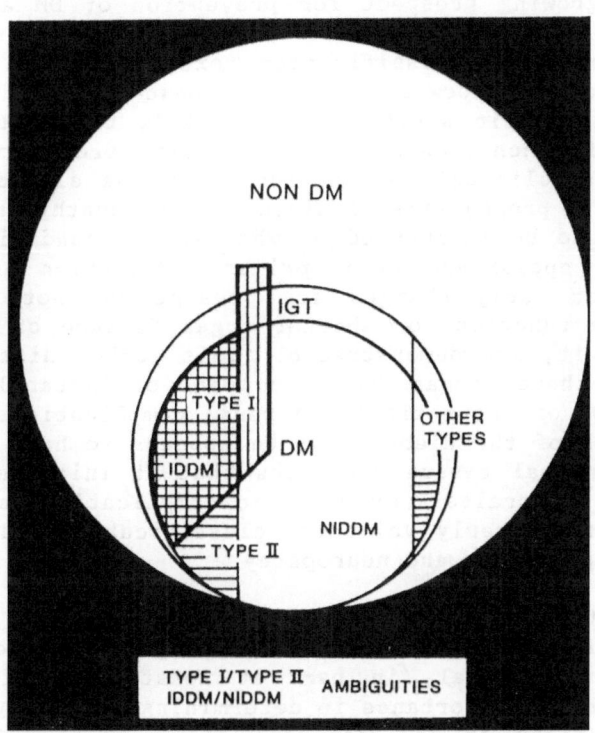

Fig. 1:   In this diagram, the area enclosed by the large circle
circumscribes the 'universe' which, largely normal in
respect of glucose tolerance (outermost area), includes a
group with impaired glucose tolerance (IGT) (area between
outermost and innermost circle) and a group with DM
(innermost circle). Horizontal shading lines identify an
area of DM which is clinically insulin-dependent (IDDM)
while vertical shading lines represent the area to which
the term Type I with its immunological and genetic
connotations might be applied. While the latter largely
coincides with IDDM, it also includes some of the non
insulin-dependent (NIDDM) area, extends into IGT and even
into the metabolically normal (non DM) area. There is
also a proportion of IID patients who could not be
classed as Type II (no genetic or immunological markers,
often later onset with many years of NIDDM deteriorating
acutely, temporarily or chronically to IDDM). There is
also a proportion of 'OTHER TYPES' of DM who are clearly
insulin-dependent but not Type I.

'STAGING' AND CLASSIFICATION

With the growing prospect for prevention of DM and its consequences, there is a strong case to be made for the introduction of a
staging component into classification, extending back into the prediabetic period and forward into the post-diagnostic (Table 3).
Preventive antidiabetic strategies are likely to be quite different
in the stage of 'unchallenged susceptibility' from those adopted in
the stage of 'subclinical dysfunction'. In the already established
diabetic patient, prophylaxis of diabetic retinopathy and nephropathy
is likely also to be influenced by whether the condition has yet to
make its first appearance (i.e. primary prevention of the complication), whether early changes are present but not yet affecting
organ or tissue function, or whether organ failure or the high risk
indicators for it, are demonstrable. This latter distinction is of
importance for there appears to be a point of 'metabolic no return'
in the evolution of the retinal and renal complications of DM beyond
which correction of the diabetic state appears to have little influence on the abnormal tissue processes that it initiated. Epidemiologically usable appraisals of diabetic complications are in need of
well defined and properly validated classificatory staging steps of
retinopathy, nephropathy and neuropathy.

Both for the diabetic state itself and for its serious long-
term consequences, it appears that the susceptibility (or resistance)
status of the individual (in part at least, probably genetically
defined) is of major importance in determining liability as it interacts with a variety of environmental determinants. In this relatively new field of susceptibility status, the interests of the
investigator, the clinician, the epidemiologist and the patient himself, coincide!

CONCLUSION AND SUMMARY

1. There are residual ambiguities between the two main current
    glycaemic definitions of the categories of DM, IGT and normal
    GT which should be resolved.

2. IGT is clearly a highly heterogeneous category and could with
    advantage be resolved into its identifiable subsets though ade-
    quate data for this is not yet available.

3. The concept of insulin dependency requires clearer definition
    for operational purposes. Biochemical parameters (e.g.
    C-peptide responses) may help.

4. Attempts to combine clinical manifestations and pathogenic
    mechanisms in a single classification (e.g. IDDM/NIDD versus

TABLE 3   Staging Classification of DM

DEFINING FEATURES IN:

STAGE	IDDM	NIDDM
1. UNCHALLENGED SUSCEPTIBILITY	HLA DR 3/4	DNA POLYMORPHISM CHROMOSOME 11
2. CHALLENGED SUSCEPTIBILITY	ICA (IgG, CF) ? CMI	LOW FIRST PEAK INSULIN RELEASE
3. SUBCLINCIAL DYSFUNCTION	REDUCED MAXIMUM INSULIN SECRETION	IGT
4. EARLY DISEASE	IGT/NIDDM	REVERSIBLE DM ('DIET RESPONSIVE')
5. CLINICAL PARADIGM	'CLASSICAL' IDDM, DKA	FIXEC DM ('DIET UNRESPONSIVE')
6. 'EARLY' COMPLICATIONS	RETINAL/RENAL MICROABNORMALITIES NEURAL CONDUCTION DEFECTS	
7. 'LATE' COMPLICATIONS	ORGAN FAILURE – BLINDNESS, URAEMIA TISSUE BREAKDOWN (NEURO/VASCULAR)	

Suggested schema for a staging classification of the two major clinical types of DM. It is recognised that both IDDM and NIDDM are
heterogeneous so the above refers only to subsets of them. Individuals will move through the staging sequence at varying rates, possibly reversible in the earlier stages. Progression from stage 6 to
stage 7 may not occur in a 'severe-complications-resistant' subset.

Type I/Type II) should be handled with care. If the term Type
I is to be retained, it should be applied to a defined pathogenic process, not to a clinical type of DM. The term Type II
is inadequately defined at present.

5.   IDDM and NIDDM, clinical descriptive terms, may be provoked by
a variety of pathogenic mechanisms (i.e. they are 'heterogeneous'). They could be subclassified by mechanism (when
known).

6.   More visibility should be given in classification to
non-Europid forms of DM (e.g. 'Tropical or 'Nutritional' DM).

7.   A staging dimension should be recognised in classifications of DM.

8.   Future classifications will benefit from the incorporation of the presence or absence of susceptibility/resistance factors to diabetes itself or to its severe long term sequelae.

9.   There remain uncertainties about the definitions and clinical implications of gestational DM (and gestational IGT) not discussed above.

10.   It should be accepted that different user groups may need different subclassification of diabetes and glucose intolerance to meet their specific requirements and so long as this is made clear and definitions are adequate this should not be a problem. However, for the present, all groups should accept the proposed glycaemic definitions of DM or IGT for the purposes of comparability.

REFERENCES

1.   National Diabetes Data Group, Classification and diagnosis of diabetes and other categories of glucose intolerance, Diabetes 28:139–157 (1979).
2.   World Health Organisation Expert Committee, Second Report on Diabetes Mellitus, Tech. Rep. Series 646, WHO, Geneva (1980).
3.   H. Keen, S. Tang Ng Fui, The definition and classification of diabetes mellitus, Clin. Endocrinol Metab. 11:279–305 (1982).
4.   K.M. West, Substantial differences in diagnostic criteria used by diabetes experts, Diabetes 24:641–664 (1975).
5.   H. Keen, R.J. Jarrett, P. McCartney, The ten–year follow-up of the Bedford Survey (1962–1972): glucose tolerance and diabetes, Diabetologia 22:73–78 (1982).
6.   T. Kadowaki, Y. Miyake, R. Hagura et al., Risk factors for worsening to diabetes in subjects with impaired glucose tolerance, Diabetologia 26:44–49 (1984).
7.   J.B. O'Sullivan, C.M. Mahan, Blood sugar levels, glycosuria and body weight related to development of diabetes mellitus, J. Am Med. Assoc. 194:117–122 (1965).
8.   R.J. Jarrett, H. Keen, J.H. Fuller, M. McCartney, Worsening to diabetes in men with impaired glucose tolerance ('borderline diabetes'), Diabetologia 16:25–30 (1979).
9.   A. Sasaki, T. Suzuki, N. Horiuchi, Development of diabetes in Japanese subjects with impaired glucose tolerance; a seven year follow-up study, Diabetologia 22:154–157 (1982).
10.   J.H. Fuller, M.J. Shipley, G. Rose, R.J. Jarrett, H. Keen, Coronary heart disease risk and impaired glucose tolerance: The Whitehall Study, Lancet 1:1373–1376 (1980).

11. R.J. Jarrett, P. McCartney, H. Keen, The Bedford Survey: Ten year mortality rates in newly diagnosed diabetics, borderline diabetes and normoglycaemic controls and risk indices for coronary heart disease in borderline diabetics, Diabetologia 22:79-84 (1982).

12. J.H. Fuller, M.J. Shipley, G. Rose, R.J. Jarrett, H. Keen, Mortality from coronary heart diease and stroke in relation to degree of glycaemia: The Whitehall Study, Br. Med. J. 287:867-870 (1983).

13. R. Stamler, and J. Stamler, Asymptomatic hyperglycaemia and coronary heart disease: a series of papers by the international collaborative group based on studies in fifteen populations, J. Chron Dis. 32:683-837 (1979).

14. P.J. Savage, P.H. Bennett, P. Gorden, M. Miller, Insulin response to oral carbohydrate in true prediabetics and matched controls, Lancet 1:300-302 (1975).

15. R.J. Jarrett, Reflections on gestational diabetes mellitus, Lancet 2:1220-1222 (1981).

15a. H. Keen, Glucose intolerance in pregnancy. Diabetologia 24:460-461 (1983).

16. M.I. Harris, W.C. Hadden, W.C. Knowler, P.H. Bennett, "International criteria for the diagnosis of diabetes and impaired glucose tolerance" (In Press) (1984).

17. L. Jovanovic, C. Peterson, The clinical utility of glycosylated hemoglobin, Am. J. Med. 70:331-338 (1981).

18. P.M. Hall, J.G.H. Cook, J. Sheldon, S.M. Rutherford, B.J. Gould, Glycosylated hemoglobins and glycosylated plasma proteins in the diagnosis of diabetes mellitus and impaired glucose tolerance, Diabetes Care 7:147-150 (1984).

19. M. Modan, H. Halkin, A. Karasik, A. Lusky, Effectiveness of glycosylated haemoglobin, fasting plasma glucose and a single post-load plasma glucose level in population screening for glucose intolerance, Amer. J. Epidemiol 119:431-444 (1984).

20. U. Di Mario, W.J. Irvine, D.Q. Borsey et al., Immune abnormalities in diabetic patients not requiring insulin at diagnosis, Diabetologia 25:392-395 (1983).

21. S. Ng Tang Fui, H. Keen , R.J. Jarrett et al., Epidemiological study of prevalence of chlorpropamide alcohol flushing in insulin dependent diabetics, non-insulin dependent diabetics and non-diabetics, Br. Med. J. 287:1509-1512 (1983).

22. R.B. Tattersall, R.M. Wilson, P. van der Minne, I. Deverill, K. Gelsthorpe, W.G. Reeves, Problems with the classification of Type I diabetes - a prospective study, Diabetic Med. (In Press) (1984).

23. S. Ng Tang Fui, H. Keen , R.J. Jarrett, W. Gossanin, P. Marsden, Test for chlorpropamide treatment in insulin-dependent and non-insulin-dependent diabetics, N. Eng. J. Med. 3009:93-96 (1983).

24. P.S. Rotwein, J. Chirgwin, M. Province et al., Polymorphism in
    the 5' flanking region of the human insulin gene: a genetic
    marker for non-insulin-dependent diabetes, N. Eng. J. Med.
    308:65-71 (1983).
25. H. Keen, J.M. Ekoe, The geography of diabetes, Brit Med. Bull
    40:359:365 (1984).
26. E. Morrison, Diabetes mellitus — a third syndrome, Phasic
    insulin dependence (PID), Int. Diab. Fed. Bull 26:6-8 (1981).

GESTATIONAL DIABETES: PROBLEMS IN CLASSIFICATION

AND IMPLICATIONS FOR LONG-RANGE PROGNOSIS

Norbert Freinkel and Boyd E. Metzger
Center for Endocrinology, Metabolism and Nutrition
Northwestern University Medical School
Chicago, Il.   U.S.A.

1.   INTERMEDIARY METABOLISM IN NORMAL PREGNANCY

Pregnancy is the quintessential anabolic event. An accretion of maternal mass consisting largely of fat characterizes the first half of pregnancy; a massive accumulation of new cells coincident with the maturation and full development of the conceptus occurs during the second.[7] As with all anabolic events, these processes are attended by major changes in insulin economy. During the latter half of pregnancy, the response to exogenous insulin is blunted; basal plasma levels of endogenous insulin increase; and glycemic challenge elicits a two to threefold greater release of insulin than under nongravid conditions.[7] The basis for the heightened resistance to insulin action has not been clarified completely. However, within the last few years, four laboratories have independently reported that it cannot be ascribed to a reduction in the number or affinity of insulin receptors.[26,36,37,41,42] In our own Unit, Baumann and colleagues compared the same normal women, pre- and postpartum, to assess these relationships[36] (Fig. 1). They demonstrated that insulin binding to monocytes and red blood cells at the time of the insulin resistance of late pregnancy is the same or slightly greater than during the luteal phase of the normal menstrual cycle. The lack of change in insulin receptors, in the absence of pre-receptor antagonists to insulin action, clearly indicts postreceptor phenomena in the insulin resistance of late normal gestation. The striking alterations in intermediary metabolism that normally occur at this time may be implicated.

The opportunity to review the metabolic realignments of normal gestation at a meeting in Toronto evokes great nostalgia because it was in Toronto in 1964, at the Fifth Congress of the International Diabetes Federation and, at a panel on pregnancy chaired by the late

47

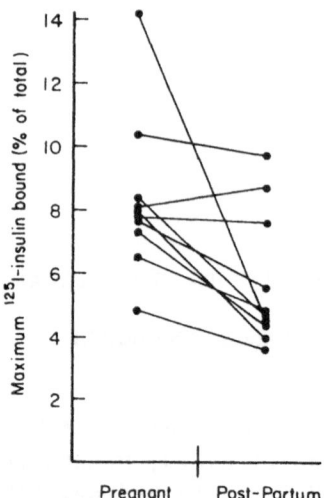

Fig. 1:   The figure depicts maximum binding of [^{125}I] insulin to
           monocytes from the same women studied during late preg-
           nancy and again postpartum (Adapted from ref. 36).

Professor Joseph P. Hoet, that we first proposed that late pregnancy
may modify the usual response to dietary deprivation.[8] At that
time, we suggested that it might be advantageous for the mother to
transfer to the metabolism of fat more rapidly and abundantly, whenever food is withheld, so that less expendable fuels such as glucose
and amino acids could be "spared" for the conceptus. We designated
this process as "accelerated starvation" and emphasized that the
"increasing placental elaboration of contrainsulin factors in parallel with the growth of the fetus provides just the right temporal
juxtaposition to make it all work".[8] During succeeding years, we
employed a variety of in vitro systems and animal models to document
that dietary deprivation in the mother does indeed elicit a quantitative and qualitative exaggeration of the starvation response, as
evidenced by a greater and more rapid: activation of lipolysis and
mobilization of fat; induction of ketonemia; decrease in maternal
glucose and gluconeogenic amino acids; catabolism of maternal
muscle; activation of gluconeogenesis; and urinary excretion of urea
and ammonia.[16,18,21,23] Others, in later studies with normal
pregnant women prior to elective abortions, demonstrated that
"accelerated starvation" is already operative by week 16-20 of human
pregnancy.[5,43] Most recently we have shown that the process can
be unmasked in normal gravida by such minimal dietary deprivation as
"skipping" breakfast so that "accelerated starvation" is a metabolic
fact of life in late gestation even under the conditions that obtain
in standard clinical practice.[25]
      In such a setting of more ready diversion to fat, normal preg-
nancy is also accompanied by changes in the fed state. Administra-

tion of oral glucose (100 g) for standard OGTT after 14-hour overnight fast in late pregnancy elicits greater and more prolonged increases in blood sugar; increments in plasma triglycerides (located chiefly in the VLDL fraction); and decrements in plasma glucagon[11] (Fig. 2). We have suggested that the sequence could "facilitate anabolism" since (a) exaggerated hyperglycemia would assure more of the ingested glucose access to the conceptus because glucose crosses the placenta in concentration-dependent fashion; b) increased plasma triglycerides could abet this objective by substituting for some of the glucose as oxidative fuel in the mother while also enabling more glucose to be retained as glyceride-glycerol or fatty acids for subsequent recall; and c) greater suppression of glucagon would hasten interruption of glucagon contributions to such ongoing hepatic aspects of accelerated starvation as glycogenolysis, gluconeogenesis and ketogenesis.[7,11]

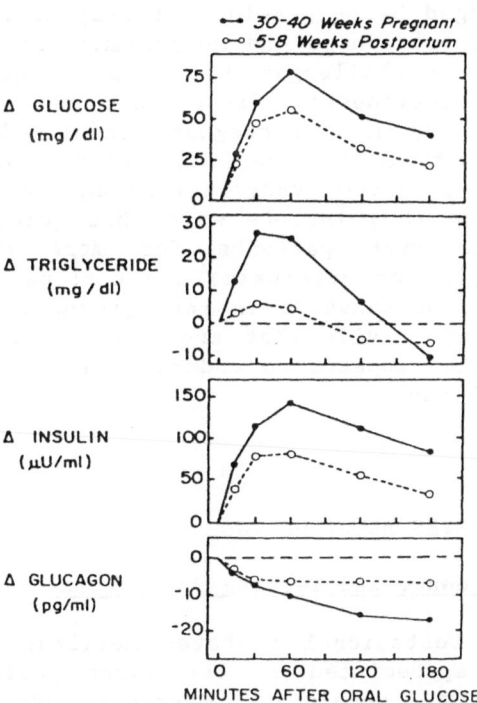

Fig. 2:   Effects of pregnancy on the response to oral glucose after overnight fast: Changes in concentrations of plasma glucose, triglycerides, immunoreactive insulin, and glucagon are expressed as net increments or decrements from basal values following the administration of oral glucose (100 g) after 14-hr overnight fast. The same women with normal carbohydrate metabolism were studied in late pregnancy and again postpartum (Adapted from ref. 11 and reproduced from ref. 7).

The proposition that such changes in the fed as well as the fasted state may alter diurnal fuel metabolism as part of normal gestation has been confirmed under conditions of meal-eating. We have evaluated the relationships by sampling circulating fuels at hourly intervals "around-the-clock" while administering liquid formula diets in three isocaloric feedings each day. Comparisons of normal gravida at 33-39 weeks of gestation and age-matched, weight-matched nongravid subjects disclosed that greater postprandial increments and preprandial decrements of plasma glucose occur with every meal during late pregnancy in keeping with the predictions of "facilitated anabolism" and "accelerated starvation" respec-tively[34] (Fig. 3). Concurrent estimates of insulin indicated that mean 24-hour values for plasma immunoreactive insulin are approx-imately twofold greater in late pregnancy and that plasma insulin immediately after meals may be increased as much as three- to four-fold.[34] Clearly, therefore, metabolic normalcy during late preg-nancy cannot be judged by nongravid criteria; oscillations of blood sugar are much more pronounced and mechanisms for chronic and acute insulin secretion are challenged to a much greater degree. Two corollaries are self-evident: first, any attempts to replicate normal fuel homeostasis in the pregnant insulin-dependent diabetic will necessitate not only more long-acting insulin for basal insulinization, but also some short-acting ad hoc insulin with each meal for fine tuning (a principle which has guided our own thera-peutic approach to such patients for more than a decade[7]). Second, any intrinsic (or extrinsic) limitations in insulin secre-tory reserve may become unmasked in late pregnancy by virtue of the augmented demands for insulin that are posed by normal pregnany at this time. The latter appears to underline the emergence of Gesta-tional Diabetes Mellitus.

2. GESTATIONAL DIABETES MELLITUS (GDM)

a) Definition, Incidence and Testing Procedures

The entity of Gestational Diabetes Mellitus (GDM) appears to have been already appreciated in the first published account of diabetes in pregnancy. Herein, J. Matthews Duncan indicated that "diabetes may come on during pregnancy" and "diabetes may occur only during pregnancy being absent at other times".[2] A more rigorous definition was adopted at the First International Workshop-Conference on Gestational Diabetes in 1979[10] and incorporated into the recommended classification of diabetes by the National Diabetes Data Group.[27] GDM was designated as "carbohydrate intolerance with onset or recognition during pregnancy".[10,27] At Prentice Women's Hospital and Maternity Center of Northwestern Memorial Hospital, we routinely screen all gravida for GDM by administering a

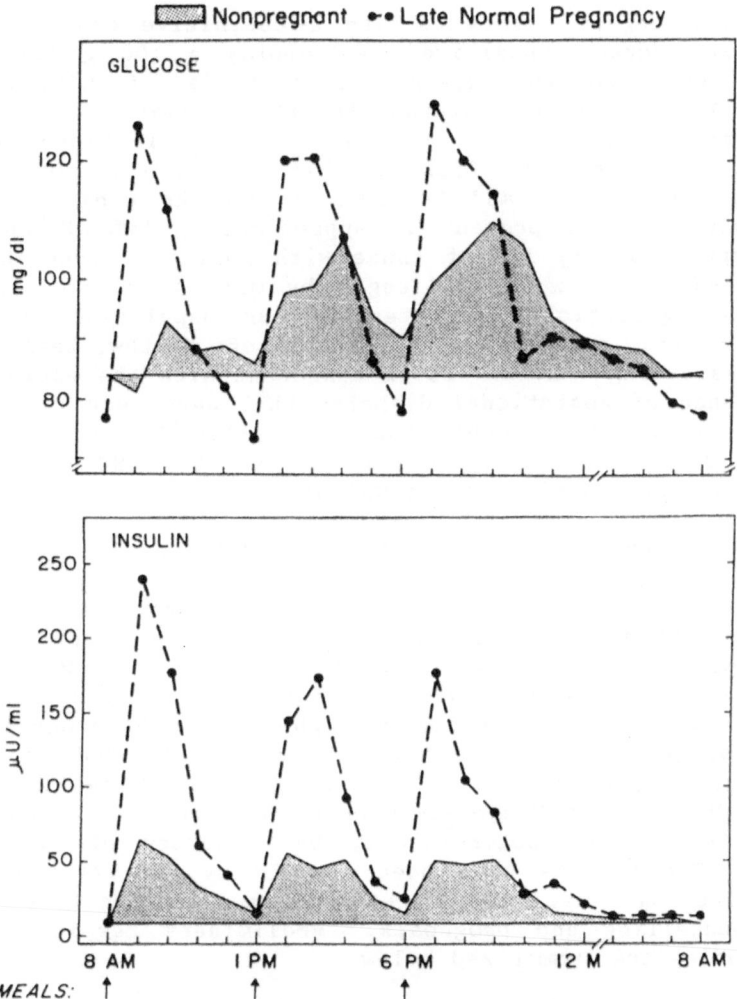

Fig. 3:   Effect of normal late pregnancy on diurnal changes in
            plasma glucose and insulin. Subjects were given 2,100
            calories/day (275 g carbohydrate; 75 g protein; 78 g fat)
            as liquid formula diets in three equal meals at the times
            denoted by the arrows (Adapted from ref. 34 and
            reproduced from ref. 7).

50 g oral load of glucose in the fasting state or 3 or more hours
postprandially. The procedure is instituted at the initial clinic
visit of those at "high risk" for gestational carbohydrate
intolerance and routinely at weeks 24-28 of gestation. The test is
repeated again at week 32 for those who screened negative but
entered with "high risk". The screening is considered positive when
plasma glucose is equal to or greater than 140 mg/dl one hour after

the 50 g challenge.[35] To establish a definitive diagnosis of GDM
in those who screen "positive", we employ a 100 g oral glucose
tolerance test and the diagnostic criteria of O'Sullivan and
Mahan.[31] Our approach conforms to the recommendations of the
National Diabetes Data Group and the First International Workshop-
Conference on Gestational Diabetes.[10,27] With it, our colleagues
Drs. Richard L. Phelps and Marilynn Fredericksen have found that
positive screening is present in approximately 14% of our gravida
and that approximately 17% of those with positive screening have a
definitive diagnosis when challenged by OGTT as above. Thus, the
incidence of gestational diabetes in our population at Prentice
Women's Hospital and Maternity Center of Northwestern Memorial
Hospital has averaged 2.4%. It is consonant with the estimates of a
2-3% incidence of gestational diabetes that have been reported from
other large metropolitan centers in the United States, and suggests
that GDM is present in approximately 60,000 - 90,000 of the 3
million annual pregnancies in the United States.[6]

b) Heterogeneity in Gestational Diabetes Mellitus

     On the basis of clinical presentations, and limited follow-up
experiences, GDM has been classically deemed to be a variant of Type
II diabetes mellitus, that is, non-insulin dependent diabetes
mellitus (NIDDM). We have been intrigued by the possibility that
GDM may include the genotypic and phenotypic heterogeneity that
seems to be present in all other forms of diabetes mellitus.[4]
Accordingly, as part of the continuing program at the Northwestern
University Diabetes in Pregnancy Center, we have been evaluating our
gravida with GDM for heterogeneity by a number of the existing
"markers". The efforts have been spurred by the recognition that
such distinctions may have profound implications for therapy,
genetic counselling and prognosis. Preliminary results from some
ongoing studies are summarized below.

     (1) Genotypic Heterogeneity: We have been examining for an
association between GDM and the HLA antigens DR2, DR3 and DR4.
Epidemiological evidence in nongravid diabetics has indicated that
the incidence of these antigens is altered in Type I (i.e. insulin
dependent) but not Type II (i.e. non-insulin dependent) diabetes
mellitus with DR2 occurring less frequently and DR3 or DR4 or both
more often.[40] In view of racial differences in HLA patterns, we
have subdivided our populations into Whites, Blacks and Hispanics
and compared each group of gravida with GDM to "glucose-tolerance
tested controls" (that is, pregnant women in whom normal gestational
glucose tolerance was documented) as well as "random controls" (that
is, nongravid HLA typed volunteers and blood donors in whom glucose
tolerance was not documented). In the 24 Caucasian, 32 Black, and
43 Hispanic gravida with GDM examined to date, we have found that
the frequencies of DR3 and DR4 are increased and DR2 diminished in
every group in comparison to racially matched "glucose tolerance

tested controls" or "random controls" and that the trend assumes statistical significance in the case of Blacks.

We have also evaluated our gravida with GDM for circulating cytoplasmic islet cell antibodies (ICA). We have found such antibodies in 11.3% of 53 gestational diabetics examined to date vis-a-vis an incidence of 1.7% in 177 control subjects (p <.01). Islet cell antibodies are another of the genotypic markers that appear to be increased in Type I but not in Type II diabetics, especially at the time of initial diagnosis.[17]

The implications of the above HLA and ICA findings (and some analogous experiences of others[19,38] are intriguing albeit still enigmatic. In the least, they suggest that there may be some genetic heterogeneity in GDM. From the available data one cannot say whether this means that some gravida with "recognition or onset of carbohydrate intolerance during pregnancy" represent a wholly separate and novel diabetic subgroup or whether the heterogenous GDM population includes some patients with evolving Type I diabetes mellitus. Traditional views concerning the acuteness of onset of insulin-dependent diabetes mellitus have been substantially modified by the recent evidence that classical Type I disease may develop slowly with immunological abnormalities and declining islet cell function preceding full-blown insulin-dependency by years.[15,39] Clearly, more long-range observations of our patients with GDM will be necessary to classify the underlying type of diabetes in some of our patients with faulty glucoregulation during pregnancy.

(2) Phenotypic Heterogeneity: We have long advocated stratification of GDM on the basis of the severity of the metabolic disturbance and have espoused subdivision on the basis of fasting plasma glucose (FPG) to make such distinctions.[12,24,28,35] Thus, we have used the following modification of the White classification to characterize patients with GDM at our Center since 1977[35]:

Class A_1: Fasting plasma glucose (FPG) within the normal range for pregnancy, i.e. less than 105 mg/dl. We have suggested that the underlying pathophysiology in Class A_1 consists principally of "underutililzation".[12]

Class A_2: FPG greater than 105 but less than 130 mg/dl, (i.e., FPG elevated for pregnancy but below the value considered diagnostic of diabetes mellitus under nongravid conditions, that is 140 mg/dl, but adjusted for the normal lowering of blood sugar in pregnancy). We have suggested that this level of FPG may reflect "underutilization" plus mild "overproduction".[12]

Class B_1: Fasting plasma glucose of 130 mg/dl or greater. Such values for FPG may connote "underutilization" as well as moderate "overproduction".[12]

We have examined metabolic profiles "around-the-clock" to assess whether such subclassifications on the basis of FPG concord with overall changes in blood sugar during meal-eating in reallife.[24] As shown in Figure 4, we have found that even Class A_1 gravida significantly exceed the normal glucose excursions during diurnal observations and that the magnitude of the deviations are significantly greater in the Class A_2 group. Thus, useful metabolic insights may be conferred by classifying GDM on the basis of fasting plasma glucose and a similar view was espoused by the National Diabetes Data Group as well as the First Workshop-Conference on Gestational Diabetes.[10,27]

We have been examining our gestational diabetics to see whether such phenotypic characteristics as age and weight are different in the various subgroups. As shown in Table 1, preliminary comparison of 148 consecutive gravida with normal glucose tolerance from our Prentice population to 127 of our Class A_1, 47 Class A_2, and 23 Class B_1 patients indicates that the gestational diabetics tend to be older and heavier, and that the obesity appears to increase in parallel with the increase in FPG. Such observations underscore the need to incorporate appropriate corrections for age and weight into

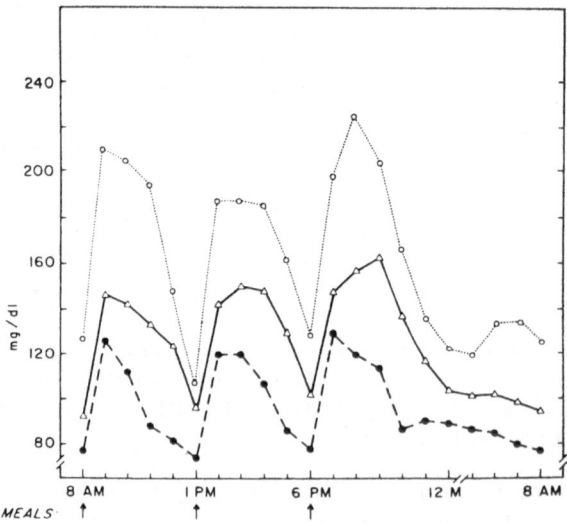

Fig. 4:   Diurnal changes in plasma glucose in late pregnancy in women with normal carbohydrate metabolism (●----●); gestational diabetes and normal fasting plasma glucose (Class A_1), (Δ-----Δ); and gestational diabetes with fasting plasma glucose greater than 105 but less than 130 mg/dl, (Class A_2), (o----o). Subjects were given liquid formula diets as described in Fig. 3 (Adapted from ref. 24).

ment of glucoregulatory factors in GDM. We have used covariance analysis to achieve this objective for our interpretation of insulin secretion in GDM. However, such statistical refinements have not modified our earlier pathophysiological conclusions[13,22]. Our analyses of insulin secretion during tests of oral glucose tolerance have indicated that all forms of GDM, are attended by an <u>absolute</u> reduction in insulin release and that this obtains in lean as well as in obese, and to a progressively more severe degree in Class A_1 vis-a-vis Class A_2 vis-a-vis Class B_1, gravida. Moreover, we have been able to demonstrate this deficit on the basis of changes in insulin (ΔI) relative to the changes in glucose (ΔG) during the first 15 min. ("acute insulin secretion"; $\Delta I/\Delta G$ 15 min.) as well as the entire 180 minutes ("chronic insulin secretion"; $\Delta I/\Delta G$ 180 min.") following oral glucose administration. Thus, our findings (like others in which phenotypic variability has not been considered[3,44]) indicate that GDM may be ascribed to some limitation in intrinsic insulin secretory capabilities. However, even here some exceptions are emerging and we have encountered a small number of gravida with seemingly normal insulin responses to oral glucose in every subgroup of GDM that we have examined to date.[13,22] Clearly, the lack of invariable insulinopenia must be viewed as another manifestation of heterogeneity.

Table 1. Gestational Diabetes Mellitus: Age and Weight*

	Control (148)	A_1 (127)	A_2 (47)	B_1 (23)
Age				
Mean	25.4±0.5	30.9±0.6	31.8±0.9	31.4±1.1
% ≥28	35	67	79	74
Weight				
Mean	109±2	102±2	136±4	157±8
% >120 PIBW	25	43	74	78

*Results are presented as Mean ± SEM. Weights refer to values prior to pregnancy and have been expressed as percent of ideal body weight (PIBW).

() = number of subjects in each group.

c) Prognostic Significance

Estimates of the frequency of glucose intolerance following GDM are few and conflicting.[20,30] The differences in reported series may result from variable criteria for the diagnosis of GDM and for failure to correct for the prevalence of confounding heterogeneity (see above). We have been instituting postpartum follow-up examinations in all of our women with GDM during pregnancy to identify the incidence of abnormalities under nongravid conditions and to see whether phenotypic and/or genotypic characteristics may confer prognostically useful information.[1] We have been designating postpartum tests as abnormal when they conform to the criteria for "impaired glucose tolerance" or "diabetes mellitus" promulgated by the National Diabetes Data Group.[27] Within that framework of reference, we have found abnormal oral glucose tolerance tests during one-year follow-up in 57% of 113 women with histories of GDM.[1] Certain phenotypic features during the index pregnancy have provided the greatest prognostic value. Thus, we have found abnormal OGTT during the first postpartum year in 95% of those with values for FPG of 130 mg/dl or greater during the pregnancy in contrast to an incidence of only 47% in those with FPG values below 130 mg/dl.[1] In the latter group, age has been predictive. Abnormal oral glucose tolerance in the first postpartum year has been encountered in two-thirds of those more than 38 years of age, but in only one-fourth of those under 28 years of age.[1] Acute secretory responsiveness has also provided useful prognostic clues. Only one-fourth of those with $\Delta I/\Delta G$ of less than 1 during the first 15 minutes following oral glucose have manifested normal oral glucose tolerance tests one year postpartum, whereas postpartum normalcy has been present in three-fourths of those with antepartum $\Delta I/\Delta G$ 15 min greater than 1.5.[1]

The foregoing experiences differ from prevailing views and suggest that long-range prognoses in GDM may be less sanguine than heretofore envisioned. Abnormalities in glucose tolerance, albeit of a subtle nature, appear to be present in a sizeable proportion of GDM patients within the first year after delivery. Hence, postpartum re-evaluation must be a routine component of standard follow-up procedure. A particularly rich harvest of abnormalities may be anticipated in the older subjects with GDM and in those whose phenotypic patterns are consistent with more pronounced limitations in insulin secretion.[1]

3. IMPLICATIONS OF GDM FOR THE OFFSPRING

a) Immediate Pregnancy Outcome

Maternal fuels constitute the building blocks from which all fetal development must take place. Appreciation of this self-evident relationship prompted the suggestion in 1978 that the metabolic aspects of pregnancy may be viewed as a "tissue culture experience".[12] This formulation stresses that the placenta and the fetus develop in an "incubation medium" that is wholly derived from maternal fuels. Since many, such as glucose, ketones, glycerol and a number of the neutral and basic amino acids appear to traverse the human placenta in concentration-dependent fashion, the oscillations in circulating maternal fuels may delimit their quantitative as well as qualitative appearance in the fetal circulation.[7,12] Furthermore, since all these fuels in the mother's circulation are responsive to maternal insulin, the ongoing insulinization of the mother may constitute the major arbiter of the whole nutrient mix to which the fetus is exposed.[7,12]

To assess the sensitivity with which these relationships may be poised, we have secured "around-the-clock" metabolic profiles for multiple fuels besides glucose in women with the least detectable defect in glucoregulation during pregnancy, i.e. Class A_1 gestational diabetics.[24] We have found that their abnormalities in fuel metabolism are not confined to glucose, but include every major class of foodstuff. Thus, besides glucose, we have documented significant aberrations in the excursions of FFA, triglycerides, and certain of the individual amino acids in maternal plasma.[12,24] The findings have prompted our thesis that the entire metabolic mixture in the fetus may be modified even in the mildest form of gestational diabetes.[12,24] As shown in Fig. 5, all fuels of maternal origin should be increasingly available, and, all may contribute to the premature stimulation of fetal islet cells and supranormal accretion of fetal mass that was initially ascribed to glucose alone in Pedersen's classical "hyperglycemia-hyperinsulinism" hypothesis.[29]

Our preliminary analyses of 46 newborn from mothers with Class A_1 gestational diabetes mellitus, in comparison to offspring from 41 matched controls with normal carbohydrate metabolism, have indicated that the former have a twofold greater frequency of age-adjusted birthweights exceeding 4,000 g, i.e. 23.9% versus 9.9%.[14] Perhaps even more striking, we have found a sevenfold greater frequency of premature maturation of fetal B cells in the offspring of even the mildest gestational diabetics (i.e. Class A_1 GDM)[14] as judged by the relationship between insulin C-peptide and ambient glucose in cord blood, that is, the C-peptide/glucose ratios.[28] Clearly, therefore, even the mildest metabolic derangements in the mother during the latter part of pregnancy may be translated into palpable impacts on developing structures in the fetus such as the adipocyte, the muscle cell, and the B-cells of the pancreas.

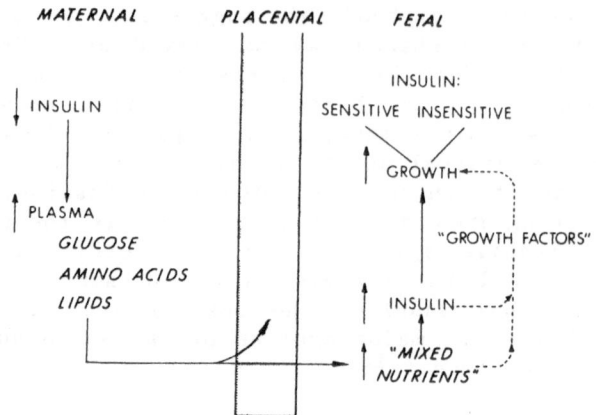

MATERNAL   PLACENTAL   FETAL

Fig. 5:   Fetal development according to the modified Pedersen
           hypothesis (Reproduced from ref. 7).

b)   <u>Long-Range Pregnancy Outcome</u>

      The above developmental changes assume heightened significance
when viewed in terms of the characteristics of the cells cited
above. Many represent terminally differentiated and poorly replicating structures so that a sizeable proportion of their lifetime
endowment is established <u>in utero</u>. Elsewhere, we have postulated
that the abnormal intrauterine environment during their period of
development and differentiation could modify genetic expression in
such cells and thereby alter their functional properties throughout
the lifetime of the offspring.[7,9,12] A long-range program has
been under way at the Diabetes in Pregnancy Center of Northwestern
University since 1977 to monitor for such putative "fuel-mediated
teratogenesis"[7,9] on a prospective basis. Although definitive
conclusions must await more prolonged follow-up, some suggestive
support is already emerging from retrospective studies of others.
Thus Pettitt et al. in the study of Pima Indians – a group in whom
incidence of non-insulin dependent diabetes mellitus is inordinately
great, have observed significantly more obesity[32] and diabetes[33]
in the offspring (up to age 19) of Pima mothers who were diabetic
during the index pregnancy than in the offspring of mothers who
remained non-diabetic or did not become diabetic until after pregnancy. The findings correlated most strongly with the manifestly
abnormal glucoregulation during the index pregnancy. They did not
correlate to an equal degree with any other phenotypic property of
the mother, including obesity. Although the data on diabetic
fathers have not yet been presented, Pettitt et al. have suggested
that the differences in the offspring during childhood and adolescence may be due to differences in maternal glucoregulation during
pregnancy rather than genetic factors[32,33] and thereby consistent

with the proposal that the intrauterine environment may exert long-range effects upon certain poorly replicating, terminally differentiated cells such as adipocytes or pancreatic B-cells.[7,9,12] As such, the findings provide compelling support for the hypothesis that "nurture, as exemplified by the intrauterine environment, may modify nature, as conditioned by genetic endowment".[7,9,12]

If the Pima Indians experiences can be corroborated in other high-risk populations, and confirmed by prospective studies in random groups, such as our Northwestern University patients, then the ramifications of gestational diabetes may well extend far beyond immediate pregnancy outcome or maternal diabetes. Indeed, gestational diabetes may well constitute the optimum arena for enlightened manipulations of the "tissue culture" that is pregnancy and for prospective efforts to influence the anthropometric and metabolic characteristics of the next generation. For those concerned with metabolic eugenics, no entity could provide a more fruitful venue for preventive approaches to such peculiarly human public health problems as diabetes mellitus or obesity.

ACKNOWLEDGEMENT

The clinical studies described in the text were performed in collaboration with many colleagues of the Diabetes in Pregnancy Center of Northwestern University-McGaw Medical Center. We are particularly grateful to such valued associates as Drs. S. Dooley, R. Depp, R. Sabbagha, J. Sciarrra, M. Socol, and R. Tamura in Obstetrics; Drs. J. Simpson and A. Martin in Genetics; Dr. J. Boehm and E. Ogata in Neonatology; Dr. R. Radvany in Surgery; and Dr. M. Vaisrub in Community Health and Preventive Medicine. We are also indebted to the nursing staff of the Clinical Research Unit at Northwestern Memorial Hospital; Ms. Concepcion Mora, Ms. Francesca Brutto, and Ms. Frances Novak for assistance in the preparation of this manuscript; and Ms. Ardean Belton for assistance with the statistical analyses. Our studies were supported in part by research grants AM10699; MRP-HD11021; RR-48; and Training Grant AM07169 from the National Institutes of Health, Bethesda, Maryland.

REFERENCES

1. D. Bybee, B.E. Metzger, N. Freinkel, R.L. Phelps, and N. Vaisrub, Gestational diabetes mellitus (GDM): Antepartum (AP) predictors of glucose tolerance during the first year postpartum (PP), Diabetes 32(Suppl.): 15A (1983).
2. J.M. Duncan, On Puerperal diabetes, Trans. Obstet. Soc. Lond. 24:256-285 (1882).

3. K. Edström, E. Cerasi, and R. Luft, Insulin response to glucose infusion during pregnancy, A prospective study of high and low insulin responders with normal carbohydrate tolerance, Acta Endocrinol. 75:87–104 (1974).

4. S.S. Fajans and J.C. Floyd, Jr, Heterogeneity of diabetes mellitus, in: "Contemporary Metabolism," Vol. 1, N. Freinkel, ed. Plenum Publishing Corp., New York 235–305 (1979).

5. P. Felig, and V. Lynch, Starvation in human pregnancy: Hypoglycemia, hypoinsulinemia, and hyperketonemia, Science 170:990–992 (1970).

6. N. Freinkel, Gestational diabetes 1979: Philosophical and practical aspects of a major public health problem, Diabetes Care 3:399–401 (1980).

7. N. Freinkel, The Banting Lecture 1980: Of pregnancy and progeny, Diabetes 29:1023–1035 (1980).

8. N. Freinkel, Effects of the conceptus on maternal metabolism during pregnancy, in: "On the Nature and Treatment of Diabetes," B.S. Leibel and G.A. Wrenshall, eds. Amsterdam, Excerpta Medica Foundation, 679–691 (1965).

9. N. Freinkel, Pregnant thoughts about metabolic control and diabetes, N. Engl. J. Med. 304:1357–1359 (editorial) (1981).

10. N. Freinkel and J. Josimovich, and Conference Planning Committee, American Diabetes Association Workshop-Conference on Gestational Diabetes, Summary and Recommendations, Diabetes Care 3:499–501 (1980).

11. N. Freinkel, B.E. Metzger, M. Nitzan, R. Daniel, B. Surmaczynska, and T. Nagel, Facilitated anabolism in late pregnancy: Some novel maternal compensations for accelerated starvation, in: Proceedings of the VIIIth Congr. Intl. Diabetes Fed. Malaisse, W.J. and J. Pirart, eds, Excerpta Medica, Amsterdam, Intl. Congr. Series No. 312, 474–488 (1974).

12. N. Freinkel, and B.E. Metzger, Pregnancy as a tissue culture experience: The critical implications of maternal metabolism for fetal development, in: "Pregnancy Metabolism, Diabetes and the Fetus," CIBA Foundation Symposium No. 63, Excerpta Medica, Amsterdam, 3–23 (discussion pp. 23–29) (1979).

13. N. Freinkel, and B.E. Metzger, Gestational diabetes in Chicago, in: Proceedings of the Satellite Symposium to the 10th IDF – Congress of Vienna, Karlsburg, East Germany (Sept. 4–6, 1979), H. Bibergeil, H. Zuhlke, and U. Poser, eds, Central Institute for Diabetes, "Gerhard Katsch," Karlsburg, 438–442 (1980).

14. N. Freinkel, B.E. Metzger, D. Cockroft, R.L. Phelps, N.J. Lewis, L. Gorman, E.S. Ogata, J.J. Boehm, R. Depp, S. Dooley, G.E. Shambaugh III, G. Baumann, A.R. LaBarbera, L.S. Phillips, and N. Vaisrub, Inquiries into maternal metabolism: Past, present and future – A progress report from the Northwestern University Diabetes in Pregnancy Center, in: Proceedings of the 11th Congr. Intl. Diabetes Fed., Nairobi, Kenya, (Nov. 10–17, 1982), E.N. Mngola, ed, Excerpta Medica, Amsterdam, 423–427 (1983).

15. A.N. Gorsuch, J. Lister, B.M. Dean, K.M. Spencer, J.M. McNally, G.F. Bottazzo, and A.G. Cudworth, Evidence for a long pre-diabetic period in type I (insulin-dependent) diabetes mellitus, Lancet 2:1363-1365 (1981).

16. E. Herrera, R.H. Knopp, and N. Freinkel, Carbohydrate metabolism in pregnancy, VI, Plasma fuels, insulin, liver composition, gluconeogenesis and nitrogen metabolism during late gestation in the fed and fasted rat, J. Clin. Invest. 48:2260-2272 (1969).

17. W.J. Irvine, C.J. McCallum, R.S. Gray, C.J. Campbell, L.J.P. Duncan, J.W. Farquhar, H. Vaughan, and P.M. Morris, Pancreatic islet-cell antibodies in diabetes mellitus correlated with the duration and type of diabetes, coexistent autoimmune disease, and HLA type, Diabetes 26:138-147 (1977).

18. R.H. Knopp, E. Herrera, and N. Freinkel, Carbohydrate metabolism in pregnancy, VIII, Metabolism of adipose tissue isolated from fed and fasted pregnant rats during late gestation, J. Clin. Invest. 49:1438-1446 (1970).

19. H. Mawhinney, D.R. Hadden, D. Middleton, J.M.G. Harley, and D.A.D. Montgomery, HLA antigens in asymptomatic diabetes, A 10-year follow-up study of potential Diabetes in Pregnancy and Gestational Diabetes, Ulster Med. J. 48:166-172 (1979).

20. J.H. Mestman, G.V. Anderson, and V. Guadalupe, Follow-up study of 360 subjects with abnormal carbohydrate metabolism during pregnancy, Obstet. Gynecol. 39:421-425 (1972).

21. B.E. Metzger, F. Agnoli, J.W. Hare, and N. Freinkel, Carbohydrate metabolism in pregnancy, X, Metabolic disposition of alanine by the perfused liver of the fasting pregnant rat, Diabetes 22:601-608 (1973).

22. B.E. Metzger, and N. Freinkel, Inquiries into the pathogenesis of gestational diabetes, in: "Treatment of Early Diabetes," R.A. Camerini-Davalos, and B. Hanover, eds, Plenum Press, New York, :201-208, (1979).

23. B.E. Metzger, J.W. Hare, and N. Freinkel, Carbohydrate metabolism in pregnancy, IX, Plasma levels of gluconeogenic fuels during fasting in the rat, J. Clin. Endocrinol. 33:869-873 (1971).

24. B.E. Metzger, R.L. Phelps, N. Freinkel, and I.A. Navickas, Effects of gestational diabetes on diurnal profiles of plasma glucose, lipids and individual amino acids, Diabetes Care 3:402-409 (1980).

25. B.E. Metzger, V. Ravnikar, R.A. Vileisis, and N. Freinkel, "Accelerated starvation" and the skipped breakfast in late normal pregnancy, Lancet 1:588-592 (1982).

26. P. Moore, O. Kolterman, J. Weyant, and J.M. Olefsky, Insulin binding in human pregnancy: Comparisons to the postpartum, luteal, and follicular states, J. Clin. Endocrinol. Metab. 52:937-941 (1981).

27. National Diabetes Data Group, Classification and Diagnosis of
     Diabetes Mellitus and other Categories of Glucose Intolerance,
     Diabetes 28:1039-1057 (1979).
28. E.S. Ogata, N. Freinkel, B.E. Metzger, R.L. Phelps, R. Depp,
     J.J. Boehm, and S. Dooley, Perinatal islet function in gesta-
     tional diabetes: Assessment by cord plasma C-peptide and
     amniotic fluid insulin, Diabetes Care 3:425-429 (1980).
29. J. Pedersen, Weight and length at birth of infants of diabetic
     mothers, Acta Endocrinol. 16:330-342 (1954).
30. J.B. O'Sullivan, Long-term follow-up of gestational diabetics,
     in: "Early Diabetes in Early Life," R.A. Camerini-Davalos, and
     H.S. Cole, eds, Academic Press, Inc., New York, :503-510 (1975).
31. J.B. O'Sullivan, and C.M. Mahan, Criteria for the oral glucose
     tolerance test in pregnancy, Diabetes 13:278-284 (1964).
32. D.J. Pettitt, H.R. Baird, K.A. Aleck, P.H. Bennett, and W.C.
     Knowler, Excessive obesity in offspring of Pima Indian women
     with diabetes during pregnancy, N. Engl. J. Med. 308:242-245
     (1983).
33. D.J. Pettitt, H.R. Baird, K.A. Aleck, and W.C. Knowler,
     Diabetes mellitus in children following maternal diabetes
     during gestation, Diabetes 31(Suppl.):66A (1982).
34. R.L. Phelps, B.E. Metzger, and N. Freinkel, Carbohydrate meta-
     bolism in pregnancy, XVII, Diurnal profiles of plasma glucose,
     insulin, free fatty acids, triglycerides, cholesterol, and
     individual amino acids in late normal pregnancy, Am. J. Obstet.
     Gynecol. 7:730-736 (1981).
35. R.L. Phelps, B.E. Metzger, and N. Freinkel, Medical management
     of diabetes in pregnancy, in: "Gynecology and Obstetrics,"
     Vol. 3, J.J. Sciarra, ed, Harper & Row, Hagerstown, MD, Ch. 13,
     :1-10 (1979).
36. G. Puavilai, E.C. Drobny, L.A. Domont, and G. Baumann, Insulin
     receptors and insulin resistance in human pregnancy: Evidence
     for a postreceptor defect in insulin action, J. Clin.
     Endocrinol. 54:247-253 (1982).
37. G. Puavalai, H.B. Levene, L.A. Domont, N. Freinkel, B.E.
     Metzger and G. Baumann, Hepatic insulin and glucagon receptors
     in pregnancy: Their role in the enhanced catabolism during
     fasting, Endocrinol. 108:1979-1986(1981).
38. P. Rubinstein, M. Walker, J. Krassner, C. Carrier, C.
     Carpenter, M.J. Dobersen, A.L. Notkins, E.M. Mark, C.
     Nechemias, R.U. Hausknecht, and F. Ginsberg-Fellner, HLA
     antigens and islet cell antibodies in gestational diabetes,
     Hum. Immunol. 3:271-275 (1981).
39. S. Srikanta, O.P. Ganda, G.S. Eisenbarth, and J.S. Soeldner,
     Islet-cell antibodies and beta-cell function in monozygotic
     triplets and twins initially discordant for type I diabetes
     mellitus, N. Engl. J. Med. 308:322-325 (1983).
40. A. Svejgaard, P. Platz, and L.P. Ryder, Insulin dependent
     diabetes mellitus, Joint report, in: "Histocompatibility
     Testing 1980," P. Terasaki, ed, UCLA Tissue Typing Lab, Los

Angeles, :638-656 (1981).

41. N. Toyoda, Insulin receptors on erythrocytes in normal and obese pregnant women: Comparisons to those in nonpregnant women during the follicular and luteal phases, Am. J. Obstet. Gynecol. 144:679-682 (1982).

42. J.C.M. Tsibris, L.O. Raynor, W.C. Buhi, J. Buggie, and W.N. Spellacy, Insulin receptors in circulating erythrocytes and monocytes from women on oral contraceptives or pregnant women near term, J. Clin. Endocrinol. Metab. 51:711-717 (1980).

43. J.E. Tyson, K.L. Austin, and J.W. Farinholt, Prolonged nutritional deprivation in pregnancy: Changes in human chorionic somatomammotropin and growth hormone secretion, Am. J. Obstet. Gynecol. 109:1080-1082 (1971).

44. S.S.C. Yen, C.C. Tsai, and P. Vela, Gestational diabetogenesis: Quantitative analyses of glucose-insulin interrelationship between normal pregnancy and pregnancy with gestational diabetes, Am. J. Obstet. Gynecol. 111:792-800 (1971.

HETEROGENEITY WITHIN TYPE II AND MODY DIABETES

Stefan S. Fajans

The Department of Internal Medicine
(Division of Edocrinology and Metabolism)
The University of Michigan
Ann Arbor, Michigan 48109 USA

ABSTRACT

The heterogeneity within Type II diabetes (NIDDM) and within Maturity-Onset type Diabetes of Young people (MODY), a subset of NIDDM which is inherited in an autosomal dominant fashion, is discussed. Aspects of the definition and phenotypic expression of MODY are reviewed. Within NIDDM there are differences in patterns of inheritance between subgroups. HLA antigen associations are not found in most NIDDM populations but exist in three specific population groups with Type II diabetes. Within NIDDM and within MODY there are differences in the magnitude of insulin responses to glucose, differences in target tissue responsiveness to insulin in vivo, and differences in receptor and post-receptor effects of insulin. Structurally abnormal variant and biologically defective insulin molecules have been found in some Type II diabetic patients and in members of certain MODY families. The presence or absence of obesity may mark heterogeneous groups of Type II diabetic patients, in addition to the importance of obesity in uncovering an insulin secretory defect by causing insulin resistance. There is heterogeneity in susceptibility to vascular disease within NIDDM and MODY. The natural history of carbohydrate metabolism and of insulin secretory responses to glucose in early Type I diabetes and in MODY with low insulin secretory responses are illustrated and similarities and dissimilarities compared and contrasted. Failure to recognize young patients with MODY may contribute to incorrect diagnosis, management, and assignment of prognosis of this form of diabetes in the young by many practicing physicians.

The recognition that Type I or insulin-dependent diabetes (IDDM) and Type II or noninsulin-dependent (NIDDM) differ from each other not only phenotypically but also in etiology and pathogenesis led the National Diabetes Data Group (NDDG) to devise the present nomenclature and classification of diabetes mellitus.[37] These were adopted by the World Health Organization.[58] As suggested by the NDDG report, the classification should be reexamined periodically to reflect improved understanding of the disease, to stimulate further research, and to be of help to practicing physicians.

Various speakers in this Symposium will address in detail the heterogeneous nature of Type I and Type II diabetes on the basis of genetic, immunologic and environmental factors and discuss similarities and dissimilarities between these two entities. I will give a simplified overview of the heterogeneity of Type II diabetes and emphasize Maturity-Onset type Diabetes of Young people (MODY), a subset of NIDDM in which there is heterogeneity in pathogenesis as well. Similarities and dissimilarities between MODY and conventional NIDDM will be reviewed on the one hand, and between MODY and Type I diabetes on the other hand. In addition, I will demonstrate that abandonment of the term MODY, or a similar term, as a subgroup within the classification of NIDDM, as adopted by the NDDG report,[37] fails to recognize this heterogeneity within NIDDM, and more importantly may contribute to incorrect diagnosis, management and prognosis of this form of diabetes in the young by many practicing physicians.

Evidence abounds for heterogeneity within Type II diabetes (Table 1). Genetic factors as expressed by patterns of inheritance differentiate subgroups within NIDDM. MODY is consistent with autosomal dominant inheritance[2,3,10,14,15,26,56,57] while most NIDDM is not inherited in this way. Further evidence for genetic heterogeneity within Type II diabetes comes from HLA antigen association. In contradistinction to Type I diabetes, HLA antigen associations have not been found in most populations with Type II diabetes. On the other hand, in three specific population groups an HLA antigen has been associated with NIDDM (Pimas, HLA-A2[59]; Xhosas, HLA-A2[6]; Fijians, HLA-Bw6.[50] No association has been found between specific HLA antigens and MODY[1,10,12,38,43,44] in spite of an earlier report to the contrary.[2]

Before proceeding, I would like to review briefly some aspects of the evolution of our definition and the phenotypic expression of MODY. In 1960 we first reported that impaired glucose tolerance, diabetic glucose tolerance and fasting hyperglycemia occurring in young patients could be normalized by sulfonylurea therapy.[17] In 1964, exactly 20 years ago here in Toronto at the Vth Congress of the International Diabetes Federation, we first used the term "maturity-onset type diabetes of young people" for the nonprogressive or slowly progressive diabetes occurring in children, adolescents and

Table 1   Heterogeneity Within Type II (NIDDM) Diabetes

---

1. Heredity - MODY vs. Other Types
    HLA Antigen Associations

    Heterogeneity Within Type II (NIDDM) Diabetes
    and Heterogeneity Within MODY

2. Magnitude of Insulin Response to Glucose
    (Low/High).

3. Insulin Resistance - Decreased Target Tissue
    Responsiveness to Insulin

    a. Receptor defects.
    b. Post-receptor defects.

4. Structurally Abnormal Variant (Mutant),
    Biologically Defective Insulin Molecule.

5. Obesity

6. Susceptibility to Vascular Disease
    (Microangiopathy, Macroangiography).

    Heterogeneity Within MODY

7. Renal Threshold for Glucose.

---

young adults, and emphasized a strong familial association of diabetes in such patients.[16] In 1974 Tattersall reported from King's College Hospital in London, three families with this type of diabetes and recognized that it appeared to be inherited in an autosomal dominant fashion.[56] In 1975, Tattersall and Fajans, on the basis of a large prospective study which has been going on in Ann Arbor since the early 1950's, differentiated between the inheritance of maturity-onset type diabetes of young people and nonprogressive or slowly progressive diabetes occurring in children, adolescents and young adults, and emphasized a strong familial association of diabetes in such patients.[16] In 1974 Tattersall reported from King's College Hospital in London, three families with this type of diabetes and recognized that it appeared to be inherited in an autosomal dominant fashion.[56] In 1975, Tattersall and Fajans, on the basis of a large prospective study which has been going on in Ann Arbor since the early 1950's, differentiated between the inheritance of maturity-onset type diabetes of young people and juvenile-onset type or Type I diabetes and first used the abbreviation "MODY".[57]

Maturity-onset type diabetes of the young, MODY, has been referred to by some as NIDDM in the young, or NIDDY.[28] However, the term NIDDY has not implied association with autosomal dominant inheritance.[25] On the other hand, the designation of NIDDM with autosomal dominant inheritance, as proposed by NDDG,[37] does not emphasize its occurrence in the young. My definition of MODY is NIDDM in the young plus autosomal dominant inheritance.[14]*

MODY is expressed phenotypically as follows. It can be suspected and recognized if NIDDM occurs in three or more generations and the pattern of inheritance conforms to autosomal dominant inheritance. MODY can be diagnosed at a young age, under 25 years of age, and frequently in early adolescence, if looked for by routine plasma glucose testing in the younger generations of families with more than one generation of NIDDM. MODY diabetes is frequently asymptomatic in younger age groups. Thus, a diagnosis of diabetes is usually not made in most members of such families until mid or late adult life, or even old age, as in other types of NIDDM. By prospective testing of young members of families with MODY it can be demonstrated that there may be very slow progression from normal glucose tolerance to impaired glucose tolerance, from impaired glucose tolerance to diabetic glucose tolerance with normal fasting plasma glucose levels (up to 18 years), and no progression or very slow progression from that state to fasting hyperglycemia (up to 21 years). The abnormality in carbohydrate metabolism is responsive to either diet therapy or diet plus oral agents for decades, even in the presence of severe fasting hyperglycemia. In obese patients, and in nonobese patients as well, it may progress in insulin-requiring diabetes (not insulin-dependent or ketotic diabetes) after many years or decades, with decreasing basal insulin levels and decreasing insulin responses to nutrients. In many MODY families microangiopathic and macroangiopathic complications occur with relatively high frequency, while members of other families who have had MODY-type diabetes of long duration may escape clinically significant complications.[14,15] When vascular complications do occur they are usually not found until middle or older age. Patients with MODY diabetes are usually nonobese, particularly in young age groups, although obesity occurs in some families. (With increasing age, mild obesity appears even in those who were initially not obese, as seen in most population groups.) A high prevalence of

_____

* Since the first of the three pedigrees with NIDDM and autosomal dominant inheritance reported from King's College Hospital[56] had the surname Mason, Pyke refers to this type of diabetes as "Mason-type" diabetes.[46] Since MODY diabetes is very heterogeneous, designation of this form of diabetes by the name of a single family which has characteristics (e.g., absence of vascular disease, presence of renal glycosuria) not shared by many other MODY families is not appropriate.

chlorpropamide-alcohol flushing has been described in many[46] but not all[14,43] diabetic members of some MODY families and it has not been found in other MODY families[31]; thus, this phenomenon is neither a genetic[14,31] nor a reliable[19] marker for MODY.

In the discussion of heterogeneity of Type II diabetes to follow, I will discuss heterogeneity within conventional NIDDM and heterogeneity within MODY together (Table 1), for the sake of brevity.

The next evidence for heterogeneity within Type II and within MODY diabetes to be discussed is the heterogeneity in the magnitude of insulin responses to administered[13,14,15,18] glucose. It is frequently stated that NIDDM is characterized by normal or elevated insulin secretory responses to glucose.[8] However, in patients with NIDDM or MODY with similar abnormalities of glucose tolerance and fasting hyperglycemia we[13,14,15,18] and others[32,47] have found a wide spectrum of insulin responses to administered glucose ranging from very low insulin responses to very high insulin responses. In MODY patients with low insulin responses there appears to be a genetically delayed and decreased insulin secretory response to nutrients from childhood.[11,14,15,26]

In some members of MODY families the insulin secretory responses to glucose are so low that they may resemble those of early Type I diabetes at any one point in time.[14,15] On the other hand, the natural history or evolution of the insulin secretory responses and the severity of metabolic abnormalities over time does make the distinction between these two types of diabetes. In Type I diabetes decompensation from an abnormal glucose tolerance test to insulin requirement (defined as inability to correct fasting hyperglycemia with diet and sulfonylurea agent), and to insulin dependence, occurs in months to a few years (usually within two years, very occasionally up to 5-6 years), while in NIDDM and MODY very slow decompensation to insulin requirement occurs over many years and even several decades.

A comparison of the natural history of carbohydrate metabolism and the insulin secretory responses to glucose in three patients with early Type I diabetes with those of five MODY patients will illustrate the above conclusion. SN was an 11 1/2 year old healthy male sibling of a classical Type I diabetic patient. At the time of a normal glucose tolerance test he had a relatively low insulin secretory response to glucose[15] (Figure 4). Carbohydrate tolerance deteriorated to diabetic glucose tolerance tests within six months, and to fasting hyperglycemia in nine months with an essentially absent insulin secretory response to glucose, and to ketotic diabetes in another three months time. He was islet-cell antibody positive at the time of normal glucose tolerance.

Table 2   Plasma Levels of Insulin and Glucose During a Glucose
           Tolerance Test at Time of Diagnosis of Type I Diabetes in
           JJ, a 27-Year Old White Male Engineer

Dec. 1981:	Normal FPG (F.H. IDDM - 5 members)						
March 1982:	Onset Polyuria, Polydipsia, 15-20 lb. Weight Loss, Fatigue, Blurred Vision						
May 1982:	Urine: 2% Glucose, ++ Ketones						
5/26/82:	F	1/2	1	1 1/2	2	2 1/2	3
PG mg/dl	267	390	497	548	598	625	591
IRI μU/ml	6	3	7	7	9	12	13

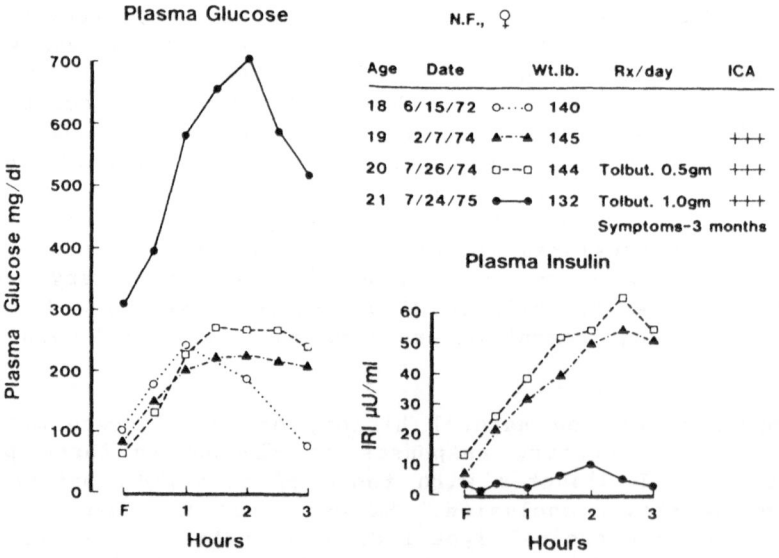

Fig. 1:   Plasma levels of glucose and immunoreactive insulin
           during glucose tolerance tests performed on a patient
           with Type I diabetes (NF). There are no MODY patients in
           the offspring of her nondiabetic father, a member of the
           RW Pedigree, Generation II (ref. 15; Figure 2; II, 4).

JJ had a five member family history of Type I diabetes in two generations (including father and two siblings) with onset of diabetes occurring in them at two, seven, nine, nineteen, and thirty-six years of age, respectively (Table 2). At the age of 27 years in December of 1981, JJ had a normal fasting plasma glucose. In May of 1982, after a 6-8 week history of symptoms and a 15-20 lb. weight loss, he had a fasting plasma of 267 mg/dl, a fasting insulin level of 6 μU/ml and an insulin response to glucose which did not increase in the first 1 1/2 hours to reach a maximum of 13 μU/ml at 3 hours.

NF is a Type I diabetic patient. Although she belongs to the RW MODY pedigree, there are no MODY patients in the offspring of her nondiabetic father from Generation II (15, Figure 2; II, 4). At the age of 18 years in June 1972, she had a glucose tolerance test showing impaired glucose tolerance (Figure 1). In February and July, 1974, she had diabetic glucose tolerance tests with delayed insulin secretory responses which rose to 55 and 65 μU/ml at 2 1/2 hours. In July 1975 she had an insulin secretory response from 4 to 10 μU/ml and had a fasting plasma glucose of 306 mg/dl while being treated with 1 gm of tolbutamide. She had been symptomatic for three months, had lost 12 lbs. in weight and was ketonuric. Her serum was strongly positive for pancreatic islet cell antibodies.

Figure 2-6 will give representative data for five MODY members of the RW pedigree studied 2-3 times yearly for periods of up to 26 years and whose serum has been persistantly negative for islet cell antibodies. In DW, diabetic glucose tolerance with normal fasting plasma glucose was found at the age of 11 years in 1958 (Figure 2). In 1962 while treated with tolbutamide he had normal glucose tolerance and a low insulin response to glucose with a single higher level of 47 μU/ml at two hours. He has had fasting hyperglycemia when off sulfonylureas for periods of two weeks since 1965. The insulin response was lower by 1970, and it was absent by 1977 in spite of a normal fasting plasma glucose while being treated with chlorpropamide (Figure 2). The fasting insulin level is 4 μU/ml, and the insulin response to glucose is so flat that it cannot be distinguished from that seen in Type I diabetes. In spite of this he was able to maintain near normal fasting and postprandial plasma glucose levels on sulfonylurea therapy for another five years (Table 3). This supports the well-described concept that sulfonylureas have extra-pancreatic effects. By March 1983, maximum chlorpropamide dosage no longer prevented fasting hyperglycemia, and the patient had lost 15 lbs. in weight (Table 3). On insulin therapy he has regained his former weight (Table 4). It is evident that his c-peptide response to a breakfast meal has diminished further. It resembles that of Type I diabetic patients more than that of typical Type II patients but is closest to that of nonketotic, insulin-requiring patients with tropical pancreatic disease.[36]

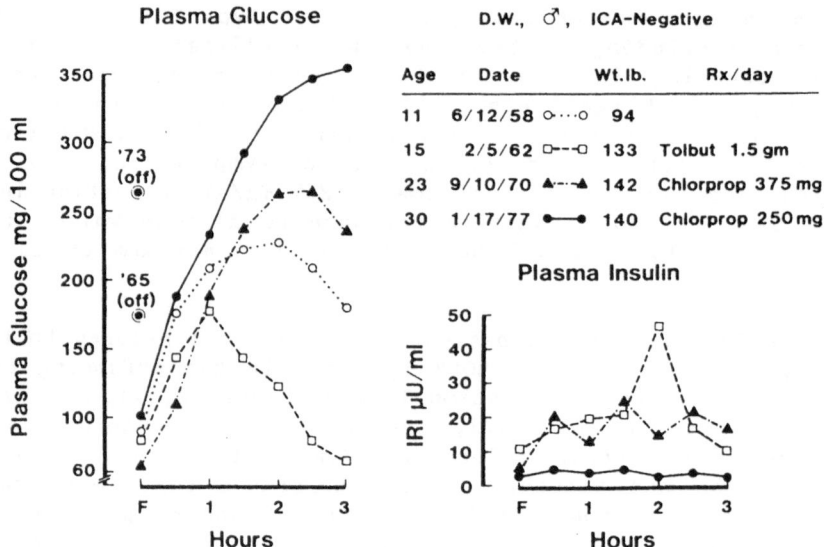

Fig. 2:   Plasma levels of glucose and immunoreactive insulin
           during glucose tolerance test in MODY family member DW,
           RW Pedigree, Generation III.

A 20-year follow-up of his 16-year old sister has been presented
previously[15] (Figure 1). Normalization of glucose tolerance as
shown in 1973 and 1977 is associated with increased peripheral
levels of plasma insulin as compared with those seen when
sulfonylureas had been discontinued for two weeks. This supports
the finding that one of the effects of sulfonylureas is increased
secretion of insulin even on a long-term basis. She had fasting
hyperglycemia off sulfonylurea after a 19-year follow-up. After 26
years, glucose tolerance is still within normal limits, but there
has been further decrease in the low insulin secretory response
while being treated with chlorpropamide (Figure 3). As a point of
reference, in 150 control subjects (mean age 23 years) without a
family history of diabetes or large newborn babies, the mean plasma
levels of insulin during glucose tolerance tests (1.75 gms
glucose/kg ideal body weight), in the fasting state and at one-half
hour intervals, were 10, 93, 103, 87, 73, 65, and 45 μU/ml.

Another example of a gradually decreasing insulin secretory
response is given for an older brother TW, who was 27-years old at
diagnosis in 1958 (Figure 4). He had fasting hyperglycemia at that
time. A subnormal insulin secretory response, shown for 1962 and
1980, gradually decreased so that by January 1984 the insulin
secretory response is minimal. Nevertheless, with an increase in
dosages of chlorpropamide to 500 mg/day, fasting hyperglycemia has
been controlled again, although not postprandial hyperglycemia

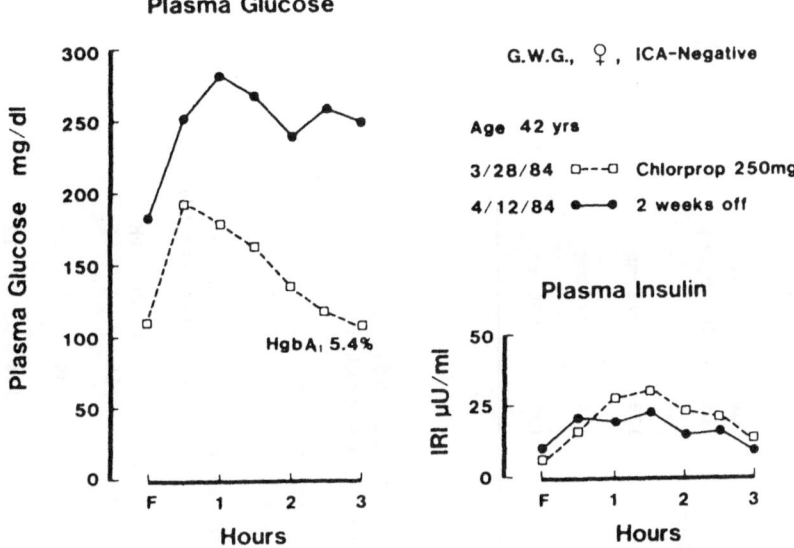

Fig. 3: Plasma levels of glucose and immunoreactive insulin during glucose tolerance tests in MODY family member GwG, RW Pedigree, Generation III.

(Table 5). Hemoglobin A_1 has decreased to the upper limit of normal. He has normal fasting levels of plasma insulin but a very low insulin secretory response to a breakfast meal.

RaF, a member of the IVth generation of this family, had mild fasting hyperglycemia with a delayed and relatively low insulin secretory response at the age of 14 years in 1967 (Figure 5). The insulin response increased when treated with 150 mg chlorpropamide with normalization of glucose tolerance as shown in 1973 However, by 1979 the insulin secretory response has become flat and hardly distinguishable from that in Type I diabetes and he had fasting hyperglycemia (Figure 5). With an increase in chlorpropamide to 350 mg/day as shown in April 1984, he had an improved insulin secretory response and a normal fasting glucose level.

In his brother RuF, aged 12 years at diagnosis in 1967, a very low insulin secretory response, indistinguishable from that of patients with Type I diabetes, improved with chlorpropamide therapy to low normal, as shown six years later in 1973 (Figure 6). Again, these data indicate that sulfonylureas not only have an extra-pancreatic effect but also influence plasma glucose and glucose tolerance by a long-term insulin secretory effect. In spite of continuation of sulfonylurea therapy, this insulin secretory response gradually diminished so that by April 1984, it is similar to what it was initially in 1967 without sulfonylurea therapy and

Table 3   Fasting and Postprandial Plasma Glucose and Insulin Levels In
           MODY Family Member, Generation III, R.W. Pedigree

D.W.: D.O.B. 10/29/46

Date	Plasma Glucose mg/dl			Plasma Insulin µU/ml			Wt. Lb.	Rx Chlorprop.
	F	1 hour	2 hour	F	1 hour	2 hour		
3/29/82	67	96	89	1	2	2	133	375 mg
10/25/82	118	138	146	3	3	5	130	375 mg
3/2/83	223	318	320	1	2	1	125	500 mg

Table 4   Plasma Glucose and C-Peptide (Fasting and Postprandial) and Hgb
           A_1 Levels in MODY Family Member, RW Pedigree, Generation III

D.W.: D.O.B. 10/29/46   (Retinopathy – Multiple Microaneurysms)

Date	Plasma Glucose mg/dl			Hgb A_1%	Plasma C-Peptide ng/ml			Wt. lb.	Insulin Humulin (U)	
	F	1 hour	2 hour		F	1 hour	2 hour		AM	PM
8/9/83	140	199	169		.59	.70	.51	135	8	12
3/7/84	118	131	116	9.8	.2	.4	.4	139	8	12
4/18/84	85	116	76	9.3	.07	.48	.17	144	8	12
6/18/84	80	106	84	6.2	.02	.17	.20	144	8	12

Table 5 Plasma Glucose and Insulin (Fasting and Postprandial) and Hgb A_1 Levels in MODY Family Member, R.W. Pedigree, Generation III

T.W. Age 53 Rx: Chlorpropamide 500 mg/day (and "reduction diet")

Date	Plasma Glucose mg/dl			Hgb A_1%	Plasma Insulin, μU/ml			Wt. Lb.
	F	1 hour	2 hour		F	1 hour	2 hour	
1/27/84	324 (chlorpropamide 250 mg/day)							157
2/24/84	139	211	258	12.6	8	18	18	154
4/6/84	122	175	190	9.1	11	14	26	158
5/11/84	95	190	200	8.0	20	27	19	160

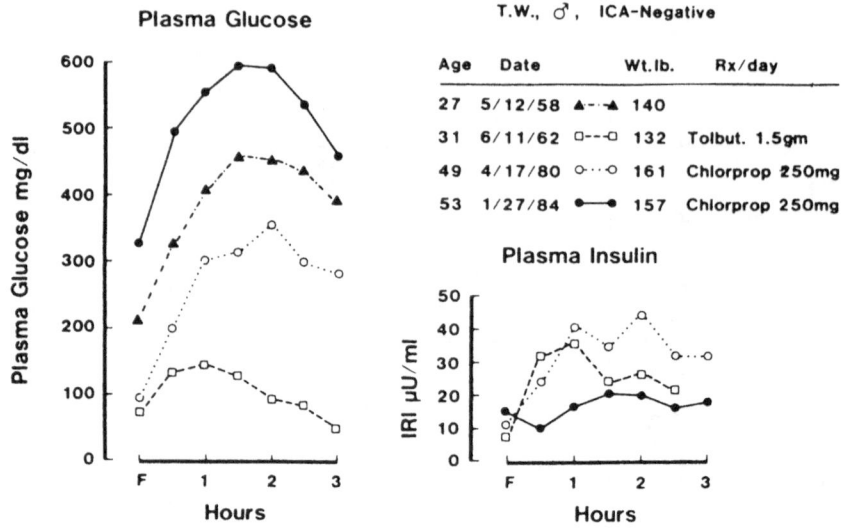

Fig. 4:   Plasma levels of glucose and immunoreactive insulin
          during glucose tolerance tests in MODY family member TW,
          RW Pedigree, Generation III.

similar to that seen in early Type I diabetes.   On June 2, 1984, he
had a fasting plasma glucose of 109 mg/dl on the same dosage of
chlorpropamide.

     It is frequently stated that nonobese Type II diabetic patients
under the age of 40 years are not good candidates for therapy with
sulfonylureas.   Nonobese MODY patients under the age of 40, indeed
under the age of 20 years, even those with low insulin responses to
glucose, can be controlled with sulfonylureas successfully with
physiological plasma glucose levels for decades.

     Some young nonobese members of MODY families first develop
carbohydrate intolerance between 9 and 12 years of age.   Normal
children have a lower insulin response to administered glucose than
adolescents and adults[35,48] implying greater insulin sensitivity
in childhood.   Thus, even a genetically-determined low insulin
response to glucose may maintain normal carbohydrate tolerance in
childhood.   With increasing body mass due to growth, insulin sensitivity decreases physiologically and a larger compensatory insulin
secretory response is required.   In MODY it can be speculated that
the inability to increase insulin levels to the higher normal
adolescent or adult levels may be at least one cause of the emerging
carbohydrate intolerance and diabetes which occurs at that time.
Examples of this phenomenon have been reported previously.[11,14]   A
16-year old boy (GG) who was reported to have normal glucose tolerance from age 7 to 10 1/2 years, had a diabetic glucose tolerance

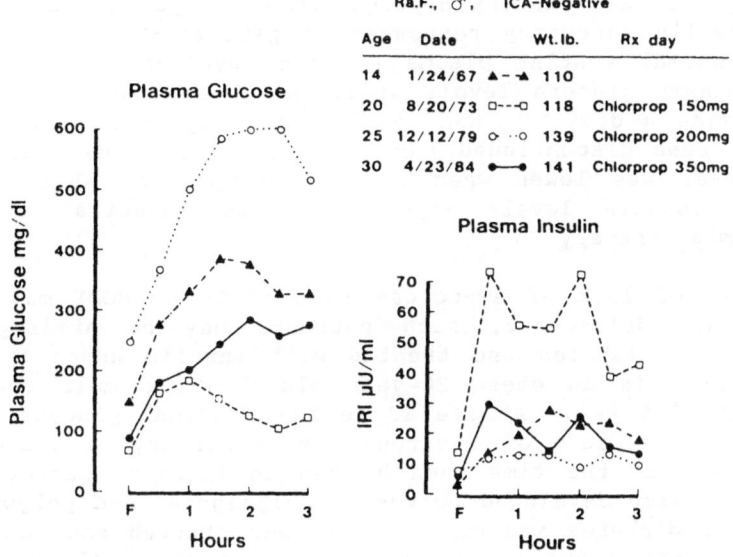

Fig. 5: Plasma levels of glucose and immunoreactive insulin during glucose tolerance tests in MODY family member RaF, RW Pedigree, Generation IV.

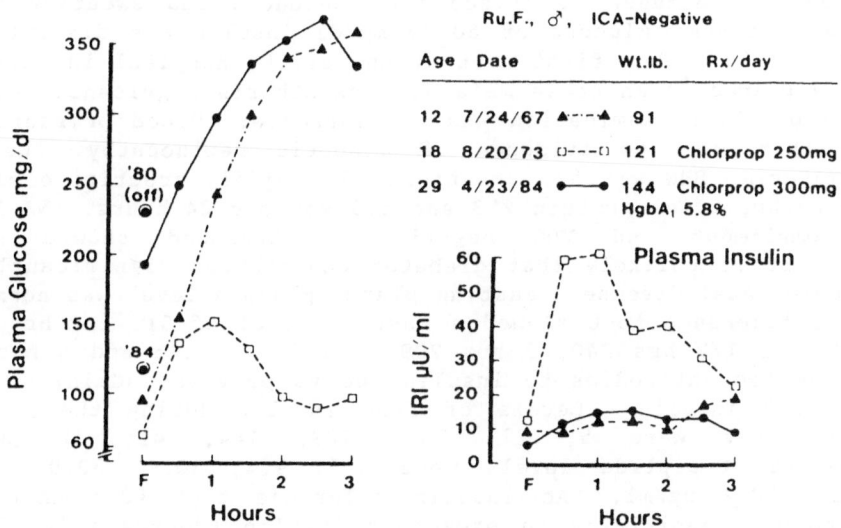

Fig. 6: Plasma levels of glucose and immunoreactive insulin during glucose tolerance tests in MODY family member RuF, RW Pedigree, Generation IV. On June 2, 1984, the patient had a fasting plasma glucose of 109 mg/dl on the same dosage of chlorpropamide as on 4/23/84.

test at age 12, and fasting hyperglycemia at age 13 years, all with similar insulin secretory responses to glucose.[14] At age 16 years he had a normal fasting plasma glucose level with elevated post-prandial plasma glucose levels while being treated with 100 mg of chlorpropamide a day. He had fasting hyperglycemia after chlorpro-pamide had been discontinued for two weeks (Table 6). The fasting insulin level was lower when off chlorpropamide, while nutrient-stimulated insulin levels appeared to be identical on or off chlorpropamide therapy.

Because of lack of awareness that NIDDM or MODY may exist in children and adolescents, such patients may be misdiagnosed as having Type I diabetes and treated with insulin unnecessarily. A recent example is an obese 26-year old Hispanic male (height 165 cm., weight 91.5 kg). At age 13 he had a normal glucose tolerance test performed because of a strong family history of diabetes. At age 14 years, at the time when he had an illness characterized by vomiting, he also developed polyuria, polydipsia, and polyphagia. A diagnosis of diabetes was made and he was started and continued on 15 units of NPH insulin for the next 12 years. All fasting and postprandial plasma glucose levels were reported to be between 110 to 140 mg/dl. He had occasional insulin reactions relieved by ingestion of carbohydrate. At the age of 24 years a diagnosis of "diabetic nephropathy" was made because of the finding of a serum creatinine of 1.8 mg/dl and hypokalemia. By age 26 years this had progressed to a serum creatinine of 4.0 mg/dl and a serum potassium of 2.4 mEq/l. Because of episodes of headache and sweating asso-ciated with plasma glucose of 60-70 mg/dl insulin was discontinued in October 1983. When first seen at University Hospital in December 1983 he appeared as an obese male with acanthosis nigricans. Other-wise the physical examination was unremarkable. Blood pressure was normal, there was no evidence of diabetic retinopathy. He had microhematuria, BUN was 51, creatinine 4.4 mg/dl, creatinine clear-ance 20 cc/hr, urine protein 2.3 and 6.9 gms per 24 hours, ANA 1:10, SPAP, compliment and VDL negative. Ultrasound showed small kidneys. It is unlikely that diabetes contributes significantly to his chronic renal disease. Fasting plasma glucose level was normal. A glucose tolerance test showed a fasting level of 91, 1/2 hr. 144, 1 hr. 240, 1 1/2 hrs 240, 2 hrs 209, 2 1/2 hrs. 115 and 3 hrs. 77 mg/dl. He had antibodies to insulin due to previous administration of beef/pork insulin. Levels of free insulin during the glucose tolerance test were 5, 27, 106, 109, 144, 41, 12 µU/ml. Corresponding C-peptide levels were 5.5, 9.4, 30.9, 30.9, 37.1, 28.2, and 18.7 ng/ml. An insulin tolerance test (0.1 units/kg) showed normal sensitivity to exogenous insulin (decrease in plasma glucose from 85 to 39 mg/dl). Five months after discontinuation of insulin therapy fasting plasma glucose levels were still normal. It appears that he has been treated with insulin unnecessarily for 12 years, because of the unawareness of his physician that NIDDM may exist in adolescence. He has a three generation family history

Table 6 Fasting and Post-Breakfast Levels of Plasma Glucose and Immunoreactive Insulin in G.G., Male MODY Family Member, R.W. Pedigree, Generation IV

Date	Age Yrs	Ht cm	Wt kg	Chlorprop Rex mg	Plasma Glucose mg/dl *Plasma Insulin μU/ml		
					F	1h pp	2h pp
3/28/84	16	171	55	100	103	193	152
					*9	*31	*16
4/12/84	"	"	"	2 wks off	146	208	132
					*4	*35	*15

(For preceeding data, see reference 14)

compatible with autosomal dominant inheritance. His father has
fasting hyperglycemia on insulin therapy, and a brother is being
treated successfully with sulfonylureas.

Some patients with NIDDM and members of some families with
MODY, without or with mild fasting hyperglycemia, have high insulin
responses to glucose as compared to normal control subjects.

Insulin resistance or decreased target tissue responsiveness to
insulin in vivo has been found in the majority of non-obese patients
with conventional NIDDM.[8] On the other hand, in many MODY families there is no evidence of significant insulin resistance. In
seven members of Generation III of the RW pedigree we found normal
insulin tolerance tests and a normal T 1/2 of insulin.[12] Insulin
requirements, when present, in diabetic members of this and other
MODY pedigrees have been relatively low (e.g., see Table 4). When
insulin resistance occurs in NIDDM it has been found to be associated with a decreased number of insulin receptors in freshly
isolated monocytes, adipocytes, and erythrocytes in some
patients.[45] In other patients with Type II diabetes with
hyperinsulinemia and in vivo insulin resistance, a defect in insulin
binding to monocyte receptors has not been identified.[51] This
indicates the existence of heterogeneity in the occurrence of
insulin binding to receptors of freshly isolated cells among
different groups of NIDDM with insulin resistance.

On the other hand, in patients who have a decreased number of
insulin receptors in freshly isolated monocytes, adipocytes, and
erythrocytes, cultured fibroblasts that are several generations
removed from the in vivo environment of the diabetic donor, do not
show a decrease in the number of insulin receptors. Normal insulin
binding, insulin internalization, insulin-mediated receptor loss and
normal fibroblast sensitivity to insulin's glucoregulatory actions
were found in these cultured fibroblasts.[24,45] These studies
provide evidence that the decrease in insulin binding in freshly
isolated cells from patients with NIDDM is a reflection of
environmental rather than intrinsic genetic cellular abnormality.[45] In members of three MODY families (one hypoinsulinemic
and two hyperinsulinemic) the number of insulin receptors on fibroblasts were normal.[20,21] In contrast, in one family consisting of
a 14 year-old patient who was diabetic, and a mother and two sisters
who were nondiabetic, hyperinsulinemia with insulin resistance
appeared to be due to a genetic deficiency of insulin receptors.[52] Insulin binding was deficient not only in the patient's
erythrocytes, monocytes, adipocytes but also in fibroblasts. The
patient's mother and two sisters had comparable, although less
severe, changes in fibroblasts. These studies demonstrate
heterogeneity in the number of insulin receptors on fibroblasts in
diabetic patients.

In NIDDM patients with insulin resistance and normal insulin binding to receptors, postreceptor defects must be the mechanism for insulin resistance when it exists. Olefsky and Kolterman have shown that in NIDDM receptor defects and postreceptor defects may coexist, a spectrum of these defects may occur, and that the mechanisms of insulin resistance in NIDDM are heterogeneous themselves.[40]

Whatever the mechanism which imparts cellular insulin resistance in patients with NIDDM, the compensatory insulin responses to nutrients must be insufficient to maintain normal carbohydrate tolerance implying an additional pancreatic defect, i.e., insufficient beta cell reserve. As an example, the diabetic patient with a congenital defect in fibroblast receptors, was also demonstrated to have an insulin secretory defect to both oral and intravenous glucose challenges.[52] The non-diabetic relatives with a defect in insulin binding to fibroblast receptors had compensatory glucose-stimulated hyperinsulinemia. Thus, the propositus' diabetes has to be explained by both a genetic defect in insulin receptors, as well as by a diminished insulin secretory capacity.

This suggests that diabetes occurs only in those patients who have a decreased pancreatic islet secretory response. Similarly, obese subjects with insulin resistance but normal carbohydrate tolerance (or glucose intolerance below levels defined as diabetes; approximately 60% of all obese subjects) have sufficient hyperinsulinemia to compensate for insulin resistance. However, when even moderate beta cell failure ensues the insulin resistance of obesity will cause diabetic glucose tolerance and diabetes.

As another cause of diabetes, the release of an insulin that is a structurally abnormal variant or mutant insulin molecule and that is biologically defective had been postulated.[7,9,15,29] It has now been found and reported in three patients.[54] In one of these three patients the abnormality in insulin structure is due to a substitution of leucine for a phenylalanine at position 25 of the B chain, while in the second patient there was a substitution of a serine for phenylalanine at B24.[22,23,54,55] The latter is a 28 year-old diabetic patient treated intermittently for 12 years by diet and oral agents. The patient had fasting hyperglycemia, hyperinsulinemia, and a strong family history of diabetes conforming to MODY-type diabetes. Sensitivity to exogenous insulin was normal, as were insulin receptors on monocytes. Insulin isolated from the patient's plasma showed decreased biological activity strongly suggesting the secretion of structurally abnormal insulin. The abnormal insulin is present in three successive generations of this family.[22] In one of our MODY families (Te) we have identified in five members (one in generation II and four in generation IV), an abnormal insulin which is more hydrophobic than normal human insulin by high performance liquid chromatography.[53]

Patients with NIDDM may have a body weight which ranges from normal to one which is excessive. The intake of excessive calories leading to weight gain and obesity and resulting in insulin resistance are important factors in the pathogenesis of NIDDM in many patients. A genetic defect in the insulin secretory response to nutrients (absolute or relative) may be brought out for the first time when increasing insulin resistance calls forth a compensatory response which cannot be met. Obesity and pathological insulin resistance are by no means essential in the evolution of NIDDM. In NIDDM patients who are not overweight, even small increases in body weight (including normal growth in childhood and adolescence) can exacerbate glucose intolerance and precipitate fasting hyerglycemia.[14,15] Nevertheless, evidence has been presented that the absence or presence of obesity may differentiate between different forms of NIDDM.[30] In an analysis of noninsulin-dependent diabetes, Köbberling found that the prevalence of diabetes in siblings was higher in nonobese than in obese human diabetic subjects. In Japanese NIDDM, Kuzuya and Matsuda also found that patients with definite obesity in the past had a lower frequency of a family history of diabetes and a lower prevalence of diabetes in their parents than did patients without obesity, supporting the concept that the presence or absence of obesity may mark heterogeneous groups of diabetics within Type II diabetes.[33]

Susceptibility to vascular disease is not uniform in all patients with Type I or Type II diabetes.[14] Similarly the typical microvascular and macrovascular complications occur in some MODY families with relatively high frequency[14,15] while most members of other families with MODY type diabetes have been reported to escape clinically significant complications.[2,34,56] This suggests heterogeneity in susceptibility or resistance to vascular disease within MODY.[14,15] These findings may be due to differences between families in the genetic component which predisposes to vascular disease, and/or due to the fact that MODY diabetes is characterized by relatively mild hyperglycemia for long periods of time in some families, and/or due to differences in the duration of hyperglycemia in diabetics at the time of the respective evaluations.

A low renal threshold to glucose has been reported in some MODY families.[56] Renal glycosuria has been known to be a dominantly inherited trait and may be an integral part of MODY diabetes in some families. It has not occurred in others; thus it may be evidence for genetic heterogeneity within MODY. In one predigree (RW) we have found a high renal threshold.

Polymorphism in the 5' flanking region of the human insulin gene has been described in diabetic patients.[4,39,41,49] Several studies have shown no linkage between the insulin gene and the inheritance of MODY[5,27,42] (Permutt et al., see this Symposium).

In summary, I have reviewed aspects of the heterogeneity of Type II diabetes and MODY. In the near future further progress will be made in delineating various subtypes; recognition of new ones will undoubtedly increase as techniques for study improve and advance.

ACKNOWLEDGEMENT

Supported in part by U.S. Public Health Service Grant AM-0888; NIH-5 MO1 RR-42 General Clinical Research Centers; and Michigan Diabetes Research and Training Center Grant 5-P60-AM20572.

REFERENCES

1. A. Arnaiz-Villena, R.B. Castellanos, J.A. Oliver, and M.A. Blanco, HLA and maturity onset diabetes of the young, Letter to the Editor, Diabetologia 24:460 (1983).

2. J. Barbosa, R. King, F.C. Goetz, H. Noreen, and E.J. Yuns, HLA in maturity-onset type of hyperglycemia in the young, Arch. Intern. Med. 138:90-93 (1978).

3. J. Barbosa, R. Ramsay, and F.C. Goetz, Plasma glucose, insulin glucagon and growth hormone in kindreds with maturity-onset type of hyperglycemia in young people, Ann. Intern. Med. 88:595 (1978).

4. G.I. Bell, S. Horita, and J.H. Karam, A polymorphic locus adjacent to the human insulin gene and diabetes mellitus, Diabetes 31:65A (1982).

5. J.I. Bell, J.S. Wainscoat, J.M. Old, C. Chlouverakis, H. Keen, R.C. Turner, and D.J. Weatherall, Maturity onset diabetes of the young is not linked to the insulin gene, Br. Med. J. 286:590-592 (1983).

6. B.R. Briggs, W.P.U. Jackson, E.D. Dutoit, and M.C. Botha, The histocompatibility (HLA) antigen distribution in diabetes in Southern African Blacks (Xhosa), Diabetes 29:68-71 (1980).

7. J.W. Conn, and S.S. Fajans, The prediabetic state, A concept of dynamic resistance to a genetic diabetogenic influence, Am. J. Med., 31:839-850 (1961).

8. R.A. DeFronzo, and E. Ferrannini, The pathogenesis of non-insulin-dependent diabetes, An Update, Medicine 61:125-140 (1982).

9. R.B. Elliott, D. O'Brien, and C.C. Roy, An abnormal insulin in juvenile diabetes mellitus, Diabetes 14:780 (1966).

10. O.K., Faber, M. Thomsen, C. Binder, P. Platz, and A. Svejgaard, HLA antigens in a family with maturity-onset type diabetes mellitus, Acta Endocrinologica 88:329-338 (1978).

11. S.S. Fajans, Etiologic aspects of types of diabetes, Diabetes Care 4:69-75 (1981).

12. S.S. Fajans, Unpublished Observations.

13. S.S. Fajans, The natural history of idiopathic diabetes mellitus, Heterogeneity of insulin responses in latent diabetes. in: "The Genetics of Diabetes Mellitus," W. Crutzfeldt, J. Köbberling, and J.V. Neel, eds., Springer-Verlag, Heidelberg, pp. 64-78 (1976).

14. S.S. Fajans, Heterogeneity between various families with non-insulin-dependent diabetes of the MODY type. in: "The Genetics of Diabetes Mellitus," J. Köbberling, and R. Tattersall, eds., Serono Symposium No. 47, Academic Press, London and New York, pp. 251-260 (1982).

15. S.S. Fajans, M.C. Cloutier, and R.L. Crowther, Clinical and etiologic heterogeneity of idiopathic diabetes mellitus, Diabetes 27:1112-1125 (1978).

16. S.S. Fajans, and J.W. Conn, Prediabetes, subclinical diabetes, and latent clinical diabetes: Interpretation, diagnosis and treatment, in: On the Nature and Treatment of Diabetes, B.S. Leibel, and G.S. Wrenshall, eds, Amsterdam, Excerpta Medica International Congress Series 84, pp. 641-656 (1965).

17. S.S. Fajans, and J.W. Conn, Tolbutamide-induced improvement in carbohydrate tolerance of young people with mild diabetes mellitus, Diabetes 9:83-88 (1960).

18. S.S. Fajans, J.C. Floyd Jr., C.I. Taylor, and S. Pek, Heterogeneity of insulin responses in latent diabetes, Trans. Assoc. Am. Phys. 87:83-94 (1974).

19. S.N.T. Fui, H. Keen, J. Jarrett, V. Gossain, and P. Marsden, Test for chlorpropamide-alcohol flush becomes positive after prolonged chlorpropamide treatment in insulin-dependent diabetics, N. Engl. J. Med. 309:93-96 (1983).

20. T. Gelehrter, V. Dilworth, B. Balka, R. McDonald, and E. Schorry, Insulin binding and insulin action in fibroblasts from patients with maturity-onset diabetes of the young, Diabetes 30:940-946 (1981).

21. T. Gelehrter, Unpublished Observations.

22. M. Haneda, K.S. Polonsky, R.M. Bergenstal, J.B. Jaspan, S.E. Shoelson, P.M. Blix, S.J. Chan, S.C.M. Kwok, W.B. Wishner, A. Zeidler, J.M. Olefsky, G. Freidenberg, H.S. Tager, D.F. Steiner, and A.H. Rubenstein, Familial hyperinsulinemia due to a structurally abnormal insulin, N. Engl. J. Med. 1288-1294 (1984).

23. M. Haneda, S.J. Chan, S.C.M. Kwok, A.H. Rubenstein, and D.F. Steiner, Studies on mutant human insulin genes: Identification and sequence analysis of a gene encoding (Ser^{B24}) insulin, Proc. Natl. Acad. Sci. USA 80:6366-6370 (1983).

24. B.V. Howard, H. Hidaka, F. Ishibashi, R.M. Fields, and P.H. Bennett, Type II diabetes and inherent cellular defects in insulin sensitivity, Diabetes 30:562-567 (1981).

25. I. Jialal, and S.M. Joubert, Obesity does not modulate insulin secretion in Indian patients with non-insulin-dependent diabetes in the young, Diabetes Care 7:77-79 (1984).

26. K. Johansen, and G. Gregersen, A family with dominantly inherited mild juvenile diabetes, Acta Med. Scand. 201:567–570 (1977).

27. C. Johnston, D. Owerbach, R.D.G. Leslie, D.A. Pyke, and J. Nerup, Mason-type diabetes and DNA insertion polymorphism. Lancet 1:280 (1984).

28. H. Keen, Problems in the definition of diabetes mellitus and its subtypes, in: "The Genetics of Diabetes Mellitus," J. Köbberling, and R. Tattersall, eds, Serono Symposium, V. 47, Academic Press, London and New York, pp. 1–11 (1982).

29. J.R. Kimmel, and H.G. Pollock, Studies of human insulin from nondiabetic and diabetic pancreas, Diabetes 16:687–694 (1967).

30. J. Köbberling, Studies on the genetic heterogeneity of diabetes mellitus, Diabetologia 7:46–49 (1971).

31. J. Köbberling, N. Bengsch, B. Brüggeboes, H. Schwarck, H. Tillil, and M. Weber, The chlorpropamide alcohol flush, Lack of specificity for familial non-insulin dependent diabetes, Diabetologia 19:359–363 (1980).

32. Kosaka, K., and Y. Akanuma, Heterogeneity of plasma IRI responses in patients with IGT, Letter to the Editor, Diabetologia 18:347–348 (1980).

33. T. Kuzuya, and A. Matsuda, Family histories of diabetes among Japanese patients with type I (insulin-dependent) and type 2 (noninsulin-dependent) diabetes, Diabetologia 22:372–374 (1982).

34. R.D.G. Leslie, A.H. Barnett, D.A. Pyke, Chlorpropamide alcohol flushing and diabetic retinopathy, Lancet 1:997–999 (1979).

35. H. Lestradet, I. Deschamps, and B. Giron, Insulin and free fatty acid levels during oral glucose tolerance tests and their relation to age in 70 healthy children, Diabetes 25:505 (1976).

36. V. Mohan, C. Snehalatha, A. Ramachandran, R. Jayashree, and M. Viswanathan, Pancreatic beta-cell function in tropical pancreatic diabetes, Metabolism 32:1091–1092 (1983).

37. National Diabetes Data Group, Classification of diabetes mellitus and other categories of glucose intolerance, Diabetes 28:1039–1057 (1979).

38. P.G. Nelson, and D.A. Pyke, Genetic diabetes not linked to the HLA locus, Br. Med. J. i:196–197 (1976).

39. J. Nerup, K. Johansen, P. Aaby Svendsen, P. Billesblle, S. Poulsen, B. Thomsen, and D. Owerbach, DNA sequences flanking the insulin gene and the genetics of diabetes syndrome, Diabetologia 23:188 (1982).

40. J.M. Okefsky, and O.G. Kolterman, Mechanisms of insulin resistance in obesity and noninsulin-dependent (Type II) diabetes, Am. J. Med. 70:151 (1981).

41. D. Owerbach, S. Poulsen, P. Billesblle, and J. Nerup, DNA sequence near the insulin gene affect glucose regulation, Diabetes 31:65A (1982).

42. D. Owerbach, B. Thomsen, K. Johansen, L.U. Lamm, and J. Nerup, DNA insertion sequences near the insulin gene are not associated with maturity-onset diabetes of young people, Diabetologia 25:18-20 (1983).

43. G. Panzram, W. Adolph, Heterogeneity of maturity onset diabetes at young age (MODY), Lancet 2:986 (1981).

44. P. Platz, B.K. Jakobsen, A. Svejgaard, B.S. Thomsen, K.B. Jensen, K. Henningsen, and L.U. Lamm, No evidence for linkage between HLA and maturity onset type of diabetes in young people, Diabetologia 23:16-18 (1982).

45. M.J. Prince, P. Tsai, and J.M. Olefsky, Insulin binding, internalization, and insulin receptor regulation in fibroblasts from Type II, non-insulin-dependent diabetes subjects, Diabetes 30:596-600 (1981).

46. D.A. Pyke, Diabetes: The genetic connections, Diabetologia 17:333-343 (1979).

47. G.M. Reaven, and J.M. Olefsky, Relationship between heterogeneity of insulin responses and insulin resistance in normal subjects and patients with chemical diabetes, Diabetologia 13:201-206 (1977).

48. A.L. Rosenbloom, L. Wheeler, R. Bianchi, F.T. Chin, C.M. Tiwary and A. Grgic, Age-related analysis of insulin responses during normal and abnormal glucose tolerance tests in children and adolescents, Diabetes 24:820 (1975).

49. P. Rotwein, R. Chyn, J. Chirgwin, B. Cordell, H.M. Goodman, and M.A. Permutt, Polymorphism in the 5'-flanking region of the human insulin gene and its possible relation to Type 2 diabetes, Science 213:1117-1120 (1981).

50. S.W. Sarjeantson, D.P. Ryan, P. Ram, and P. Zimmet, HLA and non-insulin dependent diabetes in Fiji Indians, Med. J. Aust. 1:462-463 (1981).

51. P.J. Savage, R.F. Hamman, and P.H. Bennett, Prediabetes in the Pima Indians, In: "Advances in Experimental Medicine and Biology: Treatment of Early Diabetes," edited by Camerini-Davalos, R.A., and Hanover, B., Plenum Press, New York, pp. 13-19 (1979).

52. J.A. Scarlett, O.G. Kolterman, P. Moore, M. Saekow, J. Insel, J. Griffin, M. Mako, A.H. Rubenstein, and J.M. Olefsky, Insulin resistance and diabetes due to a genetic defect in insulin receptors, J. Clin. Endo. & Metab. 55:123-132 (1982).

53. S. Seino, A. Funakoshi, A. Vinik, S.S. Fajans, Unpublished observations.

54. S. Shoelson, M. Haneda, P. Blix, A. Nanjo, T. Sanke, K. Inouye, D. Steiner, A. Rubenstein, and H. Tager, Three mutant insulins in man, Nature 302:540-543 (1983).

55. S. Shoelson, M. Fickova, M. Haneda, A. Nahum, G. Musso, E.T. Kaiser, A.H. Rubenstein, and H. Tager, Identification of a mutant human insulin predicted to contain a serine for phenylalanine substitution, Proc. Natl. Sci. USA. 80:7390-7394 (1983).

56.   R.B. Tattersall, Mild familial diabetes with dominant inheri-
      tance, <u>Quarterly J. Med</u>. 43:339 (1974).
57.   R.B. Tattersall, and S.S. Fajans, A difference between the
      inheritance of classic juvenile-onset and maturity-onset type
      diabetes of young people, <u>Diabetes</u> 24:44-53 (1975).
58.   WHO expert Committee on Diabetes Mellitus, Second Report, World
      Health Organization Tech. Rep. Ser.:646 (1980, Geneva: WHO).
59.   R.C. Williams, W.C. Knowler, W.J. Butler, D.J. Pettitt,
      J.R. Lisse, P.H. Bennett, D.L. Mann, A.H. Johnson, and
      P.I. Terasaki, HLA-A2 and type 2 (insulin dependent) diabetes
      mellitus in Pima Indians: An association of allele frequency
      with age, <u>Diabetologia</u> 21:460-463 (1981).

THE GENETICS OF TYPE I AND TYPE II DIABETES:

ANALYSIS BY RECOMBINANT DNA METHODOLOGY

M. Alan Permutt, Teresa Andreone, John Chirgwin,
Steve Elbein, Peter Rotwein, and Matthew Orland

Washington University School of Medicine
St. Louis, MO 63110 USA

ABSTRACT

Susceptibility to IDDM is linked to the HLA-D locus on the short arm of chromosome 6, a region believed to be involved in the process of communication between cells which determines immune responses. Presumably an HLA molecule encoded by this region, unable to present a particular antigenic pathogen to the immune system, is inherited. The HLA-DR locus is quite complex, however. The gene which codes for this defective molecule may be identified by a combination of use of monoclonal antibodies and cloned gene probes which specifically hybridize to various portions of this region. Investigators are searching for HLA-DR4 containing chromosomes in IDDM which show similar patterns of restriction enzyme polymorphism. Hopefully, complete structural analysis of these related sequences will provide information about the mechanisms which confer susceptibility to develop IDDM.

A strong genetic component is involved in NIDDM evidenced by a high concordance in monozygotic twins. Nevertheless, there is much evidence of genetic heterogeneity. At the present time no clear cut genetic marker has been defined. The human insulin gene has been cloned and by Southern blot hybridization analysis of peripheral leukocyte DNA, the insulin gene locus is being evaluated as a possible contributor to the genetic defect. Population studies at the present time have not identified any particular polymorphic insulin allele associated with NIDDM. Population studies are complicated by heterogeneity of NIDDM, racial and ethnic differences, and heterogeneity of insulin alleles. Linkage analysis in family studies will provide an alternative approach to population studies to determine what role if any the insulin gene plays in the

genetic component of this disease. Because NIDDM is heterogeneous
and perhaps polygenic in nature, these linkage analyses in families
with NIDDM can be extended to other genes when they are cloned such
as that coding for the insulin receptor.

The familial aggregation of diabetes has long been noted (see
ref. 1 for review). In relatives of diabetics, the prevalence
ranges from 10-30%, while it is variously estimated to be between
0.1-3% in the general population. But familial aggregation of a
trait may be caused either by genetic or environmental factors. One
approach to dissecting the contribution of these factors is the
study of concordance in twins. Pyke and associates[2] observed that
overall identical twins always show a higher concordance rate than
dizygotic twins, irrespective of their age of diagnosis. Furthermore, they noted that identical twins of younger onset are often
discordant for diabetes while identical twins of older onset are
usually concordant. In a study of 200 pairs of monozygotic
twins,[3] the concordance of Type I or insulin dependent diabetes
(IDDM) was 80 of 147 twin pairs (54%). In contrast, 48 of 53 Type
II or non-insulin dependent diabetes (NIDDM) pairs (91%) were
concordant for diabetes. Thus, while genetic factors are important
in both types of diabetics, a strong environmental component makes
genetic analysis of IDDM more complex.

I.   THE GENETICS OF INSULIN DEPENDENT DIABETES (IDDM)

The relationship between the HLA locus and IDDM

Which genes are involved in IDDM and NIDDM? At the First
International Workshop of the Genetics of Diabetes held in 1976,
Nerup et. al.[4] presented evidence that there was a relationship
between certain histocompatibility alleles and IDDM, suggesting that
inheritance is related to one or more genes on the short arm of
chromosome 6. Since that time numerous studies have confirmed that
IDDM and NIDDM are genetically separate disease entities.

The association between the HLA system and IDDM was first noted
in population studies.[5-7] Individuals with disease were HLA typed
at the A, B, and C loci. There are two classes of HLA antigens,
class I or HLA-A, B, C antigens found on the cell membrances of all
nucleated cells and class II or HLA-D antigens which are found only
on some cell types. These two classes differ in their biochemical
structure and biological function. The HLA-A, B, C antigens are
recognized serologically, and consist of two polypeptide chains, a
heavy chain carrying the HLA-A, B, or C antigenic determinant and a
light invariant chain, beta-2 microglobulin which is controlled by a
gene outside the HLA system. When non-diabetic controls of similar
race were typed at the same loci, it was noted that certain HLA
types occurred more frequently in the diabetic population. Results

are usually expressed as the relative risk, a ratio of the frequency
of a particular HLA type in the diabetic population compared to the
frequency of that HLA type in an appropriate control population.
The relative risk for IDDM with certain HLA-A and B antigens was
increased 2-3 fold.[5-8] The association between the HLA-D locus
and IDDM was subsequently found to be stronger. In a series of
Caucasian patients from Denmark, Nerup et. al.[8] found 93% of
insulin dependent diabetic patients were either DR3 or DR4 positive,
significantly more than that found in controls. Individuals with
DR3 or DR4 antigens are at 3-6 fold increased relative risk for
developing insulin dependent diabetes. Similar results have been
found in African blacks, American blacks, and in Japanese.[8]

Many population studies confirmed the strong association
between HLA and IDDM at the DR locus. A strong association between
a particular genetic marker and a disease suggests that physical
linkage between that marker and the disease susceptibility locus may
exist. A significant association refers only to a statistical evaluation. In contrast, while linkage analysis requires statistical
evaluation, when linkage occurs with a high probability it implies a
physical relationship between two loci on the same chromosome.
Family studies are required to prove linkage. In families with two
affected sibs, Cudworth and associates[9] have studied sharing of
HLA alleles. If there was no linkage between diabetes and HLA, 25%
of pairs of diabetic sibs would be expected to be HLA identical,
that is, share the same HLA genes from the mother and father, 50%
would share only one HLA allele, or be haploidentical, and 25% would
be HLA nonidentical. If the HLA locus was linked to diabetes,
Cudworth predicted an excess of HLA identical and perhaps haploidentical pairs. The exact proportions would depend on certain
variables including the closeness of linkage of the HLA loci studied
with diabetes, and the mode of inheritance of susceptibility as well
as the penetrance of the genes. A striking deviation from the
predicted expectation of no linkage was observed, with 56% being HLA
identical, 38% haploidentical, and only 6% nonidentical. This overall deviation from the expected distribution assuming no linkage was
very highly significant. Thus, an HLA identical sib of a diabetic
child is at high risk for IDDM. In a prospective study of relative
risk of developing IDDM, the estimated relative risk for HLA identical sibs of IDDM's was 88 with a 95% confidence limit of 40-197.
Thus, an 88-fold increased risk of IDDM over the general 0.1-0.3%
risk suggests that 8.8-26.4% of HLA identical sibs of IDDM's will
develop IDDM. This estimate approached the concordance rate for
identical twins with IDDM, which strongly suggests that a gene (or
genes) within the HLA locus is the major if not the sole contributor, to the genetic liability for IDDM.

Further definition of the diabetogenic gene at the HLA-D locus

Loss of pancreatic ß-cells in IDDM is often accompanied by

immunological abnormalities such as anti-islet cell antibodies.[44]
Susceptibility to IDDM is linked to the HLA-D locus which is
believed to be involved in communication between cells determining
the immune response.[45]   Presumably, an HLA molecule unable to
present a particular antigenic pathogen to the immune system is
inherited in IDDM.   How will the genes located at or near the HLA/DR
locus which code for this defective molecule be identified?   The
HLA-DR antigens are detected serologically and also consist of two
transmembrane polypeptide chains.   More than 100 monoclonal antibodies have recently raised against these antigens (reviewed in
10).   This locus is quite complex at the molecular level, and little
is known of its function.   There are three families of closely
related immune response (Ia) molecules encoded by the HLA/D region,
designated DR, SB, And DC.   Each Ia molecule is a heterodimer of two
polypeptide chains, alpha and beta encoded by two genes in the D
region.   DNA sequencing and Southern blot analysis of genomic DNA
indicate that for the DR, DC and SB families there are at least 3,
2, and 2 beta chain genes respectively per haplotype.   There are at
least 2 DC alpha chain genes.   DR, DC and SB beta chain genes are
known to be polymorphic.   While it appears that monoclonal antibodies may be capable of dissecting the complicated HLA/D system,
cross reactions between antibodies occur.   Furthermore, it would be
a considerable task to repeat typing of populations of various
racial groups with these new antisera to perhaps finding a stronger
association of a particular HLA-D region with IDDM.   An alternative
approach using cloned DNA fragments from HLA-D region is being
applied to this problem.

Use of recombinant DNA techniques to identify the diabetogenic locus
on chromosome 6.

     In 1978, the use of restriction endonuclease polymorphism as a
means of studying genetic disorders in clinical medicine was first
introduced.   Kan and associates[11] showed that a restriction endonuclease site polymorphism several thousand base pairs (bp) away
from the sickle mutation in the ß-globin gene was associated with
that particular mutation.   This was accomplished by Southern blot
analysis.   In this method peripheral blood leukocyte DNA is digested
with restriction endonucleases, the resulting fragments electro-
phoresed, then blotted to filters.   The filters are then hybridized
with radiolabeled cloned gene probes.   We know from extensive
restriction endonuclease analysis of globin and other genes that on
the average about 1 out of every 100 bases in the human genome
differs from individual to individual, i.e. is polymorphic.[12]   If
this particular polymorphic base occurs in a restriction enzyme
site, then restriction enzyme digestion and Southern blot analysis
allows identification of specific polymorphic alleles.   The
restriction enzyme polymorphism can thus serve as a genetic marker
for a single base mutation within a gene far removed from the
polymorphic site.

Owerbach et al.[14] have used a cloned cDNA for one of the HLA-DR beta chain cDNA genes to test whether differences could be found in hybridization patterns between DNA from healthy individuals and diabetic patients after digestion with restriction endonucleases. They succeeded in finding among diabetic patients an increased frequency of one particular restriction endonuclease fragment, and a decreased frequency of another fragment compared to HLA-D matched controls. To establish that these fragments associated with IDDM are linked to the HLA locus, the same group of investigators studied 22 HLA genotyped family members. Only two recombinant events were found out of over 100 family members studied suggesting tight linkage.[15] Analysis of individual haplotypes revealed that HLA/DR4 containing chromosomes were heterogeneous among controls, but the diabetics showed a similar pattern of restriction enzyme polymorphism. In this pilot study only two families had two affected sibs. They plan to extend their studies to a larger number of IDDM families with two or more affected sibs combining HLA/DR typing and analysis of restriction enzyme fragments to determine whether affected sibs share restriction fragments even if they are not HLA identical. Complete structural analysis of such related sequences from insulin dependent diabetics may provide information about the mechanisms which confer susceptibility to develop IDDM.

An example of a promising development in gene mapping of human disease is illustrated by recent studies of Huntington's disease. Using a series of unique cloned DNA fragments which hybridize to human genomic DNA, Gusella et al.[13] discovered a polymorphic region in close linkage to a gene for Huntington's disease. Now affected individuals can be identified before the onset of symptoms. Geneticists are aware, however, that they are still a long way away from the Huntington's disease gene.[16] The DNA probe used to identify the linkage was calculated to be on the order of 3-5 million base pairs from the gene, somewhere on the short arm of chromosome 4. While it may be possible to narrow down the location of the Huntington's gene which represents 0.1% of the chromosome fragment identified by the marker, there is no hint of what the gene does or what it looks like, so that finding it by existing techniques will be a difficult task. A similar situation exists in IDDM.

II. THE GENETICS OF NON-INSULIN DEPENDENT DIABETES MELLITUS

Evidence for genetic heterogeneity

The genetic factors involved in non-insulin dependent diabetes remain undefined. Again, the importance of inheritance has been emphasized by the finding of a very high concordance in monozygotic twins.[2,3] Environmental factors such as obesity and diet may confuse the contribution of genetic factors, and evidence for genetic heterogeneity is strong. Baird[17] and Kobberling[18] have noted differences in familial aggregation in NIDDM on the basis of weight of the proband. Overall 15% of sibs of diabetics were diabetic compared to 3.8% of sibs of controls. But 15% of sibs of non-obese diabetics were diabetic, compared to 7.3% of sibs of obese diabetics (P<.01). Obesity augmented this difference. Obese sibs of non-obese diabetics had over a 25% prevalence of NIDDM.

Genetic heterogeneity of NIDDM has been further suggested by the widely varying prevalence in certain ethnic groups in the Pacific[19] and in American Indians.[20] Prevalence differs depending on whether they live in a rural or urban environment, but within the urban area the prevalence rates for ethnic groups are widely different. Knowler et al.[20] have shown that the prevalence of NIDDM in Pima Indians cannot be accounted for by differences in weight or diet from Caucasian populations.

Perhaps because of the heterogeneous nature of NIDDM, no consistent pattern of inheritance has been identified. One group which may be genetically distinct is that with maturity onset diabetes of the young (MODY). The characteristic features include diagnosis of non-ketotic diabetes in children, adolescence, and young adults.[21] In contrast of other forms of NIDDM, obesity is uncommon. A strong familial association has been noted and it appears to be inherited in a fashion consistent with an autosomal dominant trait.

At the present time, no clear cut genetic marker has been defined. Linkage analysis in affected families with the HLA locus has been negative.[22] In some it has been reported that there is a high degree of positive responders to chlorpropamide-alcohol induced flushing in family members with NIDDM.[23-25] These reports have been variable however. Recently, it has been suggested that chlorpropamide-alcohol induced flushing is more closely correlated with previous chlorpropamide treatment.[26]

Use of recombinant DNA methodology to define the gene defect(s)

Because NIDDM is invariably associated with a relative insulin lack, the genetic defect(s) may involve any number of genes. One can imagine many causes of impaired insulin production and/or action. A significant reduction of B-cell mass has been reported in autopsy series of NIDDM.[27] A gene which regulates beta cell replication might be defective, or any genes which regulate bio-synthesis and/or secretion are candidates. Similarly, genes controlling insulin action might be involved or any combination of the above.

Mutations in the structural portion of the insulin gene have been identified in family members with NIDDM.[29,30] In these families affected members were identified by high levels of immunoreactive insulin in sera. Analysis of their DNA by cloning and sequencing confirmed that a mutation occurred within the structural portion of the gene coding for amino acid at B24, a serine replacement for phenylalanine which resulted in a biologically defective insulin.[30] Since mutations in structural genes might be rare, one might ask whether the relative insulin lack in more common forms of NIDDM is somehow related to a defect in insulin biosynthesis, similar to globin deficiencies characteristic of the thalassemias. In the thalassemias, mutations in promoter regions or exon-intron junctions lead to decreased or unstable globin mRNA.[31] One hypothesis which is being tested by our laboratories is that mutations in regulatory regions of the insulin gene may be associated with NIDDM. Southern blot analysis of DNA from diabetics have been used to test this hypothesis.

Insulin gene polymorphism:

a. Nature of the polymorphic region.

A region of marked length polymorphism in the 5' flanking region of the human insulin gene was identified,[32-33] approximately 500 bp from the transcription initiation site. This polymorphic region is composed of a family of tandemly repeating oligonucleotide units consisting of 12-14 base pairs.[34-35] Length variation presumably results from unequal crossing over of misaligned oligonucleotide repeats but because only a limited repertoire of haplotypes is found (see Table I), there may be some constraint on this process.

Insulin gene fragments identified in individuals were classified according to size (Table I). A common size allele accounted for approximately two-thirds of the alleles. Variant alleles both larger and smaller were present in the remaining one-third. Smaller alleles (50-200 bp) accounted for only 3%. The larger alleles ranged in size from 100-7600 bp larger than the common sized allele. A 1600 bp (1.6kb) larger allele was by far the most frequent variable allele and accounted for 90% of all the larger alleles. In a study of approximately 200 individuals, a significant association of the 1.6 kb larger allele with NIDDM but not IDDM was noted.[36] Since that report we have extended the study to approximately 400 individuals.

b. Differences in three racial groups

Three racial groups have been studied, including American Blacks and Caucasians from St. Louis, and Pima Indians in collaboration with William Knowler and associates, NIADDK, Phoenix, AZ. To facilitate analysis, we have adopted the classification of polymorphic alleles of Bell et. al.,[37] as illustrated in Table I. The common size allele is designated class 1, alleles at least 1.6 kbp

larger than the common size allele are class 3, and alleles
intermediate in size are class 2. Considering all individuals in a
racial group without regard to diabetic status, the 5' flanking
region of the insulin gene in American Blacks exhibited the most
polymorphism (Table I and II). In Blacks 56.4%, in Pimas 40%, and
in Caucasians 36% of the individuals were heterozygous (i.e. geno-
types 1/2, 1/3, or 2/3). The frequency of the three classes of
alleles differed between Blacks and Caucasians and Pimas. The class
2 allele was not observed in Pimas. The frequency of the class 2
allele (Table III) was 1.9% in Caucasians, and 10.7% in Blacks. The
frequency of the class 3 allele was 23% in Caucasian and Pimas and
28% in Blacks. The observed genotypic frequencies in the racial
groups did not deviate from the expected when tested for Hardy-
Weinberg equilibrium. This classification is convenient for
statistical analysis, but really does not adequately describe the
extent of heterogeneity of alleles. Recently using enzymes which
cut DNA into small fragments around the polymorphic area and gels,
alleles of the same class differing by only 25-50 bp can be distinguished. Furthermore, additional polymorphic sites around the
insulin gene have been used in conjunction with the 5' polymorphism
to define haplotypes. In Blacks at least 8 different haplotypes
have been found.

   c. Relationship of the 5' flanking polymorphism to
       diabetes.

     Within the Caucasian and Pima groups the frequency of the class
3 allele did not differ between non-diabetics and diabetics (Table
III). However, only 4 Pima individuals were not noted to be homozygous for the class 3 allele (Table II), and all four were
diabetic. The insulin gene polymorphism does not seem to play a
role in the pathogenesis of NIDDM in Pima Indians, nor does it
influence glucose or insulin concentrations.[46] The class 3
allele, especially when homozygous, may influence the severity of
the disease in Pimas as indicated by the need for drug treatment.
Since the frequency of the class 3 allele in Pimas is 0.235, from
the Hardy-Weinberg equilibrium the predicted frequency of homozygous
class 3 individuals is $(0.235)^2$ or 0.055. Thus, the population
size would have to be considerably enlarged to determine the
relationship of homozygous class 3 individuals with NIDDM in Pimas.
One alternative to larger population studies is linkage analysis in
families (see below).

     In the Blacks, there may be an increase in homozygosity for the
class 3 allele in the NIDDM group. Even in this group our data do
not support this conclusion at the present time. Because of the
small number of homozygous individuals in our population, we are
currently collaborating with Graeme Bell and John Karam at the
University of California in San Francisco to extend this study.

Table I.   Size of Polymorphic Alleles

	Class 1					Class 2					Class 3																		Total
	-.2	-.1	0	.1	.2	.3	.4	.6	.7	.8	1.0	1.1	1.2	1.3	1.4	1.5	1.6	1.7	1.8	1.9	2.0	2.1	2.2	2.4	2.5	3.4	4.0	5.5	
Caucasian	1	8	192							1	2				2	4	38	7	4	1	2	1	3						266
Pima	1	2	175											1	11		33	1	5	2					1				232
American Blacks	3	2	173	2	1	4	2	9	5	10	1	1	4	3	9	6	50	6	2		1		1	1	2		1	1	300
																													798

0 = common size allele (540/798 = 68%)

Table II. The Distribution of Genotype at the Insulin Gene Locus by 5-Flanking Region Polymorphism and Diabetes Status

Genotype Frequency

	1/1	1/2	1/3	2/2	2/3	3/3	Total
Caucasian							
Non-diabetic	30	2	18			4	54
IDDM	11		4			2	17
NIDDM	35	2	21		1	3	62
	76 (.571)	4 (.030)	43 (.323)		1 (.008)	9 (.068)	133
Black							
Non-diabetic	24	7	33	1	6	2	73
IDDM	4	1	2				7
NIDDM	33	10	30	1	2	7	83
	61 (.370)	18 (.110)	65 (.399)	2(.012)	8(.049)	9 (.055)	163
Pima							
Non-diabetic	30		27				57
NIDDM	35		19			4	58
	65 (.565)		46(.400)			4 (.035)	115

Class 1 alleles are the common size allele previously described,36 or the L allele of Owerbach et al.,38 class 3 alleles include a polymorphic region at least 1.6 kbp larger than class 1 alleles (U allele of Owerbach et al.,38 and class 2 alleles are intermediate in size.

Table III. Allelic Frequencies of the Polymorphic Insulin Gene

| | Number of alleles (frequency) | | |
	Class 1	Class 2	Class 3
Caucasian			
Non-diabetic	80 (.741)	2 (.019)	26 (.241)
IDDM	26 (.765)	0	8 (.235)
NIDDM	93 (.750)	3 (.024)	28 (.226)
	199 (.748)	5 (.019)	62 (.233)
Black*			
Non-diabetic	88 (.603)	15 (.103)	43 (.295)
IDDM	11 (.786)	1 (.071)	2 (.143)
NIDDM	106 (.639)	14 (.084)	46 (.277)
	205 (.629)	30 (.092)	91 (.279)
Pima			
Non-diabetic	87 (.763)	0	27 (.237)
NIDDM	89 (.767)	0	27 (.233)
	176 (.765)	0	54 (.235)

*3 x 2 analysis vs Caucasian x^2 = 18.1, df = 2, p<.001
 3 x 2 analysis vs Pima, x^2 = 24.9, df = 2, p<.001

d. Comparison with other studies.

The frequency of the 5'-flanking insulin gene polymorphism and its relationship to diabetes reported in the two other population studies is illustrated in Table IV. Bell and Karam (San Francisco) studied Caucasians and Blacks,[39] and Owerbach et al. (Cophenhagen) Danish Caucasians.[38] The aggregate data for Caucasians shows no difference in the allelic frequencies between NIDDM and that in non-diabetics. As previously noted by Bell et al.,[39] there is a significant increase of class 1 alleles in the IDDM group. A similar trend can be seen in the aggregate data for Blacks but the sample size is smaller.

The relationship between NIDDM and insulin gene polymorphism has been investigated by others. Owerbach et al. found a positive association of class 3 alleles within NIDDM in Danish Caucasians,[38] but not in Nauruans.[43] Bell et al. reported an association of class 1 alleles with IDDM in Caucasians but found no association of class 3 alleles with either type of diabetes in Asians or American Blacks.[39]

In a previous report we had noted an association of class 3 alleles in NIDDM in a racially mixed group consisting of Caucasians and Black subjects from St. Louis and Pima Indians from Arizona.[36] Because mixing racial groups might confound the association, further studies were performed in the three racial groups. Although the association was not statistically significant in any racial group considered alone, the finding in all three groups was that NIDDM was associated with class 3 alleles. It was noted however, that the observed association was much stronger in Blacks (odds ration = 2.9, comparing presence or absence of a class 3 allele and NIDDM or no diabetes than in Caucasians (odds ration = 1.4) or in Pima Indians (odds ration = 1.5). Further it was noted that the class 3 alleles were more frequent in Black subjects. These findings suggested racial differences which the study was not large enough to detect. In view of our more recent findings in Pimas and Caucasians and lack of association with NIDDM in Nauruans, it apears that with the possible exception of Black subjects, class 3 alleles do not directly predispose a person to NIDDM.

e.   Insulin gene polymorphism and other associations

Mandrup-Poulsen et al. reported on a possible association between class 3 alleles and atherosclerosis.[41] They observed the frequency of the class 3 allele to be 2.5 times more common in a group of non-diabetic patients with severe atherosclerosis demonstrated by coronary arteriography compared with a group of non-diabetic control subjects with normal coronary arteriograms and no clinically demonstrable signs of atherosclerosis. The class 3 alleles did not confer risk of atherosclerosis through conventional risk factors such as body weight, blood pressure, blood glucose, triglyceride, cholesterol or lipoproteins. In that study a total of 41 atherosclerotic patients were compared to 21 non-atherosclerotic patients. The frequency of the class 3 allele in the atherosclerotic patients was .30 which was quite similar to the frequency reported in their earlier studies and similar to the frequency reported in Caucasians by us and by Bell et. al. (see Table IV). In the 21 non-atherosclerotic patients the frequency of the class 3 allele was .12, a much lower frequency than that reported for any other non-diabetic group. A larger number of patients need to be investigated before this association can be adequately interpreted.

Jowett et al.[42] studied the relationship between polymorphism in the 5' flanking sequence of the insulin gene and its relationship to diabetic hypertriglyceridemia. Four groups were evaluated, including diabetic and non-diabetic normolipemic and hypertriglyceridemic individuals. The number of individuals studied was small but the results suggested a stronger association of class 3 alleles with hypertriglyceridemia than with NIDDM.

Table IV. Polymorphism at the Insulin Gene Locus in Caucasians
          and Blacks: Results of Population Analysis from
          St. Louis, San Francisco[39] and Copenhagen[38]

	Allelic frequency			Genetopic frequency		
	1	2	3	1/1	1/3	3/3
Caucasian						
Nondiabetic						
St. Louis	.74 (80)	.02 (2)	.24 (26)	.56 (30)	.37 (20)	.07 (4)
San Francisco	.67 (112)	.01 (1)	.32 (53)	.45 (37)	.46 (38)	.10 (8)
Denmark	.73 (76)		.27 (28)	.50 (26)	.46 (24)	.04 (2)
	.71 (268)	.01 (3)	.28 (107)	.49 (93)	.43 (82)	.07 (14)
IDDM*						
St. Louis	.77 (26)	0	.24 (8)	.65 (11)	.24 (4)	.12 (2)
San Francisco	.88 (199)	0 (1)	.12 (26)	.76 (86)	.24 (27)	(0)
Copenhagen	.85 (63)		.15 (11)	.73 (27)	.24 (9)	.03 (1)
	.84 (288)	0 (1)	.14 (45)	.74 (124)	.24 (40)	.02 (3)
NIDDM						
St. Louis	.75 (93)	.02 (3)	.23 (28)	.57 (35)	.39 (24)	.05 (3)
San Francisco	.79 (120)	0	.21 (32)	.63 (48)	.32 (24)	.05 (4)
Copenhagen	.65 (61)		.35 (33)	.47 (22)	.36 (17)	.17 (8)
	.74 (274)	.01 (3)	.25 (93)	.57 (105)	.39 (65)	.09 (15)

*Allelic frequencies of IDDM vs non-diabetic, 3 x 2 analysis, $x^2 = 23.95$, p<.001

	1	2	3	1/1	1/3	3/3
Black						
Nondiabetic						
St. Louis	.60 (88)	.10 (15)	.30 (43)	24	46	2
San Francisco	.63 (40)	.11 (7)	.27 (17)	12	18	2
	.61 (128)	.11 (22)	.29 (60)	.35 (36)	.62 (64)	.04 (4)
IDDM						
St. Louis	.78 (11)	.07 (1)	.14 (2)	4	3	0
San Francisco	.70 (7)	.10 (1)	.20 (2)	2	3	--
	.75 (18)	.08 (2)	.17 (4)	.50 (6)	.50 (6)	0
NIDDM						
St. Louis	.64 (106)	.08 (14)	.28 (46)	33	43	7
San Francisco	.50 (40)	.14 (11)	.36 (29)	11	24	5
	.59 (146)	.11 (25)	.31 (75)	.36 (44)	.55 (67)	.10 (12)

Linkage analysis in families

Population studies are complicated by (1) heterogeneity of
NIDDM, (2) racial and ethnic differences in the allelic frequencies,
and (3) heterogeneity of insulin alleles. Linkage analysis in
family studies provides an important alternative approach to population studies to determine what role if any the insulin gene plays in
the genetic component of the disease. One group which has been
studied is that with maturity onset diabetes of the young (MODY), a
type of NIDDM inherited in a fashion consistent with an autosomal
dominant trait. Linkage analysis in affected families with a number
of markers including the HLA locus has been negative.[21] In
collaboration with Dr. Stefan Fajans (Ann Arbor, MI) lack of linkage
with the insulin gene has been established in one large pedigree
with over 50 members studied.[47] Other MODY families have shown
similar lack of linkage.[40]

Linkage analysis in affected families of different racial and
ethnic origins should soon indicate whether the insulin gene is
contributing to the etiology of NIDDM. Because of its heterogeneous
and perhaps polygenic nature, it will be important to extend linkage
analysis in these families to other loci when they are cloned.
Another obvious candidate is the insulin receptor gene which is
currently being pursued by a number of investigators.

ACKNOWLEDGEMENTS

This work was supported by NIH grants AM16746 and AM31866. The
authors are grateful for the secretarial help of Pat Stewart and Pam
Rader.

REFERENCES

1. J.I. Rotter, and D.L. Rimoin, Genetics, in: "Handbook of
    Diabetes Mellitus," M. Brownlee, ed., Gorland STPM Press, New
    York (1980).
2. R.B. Tattersall, D.A. Pyke, Diabetes in identical twins, Lancet
    ii:1120-1125 (1972).
3. A.H. Barnett, C. Eff, R.D.G. Leslie, and D.A. Pyke, Diabetes in
    identical twins, Diabetologia 20:87-93 (1981).
4. J. Neurp, P. Platz, O. Ortved-Anderson, M. Christy, J. Egeberg,
    J. Lyngsoe, J.E. Poulsen, L.P. Ryder, M. Thomsen, and A.
    Svejgaard, in: "The Genetics of Diabetes Mellitus," W.
    Creutzfeldt, J. Kobberling, and J.V. Neel, eds., SpringerVerlag
    (1976).

5. M. Thomsen, P. Platz, O.O. Andersen, M. Christy, J. Lyngsoe, J. Nerup, K. Rasmussen, L.P. Ryder, L.S. Nielsen, and A. Sveigaard, MLC typing in juvenile diabetes mellitus and idiopathic Addison's disease, Transplant Res. 22:125-147 (1975).

6. N.R. Farid, and J.C. Bear, The human major histocompatibility complex and endocrine disease, Endocrine Rev. 2:50-86 (1981).

7. M. Christy, G. Green, and B. Christan, Studies of the HLA system and IDDM, Diabetes Care 2:209-214 (1979).

8. J. Neurp, M. Christy, A. Green, M. Hauge, P. Platz, L.P. Ryder, A. Svejgaard, and M.L. Thomsen, HLA and insulin dependent diabetes - population studies, in: "The Genetics of Diabetes Mellitus. Serono Symposium. Vol 47," J. Kobberling and R. Tattersall, eds., Academic Press (1982).

9. A.N. Gorsuch, K.M. Spencer, E. Wolf, and A.G. Cudworth, HLA and family studies, in: "The Genetics of Diabetes Mellitus. Serono Symposium. Vol. 47," J. Kobberling and R. Tattersall, eds., Academic Press (1982).

10. S. Shaw and A. McMichael, HLA class II antigens and monclonal antibodies, Nature 306:538-539 (1983).

11. Y.W. Kan, and A.M. Dozy, Polymorphism of DNA sequence adjacent to human ß-globin structural gene: relationship to sickle mutation, Proc. Natl. Acad. Sci. USA 75:5631-5635 (1978).

12. A.J. Jeffreys, DNA sequence variants in the $^Gy-$, $^Ay-$, and Sand ß-globin genes in man, Cell 18:1-10 (1979).

13. J.F. Gusella, N.S. Wexler, P.M. Conneally, S.L. Naylor, M.A. Anderson, R.E. Tanzi, P.C. Watkins, K. Ottina, M.R. Wallace, A.Y. Sakaguchi, A.B. Young, I. Shoulson, E. Bonilla, and J.B. Martin, A polymorphic DNA marker genetically linked to Huntington's disease, Nature 306:234-238 (1983).

14. D. Owerbach, A. Lernmark, P. Platz, L.P. Ryder, L. Rask, P.A. Peterson, and J. Ludvigsson, HLA-D region ß-chain DNA endonuclease fragments differ between HLA-DR identical healthy and insulin-dependent diabetic individuals, Nature 303:815-817 (1983).

15. D. Owerbach, B. Hagglof, A. Lernmark, and G. Holmgren, Susceptibility in insulin-dependent diabetes defined by restriction enzyme polymorphism of HLA-D region genomic DNA, Submitted to Diabetes.

16. C.R. Cantor, Huntington's disease, Charting the path to the gene, Nature 308:404-405 (1984).

17. J.D. Baird, Is obesity a factor in the aetiology of noninsulin-dependent diabetes?, in: "The Genetics of Diabetes Mellitus. Serono Symposim. Vol. 47," J. Kobberling, and R. Tattersall, eds., Academic Press (1982).

18. J. Kobberling, Genetic heterogeneities with idiopathic diabetes, in: "The Genetics of Diabetes Mellitus," W. Creutzfeldt, J. Kobberling, and J.V. Neel, eds. Springer-Verlag, Berlin (1976).

19. P.Z. Zimmet, R.L. Kirk, and S.W. Serjeantson, Genetic and environmental interactions for non-insulin-dependent diabetes in high prevalence Pacific populations, in: "The Genetics of Diabetes Mellitus. Serono Symposium. Vol. 47," J. Kobberling, and R. Tattersall, eds., Academic Press, (1982).

20. W.C. Knowler, P.J. Savage, M. Nagulesparan, B.V. Howar, D.J. Pettitt, J.R. Lisse, S.L. Aronoff, and P.H. Bennett, Obesity, insulin resistance and diabetes mellitus in the Pima Indians, in: "The Genetics of Diabetes Mellitus. Serono Symposium. Vol. 47," J. Kobberling and R. Tattersall, eds., Academic Press (1982).

21. R.B. Tattersall, and S.S. Fajans, A difference between the inheritance of classical juvenile onset and maturity onset types diabetes in young people, Diabetes 24:44-53 (1975).

22. S.S. Fajans, M.C. Coultier, and R.L. Crowther, Clincial and etiologic heterogeneity of idiopathic diabetes mellitus, Diabetes 27:1112-1125 (1978).

23. D.A. Pyke, Diabetes: The genetic connections, Diabetologia 17:333-343 (1979).

24. R.D.G. Leslie, and D.A. Pyke, D.A.: Chloropropamide-alcohol flushing: A dominantly inherited trait associated with diabetes, Br. Med. J. 2:1519-1520 (1978).

25. D.A. Pyke, and R.D.G. Leslie, Chloropropamide-alcohol flushing: A definition of its relation to non-insulin dependent diabetes, Br. Med. J. 2:1521-1522 (1978).

26. S.N.T. Fui, H. Keen, J. Jarrett, V. Gossain, and P. Marsden, Test for Chlorpropamide-alcohol flush becomes positive after prolonged chlorpropamide treatment in insulin-depedent and noninsulin dependent diabetics, New Engl. J. Med. 309:93-96 (1983).

27. N. Maclean, and R.F. Ogilivie, Quantitative estimation of the pancreatic tissue in diabetic subjects, Diabetes 4:367-376 (1955).

28. R.L. White, D. Barker, T. Holm, J. Berkowitz, M. Lepert, W. Cavenee, R. Leach, and D. Drayna, Approaches to linkage analysis in the human, in: "Banbury Report 14. Recombination DNA Applications to Human Disease," C.T. Caskey, and R.L. White, eds., Cold Spring Harbor Laboratory (1983).

29. S.C.M. Kwok, S.J. Chan, A.H. Rubenstein, R. Poucher, and D.F. Steiner, Loss restriction endonuclease cleavage site in the gene of a structurally abnormal human insulin, Biochem. Biophys. Res. Comm., 98:844-849 (1981).

30   S.C.M. Kwok, D.F. Steiner, A.H. Rubenstein, and H.S. Tager, Identification of a point mutation in the human insulin gene giving rise to a structurally abnormal insulin (Insulin Chicago), Diabetes 32:872-875 (1983).

31. S.E. Antonarakis, S.H. Orkin, T. Cheng, A.F. Scott, J.P. Sexton, S.P. Trusko, S. Charache, and A.H. Kazazian, Jr., ß-Thalessemia in American Blacks: Novel mutations in the

"TATA" box and an acceptor splice site, PNAS 81:1154-1158 (1984).

32   G.I. Bell, R. Pictet, and W.J. Rutter, Analysis of the regions flanking the human insulin gene and sequence of an Alu family member, Nucleic Acids Res. 8:4001-4008 (1980).

33. P. Rotwein, R. Chyn, J. Chirgwin, B. Cordell, H. Goodman, and M.A. Permutt, Polymorphism in the 5'-flanking region of the human insulin gene and its possible relation to Type 2 diabetes, Science 213:1117-1120 (1981).

34. G.I. Bell, M.J. Selby, and W.J. Rutter, The highly polymorphic region near the human insulin gene is composed of simple tandemly repeating sequences, Nature 295:31-35 (1982).

35. A. Ullrich, T.J. Dull, A. Gray, J.A. Philips III, and S. Peter, Variation in the sequence and modification state of the human insulin gene flanking regions, Nucleic Acids Res. 10:2226-2240 (1982).

36. P.S. Rotwein, J. Chirgwin, M. Province, W.C. Knowler, D.J. Pettitt, B. Cordell, H.M. Goodman, and M.A. Permutt, Polymorphism in the 5'-flanking region of the human insulin gene: A genetic marker for non-insulin-dependent diabetes, New Engl. J. Med. 308:65-71 (1983).

37. G.I. Bell, J.H. Karam, and W.J. Rutter, Polymorphic DNA region adjacent to the 5' end of the human insulin gene, Proc. Natl. Acad. Sci. USA, 78:5759-5763 (1983).

38. D. Owerbach, and J. Nerup, Restriction fragment length polymorphism of the insulin gene in diabetes mellitus, Diabetes 31:275-277 (1982).

39. G.I. Bell, S. Horita, and J.H. Karam, A polymorphic locus near the human insulin gene is associated with insulin-dependent diabetes mellitus, Diabetes 33:176 (1984).

40. J.I. Bell, J.S. Wainscoat, J.M. Old, C. Chlouverakis, H. Keen, R.C. Turnver, and D.J. Weatherall, maturity onset diabetes of the young is not linked to the insulin gene. Br. Med. J. 286:590-592 (1982).

41. T. Mandrup-Poulsen, D. Owerbach, S.A. Mortensen, K. Johansen, H. Meinertz, H. Sorensen, and J. Nerup, DNA-sequences flanking the insulin gene on chromosome 11 confer risk of athero-sclerosis, Lancet 1:250-252(1984).

42. N.I. Jowett, L.G. Williams, G.A. Hitman, and D.J. Galton, Diabetic hypertriglyceridaemia and related 5'-flanking polymor-phism of the human insulin gene, Br. Med. J. 288:96-99 (1984).

43. S.W. Serjeantson, D. Owerbach, P. Zimmet, J. Nerup, and K. Thoma, Genetics of diabetes in Nauru: Effects of foreign admix-ture, HLA antigens and the insulin-gene-linked polymorphism, Diabetologia 25:13-17 (1983).

44. G.F. Cahill, Jr., and H.O. McDevitt, Insulin-dependent diabetes mellitus: the initial lesion, N. Engl. J. Med. 304:1454 (1981).

45. J.F. Kaufman, C. Auffray, A.J. Korman, D.A. Shackelford, and J. Strominger, The Class II molecules of the human and murine major histocompatibility complex. Cell 36:1 (1984).

46. W.C. Knowler, D.J. Pettitt, B. Vasquez, P.S. Rotwein, T.L. Andreone, and M.A. Permutt, Polymorphism in the 5'-flanking region of the human insulin gene: Relationships with non-insulin-dependent diabetes mellitus, glucose and insulin concentrations, and diabetes treatment in the Pima Indians. J. Clin. Invest. 74:2129 (1984).

47. T. Andreone, S. Fajans, P. Rotwein, W. Skolnick, and M.A. Permutt, Insulin gene analysis in a family with maturity onset diabetes of the young. Diabetes (in press).

IMMUNOLOGICAL ASPECTS OF TYPE 1 AND

2 DIABETES MELLITUS

Ake Lernmark, Steinunn Baekkeskov, Ivan Gerling,
William Kastern, Caj Knutson, and Birgitte Michelsen

Hagedorn Research Laboratory
Niels Steensensvej 6
DK-2820 Gentofte
Denmark

ABSTRACT

IDDM occurs predominantly among individuals being class II antigen HLA-DR 3 and/or 4 positive, while NIDDM is not associated with HLA-D. Although the HLA-DR 3 or 4 specificities are prerequisites for IDDM to develop, their high frequencies (about 60%) in the background population preclude tissue typing as a predictive test, underlined by the observation that less than 50% of monozygotic twins are concordant for IDDM. The presence of a number of immune abnormalities argues that the causes of IDDM may be sought in an altered immune reaction against antigens present in the pancreatic B cells and/or in the environment. The majority of IDDM patients of short duration show both cellular and humoral autoimmunity against the pancreatic B cells. Similar phenomena may be observed in patients initially diagnosed as NIDDM and treated with oral hypoglycemic agents. It has been speculated that these patients have a retarded form of IDDM. It is possible that the combination of specific Class II antigen molecule(s) and an invading antigen (virus, bacterium, chemical etc.) presented to the immune system triggers the formation of effector cells such as B lymphocytes and cytotoxic T lymphocytes which also cross-react with the pancreatic B cells. Multiple exposures to this or related antigens throughout several years may eventually lead a sufficient loss of pancreatic B cells to cause insulin dependence.

INTRODUCTION

Although diabetes mellitus has been known to man since ancient times, it is not until the past 30 years that the heterogeneity of the syndrome has been better understood. The present classification into two major groups, insulin-dependent (IDDM or Type 1) and non-insulin dependent (NIDDM or Type 2) is tentative, since the etiology and pathogenesis of either one of these disorders have yet to be clarifed. After the discovery of the pancreatic islets by Langerhans (1869), and the observation by Minkowski and von Mering (1889), that pancreatectomy was associated with the development of diabetes, it was observed that the number of islets were both altered and diminished in the pancreas of diabetic patients. Improved techniques of microscopy allowed the detection of islet A and B cells and several pathologist researchers to describe the presence of inflammatory cells in the islets in patients with onset of diabetes at a young age. The connection between the endocrine function of the pancreas and diabetes was therefore conceptually established before the final discovery of insulin in 1921 by Banting and Best in the city of this conference.

The designation of Type 2 or non-insulin dependent (NIDDM) and Type 1 or insulin-dependent (IDDM) diabetes as separate disease entities was based on long-term clinical and laboratory observations but not on differences in etiology or pathogenetic factors. Important observations to support the notion that IDDM is a disease different from NIDDM are the presence of various autoimmune phenomena among newly diagnosed IDDM patients (Table 1). Current research efforts are therefore directed towards a better understanding of the etiology of diabetes by investigating environmental factors such as viruses or chemicals, of the pathogenesis as it relates to adverse immune reactions directed against the pancreatic B cells and of genetic factors detected by association of IDDM to genes coded for in the major histocompatibility complex on the human chromosome 6. Immunological factors involved in the pathogenesis of IDDM may involve a sequence of events leading to pancreatic B-cell destruction. In NIDDM, on the other hand, there is little evidence that immunological factors are involved in the pathogenesis. The present comparison of immunological mechanisms in diabetes represent only a brief review and the reader is therefore referred to recent more extensive accounts in these subjects.[2,3,18,39,48,54,66]

Cellular Immune Abnormalities

Inflammatory cells are often seen in the pancreas of patients with IDDM of short duration. This phenomenon has now been documented in several studies (Table 2), most recently, by quantitative morphometry.[32] In a case report,[11], evidence was presented that immune competent cells including T and B lymphocytes, in addition to macrophages seemed to constitute the lesion. The presence of

Table 1. Immune phenotype associated with Type 1 (insulin-dependent) diabetes.

A. Cellular abnormalities	References
insulitis	Gepts, 1965[34]
cellular hypersensitivity to pancreatic antigens	Nerup et al. 1971[72]
alterations among T lymphocytes decreased suppressor activity	Gupta et al. 1982[38]
decreased helper cell activity	Mascart-Lemone et al. 1982[68] Herold et al. 1984[43]
increase in Ia-positive cells	Jackson et al. 1982[49] Pozzilli et al. 1983[81]
polyclonal activation	Horita et al. 1982[44] Papadopoulos et al. 1983[79]

B. Humoral immune abnormalities	
islet cell antibodies - ICA	Bottazzo et al. 1974[7]
- ICSA	Lernmark et al. 1978[57]
- C'AMC	Dobersen et al. 1980[25]
- ADCC	Charles et al. 1983[19]
	Maruyama et al. 1984[67]
- anti-64K	Baekkeskov et al. 1982[15]
- insulin	Palmer et al. 1983[78]
organ-specific antibodies	cf. MacCuish and Irvine 1975[62]
other autoantibodies - DNA/RNA	Huang et al. 1980[45]
- tubulin	Rousset et al. 1984[85]
- insulin receptor	Maron et al. 1983[65]

C. Immunogenetic factors	
association to HLA-DR 3 and/or 4	Platz et al. 1981[80] Wolf et al. 1983[97]
association to HLA-DQ ß-chain	Owerbach et al. 1983[76]
restriction enzyme polymorphism	Cohen et al. 1984[22]

Table 2. Prevalence of insulitis in human pancreas in diabetes and
          other disorders.

	Prevalence of insulitis	References
1.	Insulin-dependent diabetes of recent onset	
	16/23 (70%)	Gepts 1965[34]
	0/13 (0%)	Doniach and Morgan 1973[27]
	6/11 (55%)	Junker et al. 1977[52]
	8/11 (73%)	Foulis and Stewart 1984[32]
	2 patients of late-onset (62 and 72 years, respectively)	LeCompte and Legg 1972[56]
2.	Non-insulin dependent diabetes	Not reported
3.	Children with fatal virus disease	Jenson et al. 1980[50]

---

inflammatory cells seems to be associated with a marked reduction in
the number of pancreatic B cells although in one report it was found
that the endocrine pancreas of children dying from viral illnesses
may contain inflammatory cells.[50] Recent analyses[84] of the
endocrine pancreas by modern quantitative morphometric techniques
demonstrate that the pancreatic size and weight as well as B cell
volume (mass) is dramatically reduced in IDDM (Table 3). This is in
contrast to the patients with NIDDM who did not show any such
alterations of the relative mass except for an increased mean value
of the A cells (Table 3). The total mass of the NIDDM endocrine
pancreas was similar to that of controls.

    Although it has not been possible to study the IDDM endocrine
pancreas systematically at the time of diagnosis, it has been
observed that IDDM islets, already at the time of diagnosis, may
show pseudoatrophic features. The process leading to invasion of
islets by inflammatory cells may therefore, perhaps at a considerable time, have been present before the clinical onset of the disease. It would therefore be important to determine to what extent
the pancreatic B cell mass is diminished in individuals susceptible
to develop IDDM. However, methods other than those currently available will be required, first, to detect a decrease in pancreatic B
cell function and, second, to distinguish whether a diminution is

Table 3.   Quantitative   morphometry   of   the   endocrine   pancreas   in
           diabetes.

		% of epithelial tissue			
		B	A	D	PP
Controls	1395 mg	1.2	0.29	0.17	0.61
NIDDM	1449 mg	1.14	0.60	0.18	0.50
IDDM	413 mg	<0.01	0.49	0.33	0.77

Data from Rahier et al. 1983[84]

due to either a decrease in function without alteration in B cell
mass or to a decrease in the total number of B cells without an
alteration in the B cell function.

Recent advances in the understanding of the function of the
immune system suggest that cell-to-cell interactions operate at
several levels of an immune response to antigen. Our knowledge
about these mechanisms involving specific pancreatic B cell antigens
in diabetes are yet only fragmentary. There are two possibilities
by which autoantibodies against pancreatic B cells may be formed.
One is that the B lymphocytes producing these antibodies are
non-specifically stimulated. In fact, in IDDM there is sign of a
polyclonal activation.[44,79] However, it is difficult to envisage
how the pancreatic B cells are specifically lost by such a
mechanism. The other is that a foreign or an own antigen
(autoantigen) is presented to the immune system by an antigen-
presenting cell (a so-called accessory cell, macrophage, dendritic
cell etc). It has also been speculated that in case the pancreatic
B cells were brought to express class II transplantation antigens
(such as HLA-D region antigens), a requirement for an antigen-
presenting cell[91,92] the B cell itself would be able to present
its own antigens.[10,14] Recent investigations indicate that
circulating islet cell antibodies detect a human islet antigen of
M_r 64000.[15] However, it is not known whether this or an
environmental antigen, mimicing the M_r 64000 protein, was
originally presented to the immune system. The M_r 64000 antigen,
is yet only defined by its reactivity with autoantibodies but not as
an antigen able to stimulate the proliferation of specific T
(helper) lymphocytes when presented in conjunction with a Class II
(HLA-D) transplantation antigen. The present lack of isolated,
defined, pancreatic B cell antigens hamper our ability to study
those cellular interactions which would initiate an immune response
to autoantigens.

Evidence for a cellular hypersensitivity to crude pancreatic antigens in IDDM but generally not in NIDDM have been obtained in the leukocyte migration inhibition test (LMT). First demonstrated by Nerup and co-workers[72,73] their findings were later confirmed by others (cf. 74) and more recently migration inhibition in IDDM was also obtained with a human fetal cloned pancreatic B cell line.[71] In general, the LMT was found at a low frequency among patients with NIDDM, however, in a recent study[4] was evidence presented, using human fetal pancreatic tissue as the antigen in the LMT test, that while 95% of the 20 IDDM patients were positive in the test, also 25% of NIDDM patients showed migration inhibition. However, in a follow up investigations it was found that those NIDDM patients being positive in the LMT test later developed an insulin-independent state.[4] These observations are reminiscent of previous observations[36,47] that immune abnormalities, usually found among newly diagnosed IDDM patients, may signify a later development of an insulin-dependent state when found in patients first diagnosed and treated as NIDDM.

Other cellular immune abnormalities in diabetes are controversial.[59] Alterations in T cell subsets have not always been reproducible and the hypothesis that the development of IDDM is associated with a T suppressor cell dysfunction has therefore been difficult to verify. Again, experiments with pancreatic B cell specific antigens are of central importance since in one study guinea-pig islets[31] and in another human insulinoma fragments[94] showed a decrease in suppressor cell activity. These experiments are of great interest also to be carried out in well-characterized NIDDM patients, who show poor diabetic control to diet or oral hypoglyceamic agents, since it is often argued that many immune abnormalities, observed in diabetes are rather explained by metabolic derangements than by specific immune abnormalities. In fact, the function of peripheral blood T lymphocytes may be affected by the levels of circulating insulin.[40]

It is concluded that NIDDM is only rarely associated with cellular immune abnormalities often observed in IDDM. However, when such phenomena do occur, they may signify a propensity to develop an insulin-dependent diabetic state.

Humoral Immune Abnormalities in Diabetes

Since the first descriptions of islet cell antibodies[7,57,61,63] a wide spectrum of assay systems to detect such antibodies have been described (Table 4). Islet cell cytoplasmic (ICA), islet cell surface (ICSA), and immuneprecipitating antibodies are highly prevalent at the time of clinical onset and their prevalence tend to decrease with increasing duration of IDDM. The different assay systems seem to detect different antigenic determinants and/or autoantibody class since the concordance rate between

Table 4. Determination of islet cell antibodies

Islet cell cytoplasmic antibodies (ICA)

Sections of frozen human blood   Indirect immunofluorescence:
group O pancreas   a) anti-human IgG (ICA-IgG)
                                     b) anti-human C3 (CF-ICA)
                                        (complement fixing)

                                     Immuneperoxidase
                                     Biotin-Avidin-peroxidase

Sections of Bouin-fixed human   Indirect immunofluorescence
pancreas   Immuneperoxidase
                                     Biotin-Avidin-peroxidase

Islet cell surface antibodies (ICSA)

Human insulinoma cells   Indirect immunofluorescence
Human fetal islet cells ^{125}I-labelled second
                                        antibody
Rodent islet cells ^{125}I-protein A
Rat islet tumor cells

Complement-dependent antibody mediated cytotoxicity (C'AMC)

Human islet cels ^{51}Cr-release
Rat islet cells   Dye exclusion
Rat islet tumor cells   Release of H-leucine
Hamster or rat islets   from prelabelled cells

Antibody-dependent cellular cytotoxicity (ADCC)

Human fetal B cells ^{51}Cr-release

Immunoprecipitating antibodies

Human islets   A M_r 64000 component detected
Rat islets   by metabolic labelling,
                                     immunoprecipitation, SDS-gel
                                     electrophoresis and autoradio-
                                     graphy

Table 5.   Autoantibodies found at an increased frequency among IDDM
           patients

Type	Antibody
1. Organ-specific	
Islets	ICA, ICSA or C'AMC Insulin
Thyroid	Thyroid microsomal Thyroglobulin
Stomach	Gastric-parietal cell Intrinsic factor
Adrenals	Adrenal cell
Pituitary	Pituitary cell
2. Non-organ specific	
Peripheral lymphocytes	Lymphocytotoxic
Nucleic acids	Single-stranded DNA Double-stranded RNA
Cell constituents	Tubulin Insulin receptor

(See text for references)

ICA and ICSA positive sera is only 50-60%.[58,96] On the other hand,
although the prevalence at onset was lower compared to ICSA determined by indirect immunofluorescence, cytotoxic or complement-
dependent antibody mediated cytotoxic (C'AMC) antibodies[30,83]
showed a good correlation to ICSA.[25] ICSA positive sera also tend
to be specific for the pancreatic B cells.[26,95] In the same vein,
the presence of antibodies against the M_r 64000 islet cell protein
correlated to ICSA-positive sera rather than to sera positive for
ICA.[15,16] Further experiments are necessary to clearly delineate
the specificity of these islet cell antibodies in terms of subclass
and recognition of antigen. In addition, the induction of these

autoantibodies are poorly known both in terms of the temporal appearance and switch from one subclass to another during the maturation of the antibody response. In a recent investigation, IDDM sera with high titers of ICA were fractionated into IgM, IgA and IgG. It was found that all ICA activity was associated with the IgG fraction despite the samples were obtained only 2-9 days following diagnosis (Gerling, unpublished obsrvations).

Efforts are made to identify islet cell antigens, their route of synthesis and their subcellular localization.[15,16,17,28] The M_r 64000 component (Table 1) may represent only one antigenic determinant reactive in the particular system used to detect this antigen. Increased sensitivity in the assays used and the precision of the immunological detection system may allow the identification of other antigens. Since IDDM patients are known to have an increased frequency of organ-specific autoantibodies (Table 5), the prevalence of different autoantibodies are expected to increase assay sensitivity as exemplified by the detection among IDDM patients of autoantibodies against tubulin,[85] insulin[78] and the insulin receptor.[65] Antigens may also include RNA or DNA[45] and determinants on lymphocytes.[43,86] The development of antigen-specific and highly sensitive and reproducible assays to detect increased levels of islet cell autoantibodies are important in view of the many recent attempts to use islet cell antibodies as predictive markers for a later onset of IDDM. However, the wide variety of autoantibodies among both IDDM patients and their first degree relatives and the more recent observations that IDDM patients show signs of a polyclonal activation[44,79] suggest that these abnormalities may be a feature of diabetic families. In fact, recent analyses among relatives to IDDM patients suggest that a variety of autoantibodies may be present among the healthy relatives who showed no sign or were not treated for any organ-specific autoimmune disorder.[4,8,45] These phenomena should be born in mind when evaluating the predictive risks for developing IDDM based on screening for islet cell antibodies alone.

Islet Cell Antibodies and the Pathogenesis of Diabetes

Islet cell antibodies have been detected in several individuals who years later developed diabetes.[33,35,37,60,89] In one study it was argued that the presence of complement fixing ICA (CFICA) was of predictive value[37] while in another the presence of ICA in conjunction with the absence of the first peak of insulin release following glucose stimulation would mark the disease.[89] Since islet cell antibodies may appear temporarily[41,88] it still remains to be clarified to what extent an islet cell antibody is of predictive value and/or of pathogenetic importance. Islet cell antibodies, either formed following a primary lesion to the pancreatic B cells or to an unknown antigen which mimic B cell determinants, would by themselves have the propensity to affect the B cells. In

the former case, the islet cell autoantibodies are expected to be
formed in response to an outflow of cellular constituents later to
be removed from circulation as immune complexes. In the latter situation, the autoantibodies may be able to cause tissue damage or
alter cellular functions either by binding to cell surface determinants, important to the function of the B cells, by being part of
a complement-dependent antibody mediated cytotoxic (C'AMC) reactions[25,83] or by arming killer cells (antibody-dependent cellular
cytotoxicity) (ADCC).[19] It was found that immunoglobulin, purified from IDDM plasma inhibits glucose-stimulated insulin release
from both perifused rat islet cells,[53] isolated rat or human
islets[1,42] or the perfused pancreas of mice following passive
transfer of immunoglobulin.[90] It can therefore not be excluded
that the presence of islet cell antibodies may contribute to a loss
of pancreatic B cells either by directly inhibiting their function
and/or ability to proliferate or indirectly by mediating immune
effector mechanisms. The possible in vivo correlates to such
reactions remain to be defined.

Islet Cell Antibodies as a Predictive Test for IDDM

It has been observed that ICA are often detected among healthy
first-degree relatives[5,8,13,25,37,75] or in patients with
NIDDM.[24,36,47] The number of such individuals who later developed
IDDM in relation to those who had the marker but did not develop
IDDM is yet too small to allow a calculation of the predictive value
of a positive ICA test for IDDM to develop. CF-ICA was first proposed to be a better predictive marker than IgG – ICA,[9] however,
recent studies suggest that there is a good correlation between a
high titre of IgG-ICA and the presence of a positive CF-ICA[12,36]
and that CF-ICA is not to be regarded as an obligate predictive
marker.[36,88] The qualitative nature and the histological evaluation procedures makes the current immunofluorescence assays for ICA,
whether CF-ICA, IgG-ICA or ICSA highly susceptible to variation in
quality of the pancreas used for sections[64] as well as to a
significant observer bias. Stringent assay definitions and
continuous control of assay reproducibility and precision will be
necessary for an islet cell antibody assay system to be of any value
for long-term studies of individuals susceptible to develop IDDM.
Approaches to control islet cell antibody assays are summarized in
Table 6. It is possible that prospective analyses of individuals
susceptible to develop IDDM by titration of ICA, ICSA or immune
precipitating antibodies,[60] combined with a test for pancreatic B
cell function such as the intravenous glucose tolerance test[33,89]
and HLA-typing, will provide more reliable means by which IDDM can
be predicted. In a recent cross-sectional study of NIDDM patients,[36]
it was found that 89 per cent of the patients who were ICA positive
required insulin therapy within a mean period of 3.7 years while it
took 8.4 years among the ICA-negative NIDDM patients. There was also
a significant excess of HLA-DR 3 and DR3/DR4 phenotypes among the

Table 6   Reproducibility, precision and sensitivity of ICA and ICSA
assays

	ICA[1]	ICSA[2,3]	C'AMC[4]
Sensitivity	40–98%	not tested	–
Specificity	96–100%	not tested	–
Inter–observer variation	12–27%	15%	–
% C.V.			
intra–assay	–	14%	18%
inter–assay	–	16%	17%

1   Marner et al.[64]
2   Lernmark et al.[58]
3   Huen et al.[46]
4   Rabinovitch et al.[83]

ICA–positive NIDDM patients with secondary oral hypoglycemic agent
failure. These authors speculated that the presence of ICA and certain HLA–DR specificities identify adult diabetics with a retarded
form of IDDM. Prospective analyses of NIDDM patients will be needed
to verify this hypothesis. It is concluded that controlled analysis
of islet cell antibodies and HLA specificities may allow a proper
diagnosis of diabetes among adult patients and that an early detection of IDDM will be advantageous for the individual patient in terms
of avoiding ketoacidosis and severe metabolic decompensation. An
early detection of processes known to result in pancreatic B cell
disappearence will also be necessary for future attempts to specifically halt an hypothetical autoimmune destruction of the insulin-
producing cells.

Immunogenetic Factors in Diabetes

     It has long been recognized that IDDM as well as NIDDM tend to
run in families, however, the mode of inheritance has not been
defined. The observations that human diseases might be associated
with HLA antigen coded for by the major histocomatibility complex
(MHC)[23] prompted similar investigations among IDDM and NIDDM
patients. First, IDDM, but not NIDDM, was found to be associated
with HLA–B8 and/or B15. Later, the association to IDDM was found to
be stronger with the serologically defined HLA–DR3 and DR4 specificities (Table 7). This observation is explained by the pronounced
linkage disequilibrium among various MHC loci which means that

Table 7. Association between IDDM and markers for HLA genes.

A.   Serological analysis*

HLA-DR specificity	Controls (%)		IDDM (%)		Relative risk	
	A	B	A	B	A	B
3/4	4	6	34	51	13.2	14.3
3	29	32	54	71	2.9	5.0
4	32	34	72	78	5.4	6.8
3 and/or 4	57	59	93	98		

B. Restriction fragment length polymorphism detected with an HLA-DC chain cDNA probe**

HLA-DR genotype	Length of fragment	Controls (%)	IDDM (%)	Relative risk
3 and/or 4	BamHI 3.7 kb	27	2	0.05

*   Data is from Platz et al. 1981[80] (Study A) and Wolf et al. 1983[97] (Study B).

**   Data from Owerbach et al.[76] The relative risk was calcu-
     lated among the HLA-DR identical control and IDDM individuals.
     The absence of the BamHI 3.7 kb fragment was associated with
     IDDM.

---

certain specificities tend to appear together in the same individual
more often than expected from the individual frequencies of the different specificities. The relative risk value indicate the strength
of the association between a disease and an HLA specificity and
reveal the increased frequency with which the disease occurs in a
group of individuals that have a specificity compared to a group
that lacks it. The HLA-DR typing of IDDM patients demonstrates that
more than 90 per cent are positive for HLA-DR3 and/or 4 compared to
nearly 60 per cent of the background population.[80,97] Detailed
reviews of the HLA-associations in diabetes are available elsewhere.[2,20,21]

    Extensive HLA-DR typing of families having two or more members
affected by IDDM demonstrates that HLA-identical siblings have an
increased risk of developing IDDM.[51,80] However, HLA-identity is
not sufficient for IDDM to develop since even among monozygotic twins
the rate of concordance, i.e. both twins developing the disease, is

only 30–50 per cent[51,82] although there was an increased risk among twins being HLA–DR 3/4.[51]

The association between certain HLA–DR specificities and IDDM argues that gene(s) conferring susceptibility to IDDM reside in the HLA–system. A diabetogenic locus would therefore be more closely linked to the DR than to the B locus. The analysis of monozygotic twins support this hypothesis but require, in addition, either an influence from environmental factors or constitutive alterations of the function of the immune system. The latter would involve structural changes of genes which are known to occur in the immunoglobulin genes following the specific differentiation of B lymphocytes. It can also not be excluded that environmental factors may influence the expression of HLA–gene products, important to the immune response, differently in monozygotic twins. It is now possible to study such alterations since molecular cloning methods have provided new means by which to determine the entire structure of the HLA–complex and of specific immunoglobulin genes. Since a better understanding of those factors which govern the development of an auto-immune disorder is of great interest, experiments are undertaken to clone and sequence[70] HLA gene fragments which have been found to be closely associated with IDDM.[76,77] Since the genes for the HLA Class II antigens are highly polymorphic molecules, the analysis of individual genes may provide both new DNA probes to be used to study the disease association, and the amino acid sequence of individual proteins predicted from the nucleotide sequence of cloned genes.

Efforts in several laboratories[69,87] have provided evidence that the heterodimeric HLA Class II molecules, composed of a heavy (α) chain (M_r 34.000) and a light (β) chain (M_r 28.000), are encoded for by several genes (Figure 1). The nomenclature is that of a recent workshop.[6,93] Using an HLA–DQ β–chain cDNA probe[55] in the Southern blotting technique to determine restriction fragment length polymorphism, it was discovered that the frequency of certain restriction enzyme fragments differed between HLA–DR identical IDDM and control individuals (Table 7). This approach, which allows an analysis of the association between HLA–genes and IDDM beyond that

	SB	DC	DR	complement genes	B	C	A
centromere							
	$\alpha\beta\alpha\beta$	$\alpha\beta\alpha\beta$	$\alpha\beta\beta\beta$				

Fig. 1   The class II antigens, comprising one α and one β chain, are expressed on the surface of cells, e.g. macrophages, dendritic cells, B lymphocytes and other which are important to the immune response. Data from.[6]

of serological HLA-determination, suggested that the HLA-DR4 specificity is heterogeneous and that not all HLA-DR4 are associated with
IDDM.[76,77] One fragment, defined by its hybridization to the HLA-
DQ ß-chain probe used after digestion of the genomic DNA with BamHI,
being 3.7 kb, was rarely found among HLA-DR4 positive IDDM
patients.[76,77] A BamHI 3.7 kb fragment present on an HLA-DR4
containing chromosome from a healthy individual without history of
diabetes in the family was cloned and its partial sequence determined.[70] This analysis strongly suggested that the Bam 3.7 kb
fragment was part of an HLA-DQ ß-chain gene. This gene has been
found to consist of 6 coding regions (exons) and 5 intervening
sequences.[69,87] The Bam 3.7 kb fragment was defined by one
restriction site located in the first and the other site in the
third intervening sequence. Further analysis of restriction fragments detected by the HLA-DQ ß-chain probe in families with or without IDDM indicated that those HLA-DR 4-positive individuals who did
not have a BamHI 3.7 kb fragment, had a BamHI 12 kb fragment instead.
Hence, HLA-DR 4 positive IDDM individuals often have a BamHI 12 kb
fragment which would be defined by the absence of a BamHI restriction
site either in the first or third intervening sequence in one of the
two HLA-DQ ß-chain genes. Experiments are in progress to determine
whether the expression of this gene in circulating monocytes and B
lymphocytes differ between HLA-DR identical control and IDDM individuals. It should, however, be kept in mind that the observed gene
polymorphism may be explained by the possibility that the HLA-DQ
ß-chain gene is more closely linked to a hypothetical diabetogenic
gene than is HLA-DR. It is likely, however, that the genetic analysis with different gene probes[22,29,76,77] will better define
individuals at risk particularly by decreasing the presence of a
genetic marker in the background population to come closer to a
frequency which is similar to the actual prevalence of the disease.

ACKNOWLEDGEMENT

    Studies in the author's laboratory was supported by the National
Institutes of Health (grants AM 26190, AM 33873) and the Juvenile
Diabetes Foundation International. Marianne Sondergaard is greatly
acknowledged for secretarial assistance.

REFERENCES

1. W.W. Alden, K.W. Taylor, and G.F. Bottazzo, Effects of immuno-
    globulin and sera from newly diagnosed Type 1 (insulin-
    dependent) diabetic patients on glucose-induced insulin release
    in human islets of Langerhans, Diabetologia 27:251A (1984).

2. D. Andreani, M. Berger, U. DiMario, G. Eisenbarth, A. Lernmark,
    and A.H. Rubenstein, eds., Immunology in diabetes '84,
    Diabetologia 27 (suppl), 65:164 (1984).

3. D. Andreani, U. DiMario, K.F. Federlin and L.G. Heding, eds., "Immunology in Diabetes," Kimpton Medical Publications, London (1984).

4. I. Balazsi, M. Horvath, Z. Rozsas, and I Karadi, Cell-mediated and humoral immune responses in Type I and Type II diabetic patients, XIth International Karlsburg Symposium (Abstr) 71 (1983).

5. C. Betterle, F. Zanette, B. Pedini, F. Presotto, L.B. Rapp, C.M. Monciotti, and F. Rigon, Clinical and subclinical organ-specific autoimmune manifestations in Type 1 (insulin-dependent) diabetic patients and their first-degree relatives, Diabetologia 26:431-436 (1984).

6. J. Bodmer, and W. Bodmer, Histocompatibility 1984, Immunol. Today 5:251-254 (1984).

7. G.F. Bottazzo, A. Florin-Christensen, and D. Doniach, Islet cell antibodies in diabetes mellitus with autoimmune polyendocrine deficiencies, Lancet ii:1279-1283 (1974).

8. G.F. Bottazzo, J.I. Mann, M. Thorogood, J.D. Baum, and D. Doniach, Autoimmunity in juvenile diabetes and their families, Br. Med. J. i:165-168 (1978).

9. G.F. Bottazzo, B.M. Dean, A.N. Gorsuch, A.G. Cudworth, and D. Doniach, Complement-fixing islet-cell antibodies in type-1 diabetes: possible monitors of active ß-cells damage, Lancet i:668-672 (1980).

10. G.F. Bottazzo, R. Pujol-Borrell, and T. Hanafusa, Role of aberrant HLA-DR expression and antigen presentation in induction of endocrine autoimmunity, Lancet ii:1115-1118 (1983).

11. G.F. Bottazzo, P. Pozzilli, R. Mirakian, B.M. Dean, and D. Doniach, Early immunological events in diabetes, in: "Immunology in Diabetes," D. Andreani, U. DiMario, K.F. Federlin and L.G. Heding, eds., Kimpton Med. Publ., London, :95-104 (1984).

12. G.J. Bruining, J. Molenaar, C.W. Tuk, J. Lindeman, H.A. Bruining, and B. Marner, Clinical time course and characteristics of islet cell cytoplasmic antibodies in childhood diabetes, Diabetologia 26:24-29 (1984).

13. K. Buschard, O.O. Andersen, B. Christau, M. Christy, H. Kromann, J. Nerup, P. Platz, A. Svejgaard, M. Thomsen, and F. Bottazzo, Islet cell antibodies a marker of subclinical diabetes. A pathogenic factor, Diabetologia 13:386 (1977).

14. S. Baekkeskov, T. Kanatsuna, L. Klareskog, D.A. Nielsen, P.A. Peterson, A.H. Rubenstein, D.F. Steiner, and A. Lernmark, Expression of major histocompatibility antigens on pancreatic islet cells, Proc. Natl. Acad. Sci. USA 78:6456-6460 (1981).

15. S. Baekkeskov, J.H. Nielsen, B. Marner, T. Bilde, J. Ludvigsson, and A. Lernmark, Autoantibodies in newly diagnosed diabetic children immunoprecipitate specific human pancreatic islet cell protein, Nature 298:167-169 (1982).

16. S. Baekkeskov, T. Dyrberg, and A. Lernmark, Autoantibodies against a M_r 64000 islet cell protein precede the onset of spontaneous diabetes, Science 224:1348-1350 (1984).

17. S. Baekkeskov and A. Lernmark, A ß-cell glycoprotein of M_r 40000 is the major islet immunogen following xenogenic immunisation, Diabetologia 27:70-73 (1984).

18. G.F. Cahill and H.O. McDevitt, Insulin-dependent diabetes mellitus: the initial lesion, N. Engl. J. Med. 304 (24):1454-1465 (1981).

19. M.A. Charles, M. Suzuki, N. Waldeck, L.E. Dodson, L. Slater, K. Ong, A. Kershnar, B. Buckingham, and M. Golden, Immune islet killing mechanisms associated with insulin-dependent diabetes: in vitro expression of cellular and antibody-mediated islet cell cytotoxicity in humans, J. Immunol. 130:1189-1194 (1983).

20. M. Christy, A. Green, B. Christau, H. Kromann, J. Nerup, P. Platz, M. Thomsen, L.P. Ryder, and A. Svejgaard, Studies of the HLA system and insulin-dependent diabetes mellitus, Diabetes Care 2:209-214 (1979).

21. W. Creutzfeldt, J. Köbberling, and J.V. Neel, The genetics of diabetes mellitus, Springer-Verlag, Berlin, Heidelberg (1976).

22. D. Cohen, O. Cohen, A. Marcadet, C. Massart, M. Lathrop, I. Deschamps, J. Hors, E. Schuller, and J. Dausset, HLA Class II ß DC DNA restriction fragments differentiate among HLA-DR2 individuals in insulin-dependent diabetes and multiple sclerosis, Proc. Natl. Acad. Sci. USA 81:1774-1778 (1984).

23. J. Dausset, The major histocompatibility complex in man. Past, present, and future concepts, Science 213:1469-1450 (1981).

24. U. DiMario, W.J. Irvine, D.Q. Borsey, J.L. Kyner, J. Weston, and C. Galfo, Immune abnormalities in patients not requiring insulin at diagnosis, Diabetologia 25:392-395 (1983).

25. M.J. Dobersen, J.E. Scharff, F. Ginsberg-Fellner, and AL Notkins, Cytotoxic autoantibodies to beat-cells in the serum of patients with insulin-dependent diabetes mellitus, N. Engl. J. of Med. 303:1493-1498 (1980).

26. M.J. Dobersen and J.E. Scharff, Preferential lysis of pancreatic B-cells by islet cell surface antibodies, Diabetes 31:449-462 (1982).

27. I. Doniach and A.G. Morgan, Islets of Langerhans in juvenile diabetes mellitus, Clin. Endocrinol. 2:233-248 (1973).

28. T. Dyrberg, S. Baekkeskov, and A. Lernmark, Specific pancreatic B cell surface antigens recognized by a xenogenic antiserum, J. Cell Biol. 94:472-477 (1982).

29. H.A. Erlich and D. Stetler, Polymorphic restriction endonuclease sites linked to the HLA-DR α-chain gene: localization and use as genetic markers in control and insulin-dependent diabetes-mellitus populations, Diabetes 33 (suppl. 1):37A (1984).

30. G.S. Eisenbarth, M.A. Morris, and R.M. Scearce, Cytotoxic antibodies to cloned rat islet cells in serum of patients with diabetes mellitus, J. Clin. Invest. 67:403-408 (1981).

31. R.S. Fairchild, J.L. Kyner, and N.I. Abdone, Specific immuno-regulation abnormality in insulin-dependent diabetes mellitus, J. Lab. Clin. Med. 99:175-186 (1982).

32. A.K. Foulis and J.A. Stewart, The pancreas in recent-onset Type 1 (insulin-dependent) diabetes mellitus: insulin content of islets, insulitis and associated changes in the exocrine acinar tissue, Diabetologia 26:456-461 (1984).

33. O.P. Ganda, S. Srikanta, S.J. Brink, M.A. Morris, R.E. Gleason, J.S. Soeldner, and G.S. Eisenbarth, Differential sensitivity to ß-cell secretagogues in "early" Type 1 diabetes mellitus, Diabetes 33:516-521 (1984).

34. W. Gepts, Pathologic anatomy of the pancreas in juvenile diabetes mellitus, Diabetes 14:619-633 (1965).

35. F. Ginsberg-Fellner, M.J. Dobersen, M.E. Witt, E.J. Rayfield, P. Rubinstein, and A.L. Notkins, HLA antigens, cytoplasmic islet cell antibodies, and carbohydrate tolerance in families with insulin-dependent diabetes mellitus, Diabetes 31:292-298 (1982).

36. H. Gleichman, B. Zörcher, B. Greulich, F.A. Gries, H.R. Henrichs, J. Bertrams, and H. Kolb, Correlation of islet cell antibodies and HLA-DR phenotypes with diabetes mellitus in adults, Diabetologia 27:90-92 (1984).

37. A.N. Gorsuch, K.M. Spencer, J. Lister, J.M. McNally, B.M. Dean, G.F. Bottazzo, and A.G. Cutworth, The natural history of type I (insulin-dependent) diabetes mellitus: evidence for a long prediabetic period, Lancet ii:1363-1365 (1981).

38. S. Gupta, S.M. Fiterig, S. Khanna, and E. Orti, Deficiency of suppressor T cells in insulin-dependent diabetes, Immunol. Lett. 4:289-294 (1982).

39. S. Gupta, ed., "Immunology of Clinical and Experimental Diabetes," Plenum Publ. Corp., New York (1984).

40. J.H. Helderman, The role of insulin in the intermediary metabolism of the activated thymic derived lymphocyte, J. Clin. Invest. 67:1636-1642 (1981).

41. K. Helmke, A. Otten, and W. Willems, Islet cell antibodies in children with mumps infection, Lancet ii:211-212 (1980).

42. K. Helmke, R. Brockhaus, M. Seitz, H. Otten, W.R. Willems, H. Laube, and K. Federlin, Virus infection: islet cell antibodies and islet cell function in Type 1 diabetes mellitus, Behring Inst. Mitt. 75:73-82 (1984).

43. K.C. Herold, A. Huen, L. Gould, H. Traisman, and A.H. Rubenstein, Alterations in lymphocyte subpopulations in Type 1 (insulin-dependent) diabetes mellitus: exploration of possible mechanisms and relationships to autoimmune phenomena, Diabetologia 27:102-105 (1984).

44. M. Horita, H. Suzuki, T. Onodera, F. Ginsberg-Fellner, A.S. Fauci, and A.L. Notkins, Abnormalities of immunoregulatory T cell subsets in patients with insulin-dependent diabetes mellitus, J. Immunol. 129 (4):1426-1429 (1982).

45. S-W. Huang, L. Hallquist Haedt, S. Rich, and J. Barbosa, Prevalence of antibodies to nucleic acids in insulin-dependent diabetes and their relatives, Diabetes 30:873-874 (1981).

46. A. Huen, M. Haneda, Z. Freedman, A. Lernmark, and A.H. Rubenstein, Quantitative determinations of islet cell surface antibodies using ^{125}Iprotein A, Diabetes 32:460-465 (1983).

47. W.J. Irvine, J.S.A. Sawers, C.M. Feck, R.J. Prescott, and L.J.P. Duncan, The value of islet cell antibody in predicting secondary failure of oral hypoglycemic agent therapy in diabetes mellitus, J. Clin. Lab. Immunol. 2:23-26 (1979).

48. W.J. Irvine, ed., "Immunology of Diabetes," Teviot Scientific Publications, Edinburgh (980).

49. R.A. Jackson, M.A. Morris, B.F. Haynes, and G.S. Eisenbarth, Increased circulating Ia-antigen-bearing T cells in type I diabetes mellitus, New Engl. J. Med. 306:785-788 (1982).

50. A.B. Jensen, H.S. Rosenberg, and A.L. Notkins, Pancreatic islet cell damage in children with fatal viral infections, Lancet ii:354-355 (1980).

51. C. Johnston, D.A. Pyke, A.G. Cudworth, and E. Wolf, HLA-DR typing in identical twins with insulin-dependent diabetes: differences between concordant and discordant paris, Br. Med. J. 286:253-255 (1983).

52. K. Junker, J. Egeberg, H. Kromann, and J. Nerup, An autopsy study of the islets of Langerhans in acute-onset juvenile diabetes mellitus, Acta. Pathol. Microbiol. Scand. (A) 85:699-706 (1977).

53. T. Kanatsuna, S. Baekkeskov, A. Lernmark, and J. Ludvigsson, Immunoglobulin from insulin-dependent diabetic children inhibits glucose-induced insulin release, Diabetes 32:520-524 (1983).

54. H. Kolb, G. Schernthaner, and A.F. Gries, eds., "Diabetes and Immunology: Pathogenesis and Immunotherapy," Hans Huber Publishers, Bern (1983).

55. D. Larhammar, L. Schenning, K. Gustafsson, K. Wiman, L. Claesson, L. Rask, and P.A. Peterson, Complete amino acid sequence of an HLA-DR antigen-like ß chain as predicted from the nucleotide sequence: similarities with immunoglobulins and HLA-A, -B, and -C antigens, Proc. Natl. Acad. Sci. USA 79:3687-3691 (1982).

56. P.M. LeCompte and M.R. Legg, Insulitis in late-onset diabetes, Diabetes 21:7621769 (1972).

57. A. Lernmark, Z.R. Freedman, C. Hofmann, A.H. Rubenstein, D.F. Steiner, R.L. Jackson, R.J. Winter, and H.S. Traisman, Islet cell surface antibodies in juvenile diabetes mellitus, N. Engl. J. Med. 299:375-380 (1978).

58. A. Lernmark, B. Hägglöf, Z.R. Freedman, W.J. Irvine, J. Ludvigsson, and G. Holmgren, A prospective analysis of antibodies reactive with pancreatic islet cells in insulin-dependent diabetic children, Diabetologia 20:471-474 (1981).

59. A. Lernmark, Cell mediated immunity in (insulin-dependent) diabetes: update 84, in: "Immunology in Diabetes," D. Andreani, U. DiMario, K.F. Federlin and L.G. Heding, eds., Kimpton Med. Publ., London, 121-132 (1984).

60. A. Lernmark, S. Baekkeskov, T. Dyrberg, I. Gerling, and B. Marner, Pathogenesis of type 1 diabetes mellitus, Proc. 7th Internat. Congr. Endocrinol., Excerpta Medica :92-96 (1984).

61. A.C. MacCuish, J. Jordan, C.J. Campbell, L.J.P. Duncan, and W.J. Irvine, Antibodies to islet-cell in insulin-dependent diabetics with coexistent autoimmune disease, Lancet ii:1529-1533.

62. A.C. MacCuish and W.J. Irvine, Autoimmunological aspects of diabetes mellitus, Clin. Endocrinol. Metab. 4:435-471 (1975).

63. N.K. MacLaren, S-W. Huang, and J. Fogh, Antibody to cultured human insulinoma cells in insulin-dependent diabetes, Lancet i:997-1000 (1975).

64. B. Marner, A. Lernmark, J. Nerup, J.L. Molenaar, C.W. Tuk, and G.J. Bruining, Analysis of islet cell antibodies on frozen sections of human pancreas, Diabetologia 25:93-96 (1983).

65. R. Maron, D. Elias, B.M. de Jongh, G.J. Bruining, J.J. van Rood, Y. Schechter, and I.R. Cohen, Autoantibodies to the insulin receptor in juvenile onset insulin-dependent diabetes, Nature 303:817-818 (1983).

66. J.M. Martin, R.M. Ehrlich, and F.J. Holland, "Etiology and Pathogenesis of Insulin-dependent Diabetes Mellitus," Raven Press, New York (1981).

67. T. Maruyama, I. Takei, I. Matsuba, A. Tsuruoka, M. Taniyama, Y. Ikeda, K. Katoaka, M. Abe, and S. Matsuki, Cell-mediated cytotoxic islet cell surface antibodies to human pancreatic B cells, Diabetologia 26:30-33 (1984).

68. F. Mascart-Lemone, G. Delespesse, H. Dorchy, B. Lemiere, and G. Servais, Characterization of immunoregulatory T-lymphocytes in insulin-dependent diabetic children by means of monoclonal antibodies, Clin. Exp. Immunol. 47:296-300 (1982).

69. C. Mawas, ed., HLA-DR research in progress, Human Immunol. 8:1-121 (1983).

70. B. Michelsen, W. Kastern, A. Lernmark, and D. Owerbach, Identification of an HLA-DQ ß-chain related genomic sequence associated with insulin-dependent diabetes, Biomed. Biochim. Acta, in press.

71. Y. Mori, I. Matsuba, T. Tanese, Y. Ikeda, and M. Abe, Cellular hypersensitivity to human pancreatic ß-cell clone in diabetes mellitus and its relationship to the presence of islet cell antibodies, Diabetologia 27:313A (1984).

72. J. Nerup, O.O. Andersen, G. Bendixen, J. Egeberg, and J.E. Poulsen, Antipancreatic cellular hypersensitivity in diabetes mellitus, Diabetes 20:424-427 (1971).

73. J. Nerup, O.O. Andersen, G. Bendixen, J. Egeberg, and J.E. Poulsen, Anti-pancreatic, cellular hypersensitivity in diabetes mellitus. Antigenic activity of fetal calf pancreas and correlation with clinical type of diabetes, Acta Allergolocica 28:233-230 (1973).

74. J. Nerup, Etiology and pathogenesis of insulin-dependent diabetes mellitus: present views and future developments, in: "Etiology and Pathogenesis of Insulin-dependent Diabetes Mellitus," J.M. Martin, R.M. Ehrlich and F.J. Holland, eds., Raven Press, New York, :275-288 (1981).

75. G. Norden, E. Jensen, I. Stilbo, G.F. Bottazzo, and A. Lernmark, B-cell function and islet cell and other organ-specific autoantibodies in relatives to insulin-dependent diabetic patients, Acta. Med. Scand. 213:199-203 (1983).

76. D. Owerbach, A. Lernmark, P. Platz, L.P. Ryder, L. Rask, P.A. Peterson, and J. Ludvigsson, HLA-D region ß-chain DNA endonuclease fragments differ between HLA-DR identical healthy and insulin-dependent diabetic individuals, Nature 303:815-817 (1983).

77. D. Owerbach, B. Hägglöf, A. Lernmark, and G. Holmgren, Susceptibility to insulin-dependent diabetes defined by restriction enzyme polymorphism of HLA-D region genomic DNA, Diabetes 33:958-965 (1984).

78. J.P. Palmer, C.M. Asplin, P. Clemons, K. Lyen, O. Tatpati, P.K. Raghu, and T.L. Paquette, Science 222:1337-1339 (1983).

79. G. Papadopoulos, J. Petersen, V. Andersen, A. Lernmark, B. Marner, J. Nerup, and C. Binder, Spontaneous in vitro immunoglobulin secretion at the diagnosis of insulin-dependent diabetes, Acta. Endocrinol. 105:521-527 (1984).

80. P. Platz, B.K. Jakobsen, M. Morling, L.P. Ryder, A. Svejgaard, M. Thomsen, M. Christy, H. Kromann, J. Benn, J. Nerup, A. Green, and M. Hauge, HLA-D and DR-antigens in genetic analysis of insulin-dependent diabetes mellitus, Diabetologia 21:108-115 (1981).

81. P. Pozzilli, O. Zuccarini, M. Iavicoli, D. Andreani, M. Sensi, K.M. Spencer, G.F. Bottazzo, P.C. Beverly, J.L. Kyner, and A.G. Cudworth, Monoclonal antibodies defined abnormalities of T lymphocytes in Type I (insulin-dependent) diabetes, Diabetes 32:91-94 (1983).

82. D.A. Pyke and P.G. Nelson, Diabetes mellitus in identical twins, in: "The genetics of Diabetes Mellitus," W. Creutzfeldt, J. Köbberling and J.V. Neel, eds., Springer-Verlag, Heidelberg, :194-202 (1976).

83. A. Rabinovitch, P. MacKay, J. Ludvigsson, and A. Lernmark, A prospective analysis of islet cell cytotoxic antibodies in insulin-dependent diabetic children: transient effects of plasma-pheresis, Diabetes 33:224-228 (1984).

84. J. Rahier, Goebbels, and J.C. Henquin, Cellular composition of the human diabetic pancreas, Diabetologia 24:366-371 (1983).

85. B. Rousset, B. Vialettes, F. Bernier-Valentin, P. Vague, M. Beylot, and R. Mornex, Anti-tubulin antibodies in recent onset Type 1 (insulin-dependent) diabetes mellitus: comparison with islet cell antibodies, Diabetologia 27:427-432 (1984).

86. S. Serjeantson, J. Theophilus, P. Zimmet, J. Court, J.R. Crossley, and R.B. Elliott, Lymphocytotoxic antibodies and histocompatibility antigens in juvenile-onset diabetes mellitus, Diabetes 30:26-29 (1981).

87. D.A. Shackelford, J.F. Kaufman, A.J. Korman, and J.L. Strominger, HLA-DR antigens: structure, separation of subpopulations, gene cloning and function, Immunol. Rev. 66:133-187 (1982).

88. K.M. Spencer, A. Tarn, B.M. Dean, J. Lister, and G.F. Bottazzo, Fluctuating islet cell autoimmunity in unaffected relatives of patients with insulin-dependent diabetes, Lancet i:764-766 (1984).

89. S. Srikanta, O. Gunda, G. Eisenbarth, and J.S. Soeldner, Islet cell antibodies and beta cell function in monozygotic triplets and twins initially discordant for type 1 diabetes mellitus, New Engl. J. Med. 308:322-325 (1983).

90. A. Svenningsen, T. Dyrberg, I. Gerling, A. Lernmark, P. MacKay, and A. Rabinovitch, Inhibition of insulin release after passive transfer of immunoglobulin from insulin-dependent diabetic children to mice, J. Clin, Endocrinol. and Metab. 57 (6):1301-1304 (1983).

91. D.W. Thomas, U. Yamashita, and E.M. Shevach, The role of Ia antigens in T cell activation, Immunol. Rev. 35:97-120 (1977).

92. E. Thorsby, E. Berle, and H. Nousiainen, HLA-D region molecules restrict proliferative T cell responses to antigen, Immunol. Rev. 66:39-56 (1982).

93. Nomenclature for factors of the HLA system 1984, Tissue Antigens 24:73-80 (1984).

94. D. Topliss, J. How, M. Lewis, V. Row, and R. Volpé, Evidence for cell-mediated immunity and specific suppressor T lymphocyte dysfunction in graves' disease and diabetes mellitus, J. Clin. Endocrinol. and Metab. 57 (4):700-705 (1983).

95. M. Van de Winkel, G. Smets, W. Gepts, and D.G. Pipeleers, Islet cell surface antibodies from insulin-dependent diabetics bind specifically to pancreatic B-cells, J. Clin. Invest. 70:41-49 (1982).

96. B. Vialettes, C. C Di Campo-Rougerie, V. Lassman, and P. Vague, Presse Med. 22:2303-2306 (1983).

97. E. Wolf, K.M. Spencer, and A.G. Cudworth, The genetic susceptibility to type 1 (insulin-dependent) diabetes: analysis of the HLA-DR association, Diabetologia 24:224-230 (1983).

INSULIN-STIMULATED GLUCOSE DISPOSAL IN
PATIENTS WITH TYPE I (IDDM) AND TYPE II (NIDDM)
DIABETES MELLITUS

Gerald M. Reaven

Department of Medicine
Stanford University School of Medicine and Geriatric
Research
Education and Clinical Center
Veterans Administration Medical Center
Palo Alto, California, U.S.A.

INTRODUCTION AND HISTORICAL BACKGROUND

In 1933 Himsworth and Kerr[8] used the plasma glucose response
to an oral glucose plus intravenous insulin challenge to divide
patients with diabetes mellitus into two types — designated as being
either insulin sensitive or insulin insensitive. Based upon the
available clinical information, patients classified by Himsworth as
being insulin sensitive seem most comparable to individuals who
would be designated as having insulin-dependent diabetes (IDDM) by
today's criteria.[12] In contrast, the group of patients who would
be classified today as having noninsulin-dependent diabetes mellitus
(NIDDM) share the characteristics of those designated by Himsworth
as being insulin insensitive. Several years ago,[16] we reviewed
available information as to the ability of insulin to stimulate glucose uptake in patients with diabetes mellitus. At that time we
indicated that resistance to insulin-stimulated glucose uptake
characterizes patients with NIDDM, but that it could also exist in
patients with IDDM. However, in the latter instance the resistance
appeared to be related to degree of metabolic control, and it seemed
to us that insulin sensitivity was normal in patients with IDDM
well-controlled on insulin. Interest in the role played by insulin
resistance in the pathogenesis of diabetes mellitus has increased
greatly since publication of our earlier review. This has been
associated with the development of new techniques for the assessment
of insulin-stimulated glucose uptake in patients with diabetes,
resulting in the appearance of a considerable amount of new
information as to the characteristics of insulin action in patients

129

with both NIDDM and IDDM. The purpose of this presentation will be to critically review available data, and to use this information in an attempt to define the effects of IDDM and NIDDM on insulin-stimulated glucose disposal.

INSULIN-STIMULATED GLUCOSE UPTAKE IN IDDM

IDDM is characterized by absolute hypoinsulinemia, and efforts have been made to use animal models rendered insulin deficient in order to gain insights into this syndrome. It is always dangerous to extrapolate from animal models, and it is obvious that there are great differences between a human being with IDDM and a rat with streptozotocin-induced insulin deficiency. On the other hand, there is considerable information concerning the impact of insulin defi-ciency on insulin-stimulated glucose uptake in both dog and rat, and these data seem worthy of review. Thus, in this section an attempt will be made to document the effects on insulin-stimulated glucose uptake in both experimentally-induced insulin deficiency in animal models and in patients with IDDM. Furthermore, an effort will be made to relate these data to the pathogenesis of IDDM.

Animal Studies

Evidence published from our group[15] has demonstrated that resistance to insulin-stimulated glucose disposal can develop in dogs secondary to alloxan-induced insulin deficiency. However, insulin resistance did not occur unless the alloxan-induced diabetes was severe in magnitude. Furthermore, insulin treatment restored insulin-stimulated glucose uptake to normal in dogs with severe alloxan-induced diabetes. Essentially identical findings have been more recently reported by Caruso et al.,[2] supporting the view that insulin resistance develops when dogs are made insulin deficient and that the resistance disappears following control of hyperglycemia with insulin.

The appearance of resistance to insulin-stimulated glucose secondary to experimentally-induced insulin deficiency is not limited to dogs, as the same phenomenon has been described in asso-ciation with streptozotocin-induced diabetes in the rat.[3] Further-more, in this animal model of IDDM it has been shown that the ability of insulin to maximally stimulate glucose transport by isolated adipocytes is also markedly reduced.[9,10] Thus, there is considerable evidence that experimentally-induced insulin deficiency in animals leads to a reduction in insulin-stimulated glucose uptake, and that the insulin resistance disappears following insulin replacement and control of hyperglycemia.

Studies on Humans with IDDM

The clinical situation which most closely resembles experimentally-induced insulin deficiency in animals is that of patients with diabetes secondary to chronic pancreatitis. We quantified insulin-stimulated glucose disposal in such a group of patients several years ago,[5] and could not document the presence of insulin resistance. However, it should be pointed out that these patients had hyperglycemia which was relatively modest in magnitude (mean fasting glucose = 142 mg/dl), consistent with the view that resistance to insulin-stimulated glucose uptake in subjects with insulin deficiency is directly related to the degree of hyperglycemia. Support for this point of view can be derived from the findings of Ginsberg[6] who could not demonstrate any difference in the ability of insulin to stimulate glucose uptake in normal subjects and insulin-treated patients with IDDM. On the other hand, Ginsberg also commented upon the degree of variability in values for insulin-stimulated glucose disposal in patients with IDDM, and he could document a significant relationship between degree of insulin resistance and height of fasting plasma glucose concentration. The close link between the presence of insulin resistance in patients with IDDM and degree of metabolic control has been most clearly shown by Revers and associates,[18] who demonstrated the presence of insulin resistance in poorly-controlled patients as contrasted to normal insulin-stimulated glucose uptake in well-controlled patients. These latter results are consistent with the findings of Yki-Jarvinen and Koivisto,[20] who showed that reduced values for insulin-stimulated glucose uptake in patients with IDDM could be significantly increased by six weeks of insulin pump therapy. However, and in contrast to the studies of Revers et al.,[18] insulin action only returned to approximately 75% of normal in the patients described by Yki-Jarvinen.[20] On the other hand, glycosylated hemoglobin only fell from 10.1 to 8.7% in patients studied by Yki Jarvinen, whereas the well-controlled insulin-treated patients with normal insulin action described by Revers and associates had a mean hemoglobin A_1C level of 7.2%. Thus, the ability of the latter authors to return insulin action to absolutely normal levels is likely due to the fact that they also achieved a greater degree of metabolic control.

Other studies[4,13] have documented the presence of reduced insulin action in patients with IDDM, but they have not investigated the effect of better control of diabetes on insulin-stimulated glucose disposal. However, in one instance[4] a correlation between insulin-stimulated glucose uptake and severity of fasting hyperglycemia was noted.

In summary, resistance to insulin-stimulated glucose uptake has been documented in animals with experimentally-induced insulin deficiency and in patients with IDDM. In both animals and humans, the degree of insulin resistance seems to be a function of the magnitude of hyperglycemia. Finally, if euglycemia can be restored by insulin treatment, the insulin resistance tends to disappear. As a corollary, it seems necessary to conclude that the presence of resistance to insulin-stimulated glucose disposal in IDDM is secondary to poorly-controlled diabetes. Thus, although loss of insulin action in patients with poorly controlled IDDM may have a significant clinical effect, it seems unlikely that the insulin resistance is playing a pathogenetic role in this syndrome.

INSULIN-STIMULATED GLUCOSE UPTAKE IN NIDDM

The pathogenesis of NIDDM remains relatively obscure, and there is no animal model which seems to be as relevant to the pathophysiology of NIDDM as does the insulin deficient dog and rat to the situation in patients with IDDM. On the other hand, there is compelling evidence in humans that resistance to insulin-stimulated glucose uptake is a characteristic finding in patients with NIDDM.[1,4,5,7,11,16,17,19] However, the relationship of this insulin resistance to the syndrome of NIDDM appears to be quite different from that which seems to exist between these two variables in patients with IDDM.

In the first place, the correlation between magnitude of insulin resistance and severity of diabetes is not nearly as simple in NIDDM as it is in IDDM. Specifically, evidence has been published[14] demonstrating that glucose uptake is markedly reduced in patients with impaired glucose tolerance (IGT), despite the modest abnormality of glucose metabolism present in this syndrome. In addition, it has been shown[1] that a relatively dramatic decrease in insulin-stimulated glucose uptake occurred as glucose tolerance deteriorated from normal to mild NIDDM (fasting plasma glucose less than 120mg/dl). In contrast, there seemed to be little further decline in insulin-stimulated glucose uptake as glucose tolerance deteriorated further, and degree of insulin resistance was not correlated with magnitude of fasting hyperglycemia.

A second important difference between the insulin resistance present in NIDDM and IDDM is the change that occurs with insulin treatment. In two studies,[7,11] institution of excellent metabolic control in patients with NIDDM had essentially no impact on insulin-stimulated glucose uptake, and the patients were as insulin resistant after therapy as before. However, we were able to demonstrate that insulin-stimulated glucose uptake could be significantly improved by six weeks of excellent diabetic control with multiple injections of insulin.[17] On the other hand, the degree of improvement was modest in magnitude, and insulin-stimulated glucose uptake remained markedly reduced as compared to normal individuals. The most substantial effect of insulin treatment on the insulin resistance of patients with NIDDM has been shown by Scarlett et al.,[19] but even in this instance the improvement was only approximately halfway back to normal values. Thus, there seems to be general agreement that control of hyperglycemia with insulin does not return insulin-stimulated glucose uptake to normal in patients with NIDDM. This conclusion is in marked contrast to the situation in IDDM, and this difference is of great importance when thinking about the pathogenesis of the two syndromes.

MECHANISM OF INSULIN RESISTANCE IN DIABETES MELLITUS

The simplest way to produce resistance to insulin-stimulated glucose uptake is to destroy beta cell function in an experimental animal. Since it is quite clear that insulin treatment restores insulin action to normal, it is tempting to speculate that insulin deficiency, per se, is the cause of insulin resistance in diabetes. However, the situation seems to be more complex than it might appear at first. For example, insulin resistance can exist in patients with IDDM, despite the fact that these individuals are being treated with exogenous insulin. Indeed, improvement in insulin-stimulated glucose uptake secondary to the use of insulin pump therapy in patients with IDDM was actually associated with a reduction of daily insulin dose.[20] Thus, insulin deficiency, by itself, cannot account for the presence of insulin resistance in IDDM. The view that insulin deficiency is the cause of insulin resistance is even less satisfactory in NIDDM. For example, patients with IGT are both hyperinsulinemic and insulin resistant.[14] Furthermore, since day-long circulating plasma insulin concentrations in patients with severe NIDDM are normal in absolute terms,[17] the decrease in insulin-stimulated glucose uptake seen in these subjects cannot be a simple function of lack of insulin. Thus, it seems necessary to postulate that insulin resistance can occur in hyperglycemic states, secondary to the abnormal carbohydrate metabolism, rather than to a lack of insulin per se. In the case of IDDM, it appears that this is the sole cause of the insulin resistance present in this syndrome: the degree of insulin resistance is directly related to the severity of hyperglycemia, and is absent when patients are well-controlled. This type of insulin resistance, i.e., secondary to uncontrolled diabetes, can also develop in patients with NIDDM. However, in this instance there is relatively little correlation between degree of insulin resistance and magnitude of hyperglycemia; specifically resistance to insulin-stimulated glucose uptake is present in patients with only minimally impaired glucose tolerance and persists even when patients with NIDDM are in excellent diabetic control.

SUMMARY AND CONCLUSIONS

In conclusion, there is considerable data documenting the presence of resistance to insulin-stimulated glucose uptake in patients with either IDDM or NIDDM. However, the characteristics of this metabolic abnormality are quite different in the two syndromes. In the case of IDDM the insulin resistance appears to be secondary to the state of altered carbohydrate homeostasis, is directly proportional to the severity of fasting hyperglycemia, and can be abolished by achievement of metabolic control. As a corollary, it seems reasonable to suggest that resistance to insulin-stimulated glucose uptake is not a primary defect in the pathogenesis of IDDM. Nevertheless, the presence of insulin resistance in the poorly-controlled patient with IDDM may be of great clinical relevance, and contribute to the difficulty in effective treatment of this syndrome.

In contrast, resistance to insulin-stimulated glucose uptake does not seem to be a simple function of severity of hyperglycemia in patients with NIDDM, and significant insulin resistance can exist in these patients in association with only mild carbohydrate intolerance. Furthermore, although the decline in insulin-stimulated glucose disposal present in patients with significant fasting hyperglycemia can be increased by instituting excellent metabolic control with exogenous insulin, it cannot be restored to normal. These observations suggest that some component of the insulin resistance in NIDDM is similar to that in IDDM, and is secondary to the state of poor metabolic control. On the other hand, it also suggests that another component of the insulin resistance in NIDDM is primary, and most likely related to the pathogenesis of this syndrome. Obviously, there is a great need to define the mechanism of this unexplained portion of the insulin resistance of NIDDM.

REFERENCES

1. C. Bogardus, S. Lillioja, B. Howard, G.M. Reaven, and D. Mott, Relationships between insulin secretion, insulin action and fasting plasma glucose concentration in non-diabetic and non-insulin-dependent diabetic subjects, J. Clin. Invest. (in press).
2. G. Caruso, J. Proietto, A. Calenti, and F. Alford, Insulin resistance in alloxan diabetic dogs: evidence for reversal following insulin therapy, Diabetologia, 25:273-279 (1983).
3. E. Dall'Aglio, F. Chang, H. Chang, D. Wright, and G.M. Reaven, Effect of exercise training and sucrose feeding on insulin-stimulated glucose uptake in rats with streptozotocin-induced insulin-deficient diabetes, Diabetes, 32:165-168 (1983).

4. R.A. DeFronzo, D. Simonson, and E. Ferrannini, Hepatic and peripheral insulin resistance: a common feature of Type 2 (non-insulin-dependent) and Type 1 (insulin-dependent) diabetes mellitus, Diabetologia, 23:313-319 (1982).

5. H. Ginsberg, G. Kimmerling, J.M. Olefsky, and G.M. Reaven, Demonstration of insulin resistance in untreated adult onset diabetic subjects with fasting hyperglycemia, J. Clin. Invest, 55:454-461 (1975).

6. H.N. Ginsberg, Investigation of insulin sensitivity in treated subjects with ketosis-prone diabetes mellitus, Diabetes, 26:278-283 (1977).

7. H. Hidaka, M. Nagulesparan, I. Klimes, R. Clark, H. Saski, S.L. Aronoff, B. Vasquez, A.H. Rubenstein, and R.H. Unger, Improvement of insulin secretion but not insulin resistance after short term control of plasma glucose in obese Type II diabetics, J. Clin. Endocrinol. Metab., 54:217-222 (1982).

8. H.P. Himsworth, and R.B. Kerr, Insulin-sensitive and insulin-insensitive types of diabetes mellitus, Clin. Sci., 4:119-152 (1939).

9. E. Karnieli, P.J. Hissin, I.A. Simpson, L.B. Salans, and S.W. Cushman, A possible mechanism of insulin resistance in the rat adipose cell in streptozotocin-induced diabetes mellitus. Depletion of intracellular glucose transport systems, J. Clin. Invest., 68:811-814 (1981).

10. M. Kobayashi, and J.M. Olefsky, Effects of streptozotocin-induced diabetes on insulin binding, glucose transport, and intracellular glucose metabolism in isolated rat adipocytes, Diabetes, 28:87-95 (1979).

11. A. Nankervis, J. Proietto, P. Aitken, M. Harewood, and F. Alford, Differential effects of insulin therapy on hepatic and peripheral insulin sensitivity in Type 2 (non-insulin-dependent) diabetes, Diabetologia, 23:320-325 (1982).

12. National Diabetes Data Group, Classification and diagnosis of diabetes mellitus and other categories of glucose intolerance, Diabetes, 28:1039-1057 (1979).

13. A. Pernet, E.R. Trimble, F. Kuntschen, P. Damoiseaux, J.-Ph. Assal, C. Hahn, and A.E. Renold, Insulin resistance in Type 1 (insulin-dependent) diabetes: dependence on plasma insulin concentration, Diabetologia, 26:255-260 (1984)

14. G.M. Reaven, and J.M. Olefsky, Relationship between heterogeneity of insulin responses and insulin resistance in normal subjects and patients with chemical diabetes, Diabetologia, 13:201-206 (1977).

15. G.M. Reaven, W.S. Sageman, and R.S. Swenson, Development of insulin resistance in normal dogs following alloxan-induced insulin deficiency, Diabetologia, 13:459-462 (1977).

16. G.M. Reaven, and J.M. Olefsky, Role of insulin resistance in the pathogenesis of diabetes mellitus, in: "Advances in Metabolic Disorders," Vol. 9, Academic Press, New York (1978).

17. G.M. Reaven, Y-D.I. Chen, A.M. Coulston, M.S. Greenfield, C.
     Hollenbeck, C. Lardinois, G. Liu, and H. Schwartz, Insulin
     secretion and action in noninsulin-dependent diabetes
     mellitus.   Is insulin resistance secondary to hypoinsulinemia?
     Am. J. Med., 75 (Proceedings 5B):85-93 (1983).
18. R.R. Revers, O.G. Kolterman, J.A. Scarlett, R.S. Gray, and J.M.
     Olefsky, Lack of in vivo insulin resistance in controlled
     insulin-dependent, Type I, diabetic patients, J. Clin.
     Endocrinol. Metab., 58:353-358 (1984).
19. J.A. Scarlett, O.G. Kolterman, T.P. Ciarldi, M. Koa, and J.M.
     Olefsky, Insulin treatment reverses the postreceptor defect in
     adipocyte 3-O-methylglucose transport in type II diabetes
     mellitus, J. Clin. Endocrinol. Metab., 56:1195-1201 (1983).
20. H. Yki-Jarvinen, and V.A. Koivisto, Continuous subcutaneous
     insulin infusion therapy decreases insulin resistance in Type 1
     diabetes, J. Clin. Endocrinol. Metab., 58:659-666 (1984).

PATHOPHYSIOLOGY OF INSULIN

SECRETION IN DIABETES MELLITUS

W. Kenneth Ward, James C. Beard, Jeffrey B. Halter, and Daniel Porte, Jr.

From the Department of Medicine, University of Washington, Division of Endocrinology and Metabolism, and Geriatric Research, Education, and Clinical Center Veterans Administration Medical Center Seattle, Washington 98108, U.S.A.

ABSTRACT

In normal man, glucose serves to regulate basal insulin secretion by its participation with insulin in a feedback loop. In addition, glucose stimulates insulin secretion directly and potentiates insulin responses to nonglucose stimuli such as amino acids, β-adrenergic stimuli, and gut hormones. Maximal glycemic potentiation of the acute insulin response to IV arginine occurs at a glucose level of approx. 450 mg/dl.

In patients with noninsulin dependent diabetes mellitus (NIDDM), basal insulin levels have usually been reported as normal, but if plasma glucose is lowered to normal levels, a deficiency of basal insulin becomes apparent. In addition, the first phase (0-10 min) insulin response to IV glucose is absent in virtually all patients with overt NIDDM. In contrast, the second-phase (> 10 min) response is often preserved in NIDDM due to its maintenance by ambient hyperglycemia. Similarly, insulin responses to nonglucose stimuli such as arginine often appear normal in NIDDM because of potentiation by hyperglycemia. However, insulin responses to arginine are lower than those of nondiabetic controls when compared at multiple matched glucose levels. Indeed, maximal potentiation by glucose of the insulin response to arginine is markedly subnormal in NIDDM, suggesting a loss of functional B cell secretory capacity.

In patients with long-standing insulin-dependent diabetes mellitus (IDDM), basal insulin secretion and insulin responses to

all stimuli are virtually absent. However, in a remission phase, or
in IDDM of short duration, basal insulin secretion and insulin responses to nonglucose stimuli may be relatively preserved. Therefore, islet dysfunction in IDDM and NIDDM, while etiologically
different, share some common pathophysiological features.

INTRODUCTION

As will be presented in this review, the development of appropriately controlled studies of islet function has provided convincing evidence that islet B-cell function is abnormal in patients
with noninsulin-dependent diabetes mellitus (NIDDM) as well as in
patients with insulin-dependent diabetes mellitus (IDDM). Since
these studies are based on an understanding of normal islet
function, normal islet B-cell physiology is discussed prior to
pathophysiology.

I.   Normal Physiology of Insulin Secretion

Basal Insulin Secretion

The basal insulin secretion rate is primarily regulated by
glucose and is directly related to glucose level when all other
factors are held constant. Basal insulin secretion is also regulated by other factors including parasympathetic and sympathetic
neural tone, other substrates such as amino acids, and hormones such
as cortisol and growth hormone[28] (see Table 1).

Since glucose, of all the substances regulating the islet, is
most affected by the secretion of insulin and glucagon, it is glucose which provides for the primary feedback loop which maintains
insulin and glucose levels constant in the basal state. Other regulators of islet function (see Table 1) are less affected, if at all,
by insulin and glucagon concentrations in the physiologic range.
Thus, they are modulators of the balance point of basal insulin
secretion in an open loop system, as opposed to the closed feedback
loop which characterizes the glucose-insulin relationship.

Glucose Stimulation of Insulin Secretion

In addition to its role in the regulation of basal insulin
secretion, glucose is an important stimulus of insulin secretion.
An abrupt rise in plasma glucose level above 100 mg/dl causes a
biphasic insulin response[29,52] (Fig. 1). The acute (first phase)
insulin response to glucose is important to intravenous glucose
tolerance and consists of a rapid rise in insulin level which begins
1 to 3 min after glucose level is raised followed by a subsequent
return towards baseline which is completed 6-10 min after the stimulus. The acute insulin response to glucose is directly related to

Table 1.   Non Glucose Regulators of Insulin Secretion (from ref. 67)

Nutrients	EFFECT ON B-CELL	REFERENCE
amino acids (particularly arginine, leucine, phenylalamine)	stimulatory	24
glycerol	†	--
ketones	*	20
Hormones		
growth hormone	stimulatory[+]	21
glucagon	stimulatory	1,59
GIP	stimulatory	66
secretin	stimulatory	15,31,40
cholecystokinin	stimulatory	15
gastrin	stimulatory	15,55
VIP	stimulatory	60
adrenocorticosteroids	inhibitory[††]	37
somatostatin	inhibitory	10
epinephrine	inhibitory**	4
norepinephrine	inhibitory**	53
prostaglandin E	inhibitory	46,56
Neural Mechanisms		
beta-adrenergic	stimulatory	31
parasympathetic (vagal)	stimulatory	36
alpha-adrenergic	inhibitory	56

†   glycerol causes secretion of insulin indirectly upon its conversion to glucose.

*   Ketones (i.e., acetoacetate) stimulate insulin secretion in dogs but not significantly in man.

††   Although the direct B-cell effect is inhibitory, corti-costeriods may indirectly stimulate insulin secretion by causing insulin resistance and hyperglycemia (3).

+   Inhibitory effects have also been reported.

**   α(inhibitory effects usually predominate over B (stimulatory) effects.

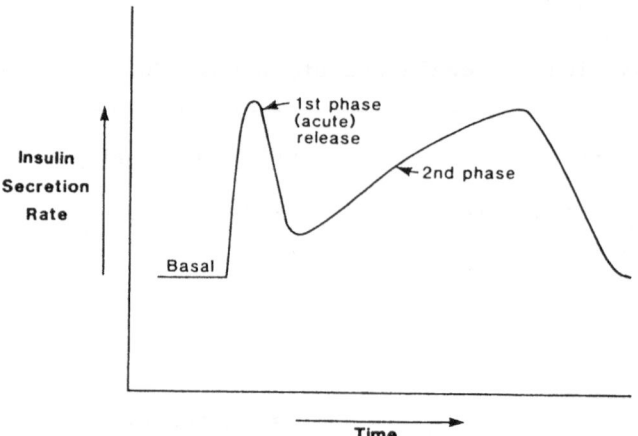

Fig. 1   The biphasic insulin response to a constant glucose stim-
            ulus. A theoretical response to a square-wave (con-
            stant) change in glucose level is shown. The peak of the
            first phase in man is between three and five minutes and
            lasts ten minutes. The second phase begins at two min-
            utes but is not evident until ten minutes have passed.
            It continues to increase slowly for at least 60 minutes
            or until the stimulus stops (from reference 67).

the rate and amount of glucose delivered,[9] with a 20 gm intravenous bolus being a maximal stimulus in man. It has been hypothesized that a small, rapidly releasable B-cell insulin pool is
responsible for the acute insulin response to glucose.[52]
Following the acute response, there is a second phase insulin response which rises more gradually and is directly related to the
degree and duration of glucose level elevation. It persists for the
duration of hyperglycemia (Fig. 1).[12,38] It is thought that
second-phase insulin secretion is partially dependent upon new
biosynthesis of insulin.[11]

        When compared to equal amounts of intravenously administered
glucose, orally-administered glucose causes a greater rise in
insulin output,[17] an effect likely caused in part by the release
of gastrointestinal peptides induced by oral glucose. Gastrointestinal polypeptide (GIP), for example, augments the effect of
hyperglycemia to stimulate insulin release, although in the absence
of concomitant hyperglycemia, GIP does not cause insulin
release.[66] Other gut peptides and neural effects of oral
carbohydrate such as the vagal response to feeding[36] are probably
also important in enhancing insulin secretion after oral glucose.

        For several reasons, oral glucose tolerance testing is an
inexact and poorly-reproducible method of quantifying pancreatic

insulin secretion. First, as mentioned, insulin responses to oral glucose are influenced by gut factors and neural responses to nutrient ingestion which may vary in magnitude among individuals and from time to time. Second, gastric emptying and gastrointestinal motility, which also vary among individuals, influence the rate of rise of plasma glucose level and thus, the rate of B-cell stimulation. Third, because the rise in amount of insulin secreted after an oral glucose load depends on the degree of plasma glucose elevation, comparisons of insulin secretion among different subjects are difficult. For these reasons, we do not use the oral glucose tolerance test to quantify and compare B-cell function.[67]

Nonglucose Regulation of Insulin Secretion

Nutrients other than glucose, particularly amino acids, also stimulate insulin release. Arginine appears to be the most potent amino acid stimulus of insulin secretion[24] and is commonly used experimentally. Although amino acids do stimulate insulin release to a modest degree in the presence of normal plasma glucose levels, they stimulate much greater insulin output when accompanied by hyperglycemia.[42,30] As is the case for the second phase insulin response to glucose, the magnitude of the acute (2-10 min after injection) insulin response to a nonglucose secretagogue such as arginine or the ß-adrenergic agonist isoproterenol is directly related to the ambient level of circulating glucose[30] (Fig. 2). We have termed such an effect of hyperglycemia to augment the acute insulin response to a nonglucose secretogogue "glucose potentiation." The magnitude of the acute insulin response to nonglucose stimuli is a nearly linear function of plasma glucose level over the glucose range of approximately 80 to 300 mg/dl. Maximal hyperglycemic potentiation of insulin responses to nonglucose stimuli occurs at a plasma glucose level of approximately 450 mg/dl, since raising plasma glucose above this level causes no further elevation of the acute insulin response to arginine[68] (Figure 3). Thus, an acute insulin response to a nonglucose stimulus obtained at a plasma glucose greater than 450 ml/dl is maximal in the sense that it represents maximal potentiation by glucose. Our present concept of the meaning of this maximal acute insulin response is that it serves as an estimate of glucose-regulated B-cell secretory capacity.

In addition to glucose and amino acids, many other signals such as gut hormones, stress hormones, and nutrients affect insulin secretion by the B-cell (see Table 1).

II. Pathophysiology of Insulin Secretion in Noninsulin Dependent Diabetes Mellitus (NIDDM)

Basal Insulin Secretion

Basal insulin levels in patients with NIDDM have usually been

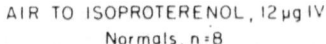

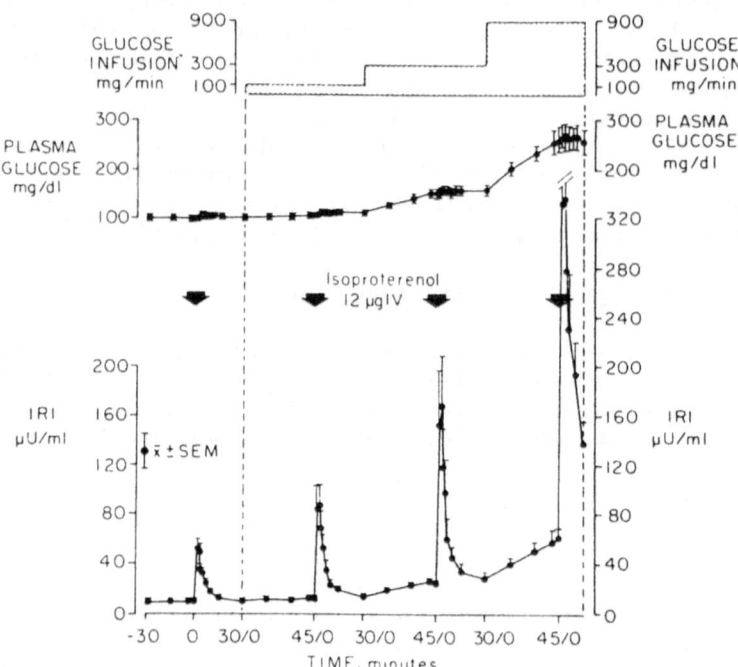

Fig. 2   Potentiation of insulin secretion to the nonglucose
            stimulant, isoproterenol, by glucose. The prestimulus
            plasma glucose level was raised by a stepwise glucose
            infusion of 100, 300 and 900 mg/min. Each elevation in
            the plasma glucose level resulted in a significant
            increase of the insulin response (from reference 30).

reported as normal,[41,2,27,50] although elevated[22,34] and diminished[35] levels have also been found. However, such comparisons
are not entirely straightforward. To accurately compare basal
insulin levels in patients with NIDDM with those of normal subjects,
the plasma glucose concentration must be taken into account. Such
comparisons have been made in two ways. When normal subjects have
been infused with glucose to match their glucose levels to those of
diabetics, their resulting steady-state insulin levels have been
found to be considerably higher.[30] Similarly, when diabetics have
received insulin infusions (followed by an insulin washout period)
in order to achieve normoglycemia, steady-state insulin levels have
been found to be lower than those of weight-matched controls.[65]
Such glycemia-matched comparisons appear to unmask a deficiency of
basal insulin output in patients with NIDDM. Thus, we believe that
a fundamental decrease of B-cell responsiveness to glucose level

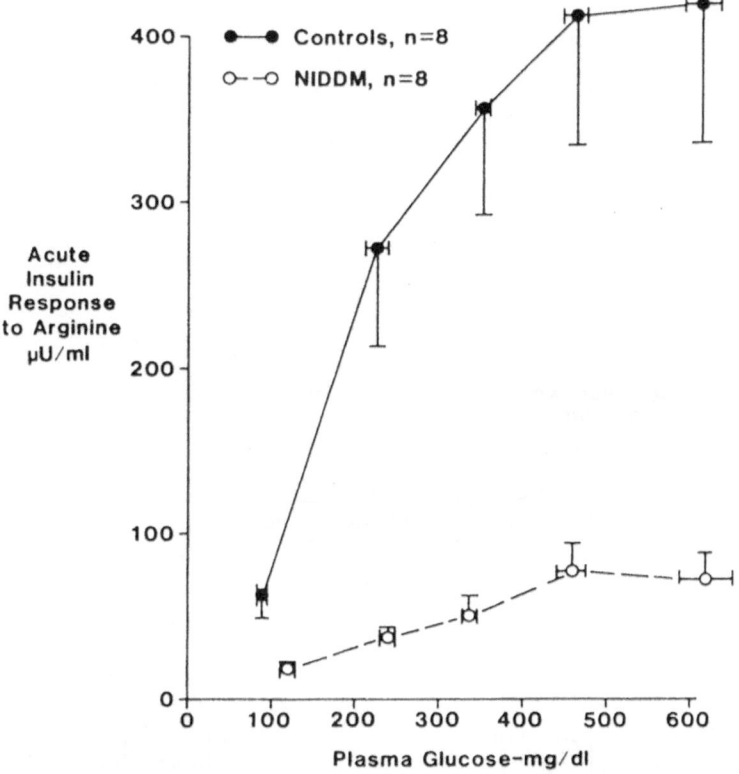

Fig. 3   A comparison of acute insulin responses to 5g IV arginine (mean 2-5 min insulin increment) at 5 matched plasma glucose levels in 8 patients with NIDDM and in 8 controls of similar age and body weight. Note that the maximal insulin response, a measure of insulin secretory capacity, tends to be much lower in the diabetic group. The lowest glucose level in diabetics was attained by an insulin infusion (from reference 68).

exists in NIDDM, but that the resultant hyperglycemia compensates by stimulating basal insulin secretion to a point where insulin levels appear normal.

The importance of glucose level to interpretation of basal insulin secretion is illustrated in Figure 4. The normal feedback loop is shown in Figure 4a. We hypothesize that a primary B-cell lesion in NIDDM results in decreased insulin output (Fig. 4b). As this impairment develops, however, the plasma glucose level rises, thereby stimulating basal insulin output to nearly normal levels (Fig. 4c). Thus, hyperglycemia compensates for impaired basal insulin secretion in NIDDM. If tissue resistance to insulin action

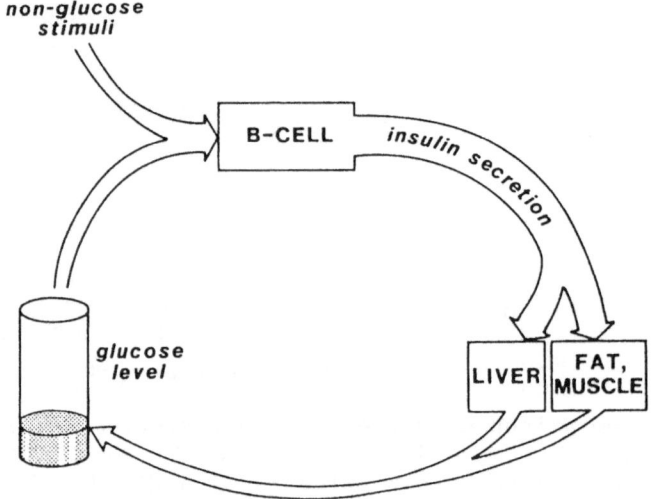

Fig. 4a   Normal basal feedback loop for insulin and glucose.
            Insulin secretion, through effects on liver, fat and
            muscle, modulates blood sugar. Blood sugar level, via
            interaction with nonglucose stimuli, feeds back to the
            islet to maintain insulin output.

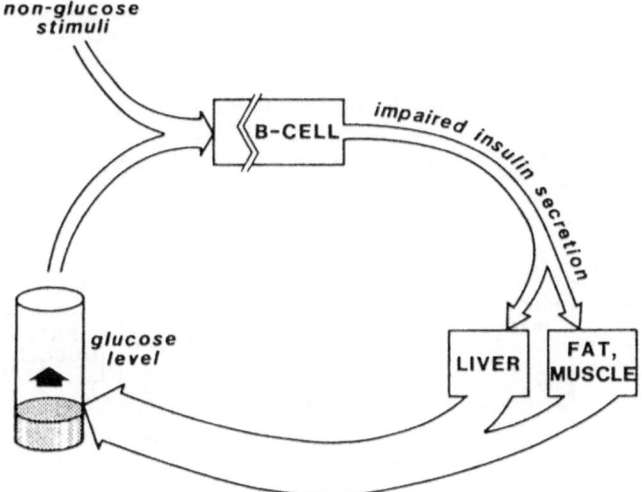

Fig. 4b. Hypothetical initial B-cell lesion of NIDDM. The impairment of insulin output would tend to lead to overproduction and underutilization of glucose, which would
cause the glucose level to rise. A major reduction of
insulin level would only be observed in this situation if
glucose level remained normal.

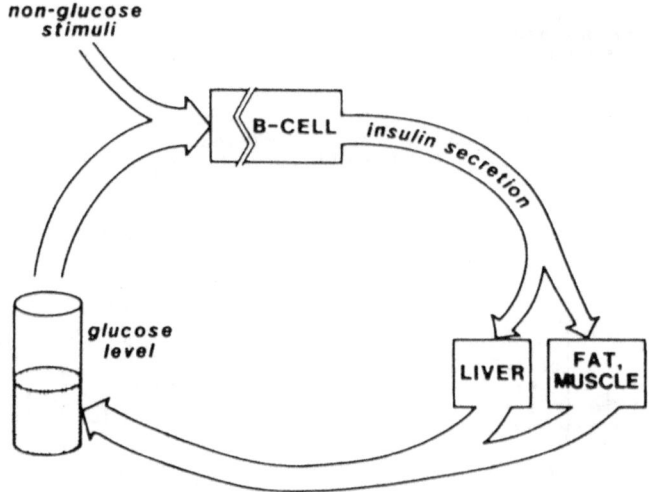

Fig. 4c.   Effect of hyperglycemia to compensate for the B—cell
            defect in NIDDM. Insulin deficiency from an initial
            islet lesion leads to hyperglycemia which, in turn, stim-
            ulates insulin secretion. Thus, resulting basal insulin
            output is partially restored, and insulin levels are only
            slightly diminished. As a result of increased insulin
            output, glucose production and utilization return toward
            normal.

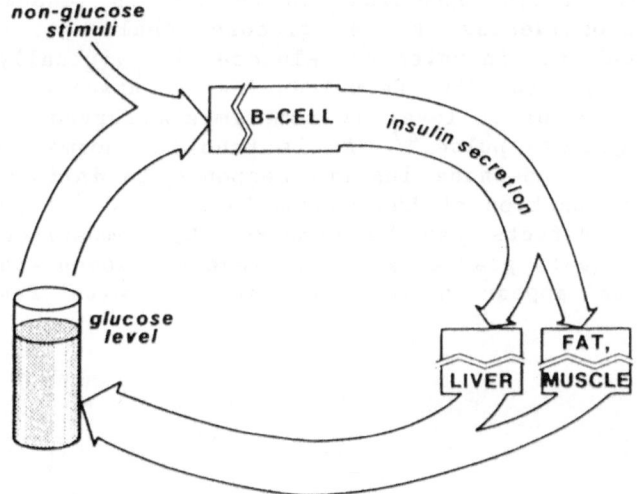

Fig. 4d.   Control of B-cell function in NIDDM when accompanied by
            tissue insensitivity to insulin, which leads to further
            hyperglycemia. In response to this further elevation in
            glucose level, the islet may secrete normal or even
            supranormal amounts of insulin despite the presence of
            impaired B-cell function (from reference 67).

develops under such circumstances, the plasma glucose level will
rise even further to stimulate sufficient basal insulin output to
overcome the insulin resistance (Fig. 4d). Therefore, despite the
presence of impaired islet function, some patients with NIDDM and
insulin resistance may have higher basal insulin levels than normal
subjects who are more sensitive to insulin. Thus, maintenance of
apparently normal or even high basal insulin levels by the
glucose-islet feedback loop in patients with NIDDM does not
necessarily indicate that B-cell function is normal.[67]

Glucose Stimulation of Insulin Secretion

Pancreatic islet function in NIDDM is characterized by
decreased responsiveness to a glucose challenge. First-phase
insulin release to intravenous glucose is virtually absent in
NIDDM[6] (Fig. 5), and in fact, an early absolute decrease in
insulin below the basal level is sometimes observed after administration of a glucose pulse.[47] As is true for normal subjects, the
height of the second-phase insulin response to intravenous glucose
is, in part, a function of the concomitant degree of hyperglycemia.
Thus, although defects can be unmasked by comparisons to normal
subjects at equal plasma glucose levels, second-phase insulin
responses often appear normal in patients with fasting plasma

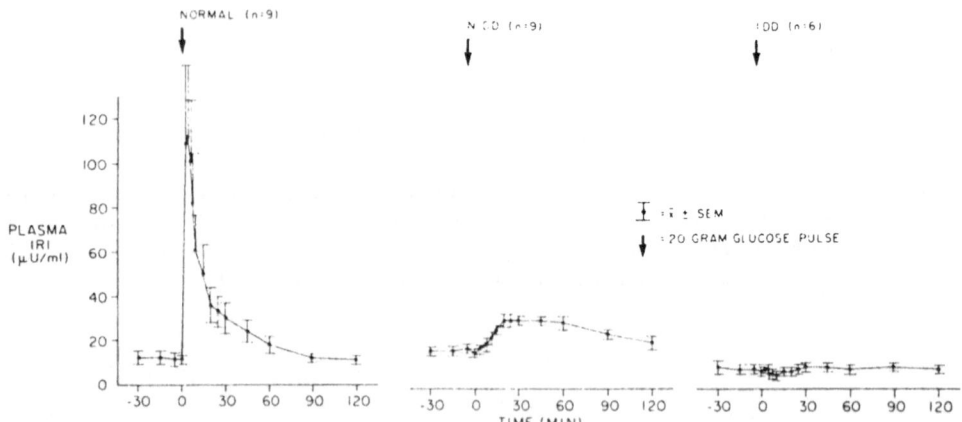

Fig. 5   Insulin release in response to IV glucose in normal,
           noninsulin-dependent diabetics (NIDD), and insulin-
           dependent diabetics (IDD). Mean fasting plasma glucose
           levels: normal subjects 85 ± 3 mg/dl; NIDD: 160 ± 10
           mg/dl; and IDD: 325 ± 33 mg/dl. Note the lack of
           first-phase insulin response and the preservation of
           second-phase response in NIDD's and the total lack of any
           response to glucose in the IDD subjects (from ref. 51).

glucose levels of less than 200 mg/dl[51] (Fig. 5). However, because of glycosuria, plasma glucose levels cannot rise indefinitely to compensate for impaired insulin secretion. Thus, patients with fasting plasma glucose levels of greater than 250 mg/dl are usually more insulin deficient and often possess decreased second-phase insulin responses to glucose.[51] These subjects have been called decompensated because glycosuria prevents the rise in glucose level which would be necessary to restore second phase insulin secretion to normal.

Assessment of B-cell function in patients with NIDDM by use of oral glucose tolerance testing poses several problems. As previously mentioned, it is impossible to accurately interpret such testing when factors such as gastric emptying, gut peptide secretion, and plasma glucose level are not controlled. The finding that some patients with NIDDM demonstrate a delayed but exaggerated insulin response to oral glucose may actually be due to a deficient early response leading to greatly increased glucose levels and an exaggerated stimulus to the islets later in the test. Nevertheless, it is generally agreed that patients with fasting hyperglycemia greater than 200 mg/dl have absolutely subnormal insulin levels after an oral glucose tolerance test despite major post-load rises in the glucose level.[54]

Nonglucose Stimulation of Insulin Secretion

Acute insulin responses to intravenous injections of nonglucose stimuli such as isoproterenol or arginine are of normal magnitude in most diabetics with a fasting plasma glucose of less than 200 mg/dl (Fig. 6). However, the elevated plasma glucose level of patients with NIDDM enhances insulin responses to such nonglucose stimuli. When the plasma glucose level of patients with NIDDM is lowered to normal by use of an insulin infusion, the acute insulin response to a nonglucose stimulus is found to be lower than normal.[30]

We recently compared insulin responses to arginine in NIDD's and controls at 5 matched plasma glucose levels ranging from approximately 100 to 620 mg/dl (Figure 3). The diabetics reached a maximal insulin response at a glucose level of approximately 450 mg/dl, as did the controls. However, the maximal acute insulin response (AIR_{max}) in the NIDD's, 83 ± 21 was much lower than the AIR_{max} in the controls, 450 ± 93 µU/ml. In contrast, the glucose level at half-maximal responsiveness, a measure of B-cell sensitivity to glucose, was similar in controls and NIDD's.[68] Such a finding of a reduced insulin secretory capacity in NIDDM is most consistent with either a structual or functional loss of B-cell mass as opposed to earlier views which suggested that glucose sensing, but not B-cell secretory capacity, was abnormal in NIDDM.[8]

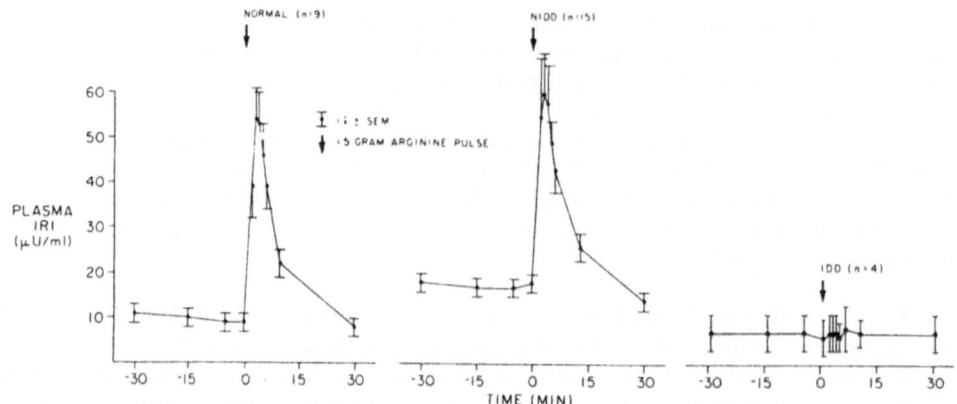

Fig. 6   Insulin responses to the nonglucose stimulant, arginine,
          in normal, noninsulin—dependent diabetics (NIDD), and
          insulin—dependent diabetics (IDD).   Insulin responses
          were similar in NIDD and control subjects, but were unde-
          tectable in IDD subjects. Mean fasting plasma glucose
          levels were 85 & 3 mg/dl in normals, 172 & 9 mg/dl in
          NIDD's and 350 & 30 mg/dl in IDD's (from ref. 51).

Interaction Between Impaired Insulin Secretion and Insulin Resistance in NIDDM

     The degree of hyperglycemia in a patient with NIDDM is
determined by an interaction between that patient's B-cell
sensitivity to glucose and the degree of tissue sensitivity to
insulin.   In the presence of otherwise normal islet function,
isolated insulin resistance does not generally lead to significant
hyperglycemia.   In support of this conclusion is the observation
that the vast majority of markedly obese persons are not hyperglycemic.   An explanation for this finding is recent evidence which
suggests that the normal pancreatic islet is capable of increasing
its responsiveness to glucose when necessary.   For example, in
response to 20 hours of mild hyperglycemia caused by a glucose
infusion[70] or to insulin resistance produced by 48 hours of oral
dexamethasone in normal subjects,[3] consistent elevations in slopes
of glucose potentiation were observed.   Cerasi et al. have shown
that when given very high rate glucose infusions for 2 to 3 hours,
normal persons will demonstrate enhanced insulin responses to a
later challenge with intravenous glucose, even when glucose levels
under both conditions are similar at the time of the tests.[7]
Thus, it appears that normal pancreatic islets possess an adaptive
capability which allows normal persons to minimize hyperglycemia as
they become insulin resistant, for example by weight gain.

On the other hand, severe loss of B-cell function will cause hyperglycemia irrespective of degree of insulin sensitivity. However, loss of greater than 70-90% of B-cell mass may be necessary for such decompensation, since some persons can tolerate a 70-90% pancreatectomy without developing overt diabetes mellitus.[71,41] An important but yet unanswered question relates to the importance of lesser degrees of B-cell loss, for example between 40% and 80%. Indeed, Turner has predicted that significant hyperglycemia would result from a 50% decrease of B-cell function if there is concomitant marked insulin resistance.[64]

Turner et al. predict that tissue insensitivity to insulin becomes an even more important determinant of plasma glucose level when a major (greater than 75%) loss of B-cell function exists.[64] Such a prediction is consistent with the common observation that a decrease in insulin sensitivity (e.g., weight gain) will cause a small rise in glucose level in a non-diabetic person but may cause a large rise in glucose level in a patient with NIDDM. Similarly, an improvement in tissue insulin sensitivity (e.g., weight loss) often markedly lowers glucose level in a hyperglycemic obese person,[23] but will only slightly lower glucose level in a euglycemic obese individual. Taken together, these observations suggest that in persons with major loss of B-cell function, insulin resistance becomes an important determinant of the degree of hyperglycemia. However, when insulin resistance coexists with normal islets (which appear capable in increasing responsiveness to glucose level), little if any hyperglycemia results. A need for more direct experimentation in this area exists.

Nature of the B-cell Lesion

It is not clear whether the B-cell lesion in NIDDM is a loss of B-cell number, a dysfunction of a normal number of B-cells, or both. Although direct quantitation of B-cell mass in patients with NIDDM is technically difficult because of post-mortem changes, amyloid and glycogen deposition, a 40% to 60% mean decrease in islet or B-cell mass has been reported in limited numbers of patients with NIDDM as compared to nondiabetic subjects.[73,58,25] As mentioned previously, such a degree of B-cell loss is probably insufficient to cause fasting hyperglycemia,[71,41] although this has not been adequately tested in humans. Thus, it appear likely that dysfunction of the remaining B-cells compounds the loss in cell number and contributes to the defect in responsiveness to glucose level observed in vivo.

In order to clarify possible B-cell regulatory mechanisms in NIDDM, models of islet dysfunction have been created in normal humans using prolonged somatostatin administration,[69] and in rats by pancreatectomy or neonatal administration of streptozotocin.[39] In normal humans in whom mild insulin deficiency was created by administration of somatostatin with glucagon replacement, resulting meta-

bolic parameters were quite similar to those of NIDDM: fasting
hyperglycemia, near-normal basal insulin levels, markedly impaired
first and second phase responses to glucose, and a preserved insulin
response to the nonglucose stimulant isoproterenol.[69] Such similarities suggest that dysfunction of a normal number of B-cells can
mimic the matabolic features of NIDDM. Partially pancreatectomized
rats also display similar insulin secretory characteristics.[39]
Thus, a decrease in B-cell responsiveness to glucose with relative
preservation of responsiveness to nonglucose stimuli appears to
result from either B-cell loss or B-cell dysfunction. These findings suggest that the abnormalities of B-cell function characteristic of NIDDM could represent a nonspecific result of a variety of
B-cell lesions and support the concept that there may be considerable heterogeneity in the pathogenesis of NIDDM.

While patients with NIDDM possess major defects in insulin
responses to intravenous and oral glucose and in glycemic potentiation to nonglucose stimuli, these defects should not be considered completely irreversible. In fact, blockers of prostaglandin
synthesis[46,56] of alpha-adrenergic activity,[57] and of opiate
action[26] have all been reported to increase (but not normalize)
pancreatic insulin secretion.

III. Pathophysiology of Insulin Secretion in Insulin Dependent Diabetes Mellitus (IDDM)

Overt insulin-dependent diabetes mellitus (IDDM) is characterized by severe insulin deficiency. In long-standing IDDM, not only
are basal insulin and C-peptide levels in plasma and urine lower
than normal, but insulin and C-peptide secretory responses to glucose and non-glucose stimuli are virtually absent[72,49,19,33] (see
Figures 5 and 6). Such a near-complete deficiency of insulin
responses to all stimuli in IDDM constitutes a fundamental difference from NIDDM, where partial responses to non-glucose stimuli are
often preserved.[30]

Although B-cells in patients with long-standing IDDM respond
poorly to all stimuli, the situation in the prediabetic period or
during remission ("honeymoon phase") appears to be different. As
B-cell function slowly deteriorates before the onset of overt hyperglycemia, the insulin secretory response to glucose first declines,
then becomes nonexistent.[14,62,32] Only later, as fasting hyperglycemia develops, do responses to non-glucose stimuli such as
arginine decline.[14,32] Thus, the prediabetic or honeymoon phases
of IDDM are similar to NIDDM in that the insulin response to glucose
may be absent when the response to arginine is relatively preserved. In fact, it appears that some endogenous insulin secretion
is often present for a short time after the diagnosis of overt IDDM.
Drash et al. reported that in newly-diagnosed, untreated IDD
patients, plasma insulin was only modestly reduced as compared to

controls (10 vs 15 μU/ml).[13] In addition, other investigators have reported that partial preservation of B-cell function, as measured by basal C-peptide levels, is common in patients whose duration of IDDM is less than 2 years.[33,18,19] Although it has also been reported that patients with IDDM of short duration can increase C-peptide secretion in response to meals and to glucagon,[33,18,19] others have reported that insulin secretory responses to glucose and to nonglucose stimuli are absent in newly-diagnosed IDD's[13,49] (see Figures 5 and 6). Patients with long-standing IDDM tend to have very low basal plasma C-peptide levels and absent secretory responses to stimuli.[72,49,19,33]

Some evidence has suggested that preservation of endogenous B-cell function in IDD's is associated with smoother metabolic control. In a study of 46 IDD patients, Shima et al. demonstrated a correlation between the plasma C-peptide response to oral glucose and the stability of glycemic control, as determined by the standard deviation of multiple fasting plasma glucose levels.[61] Other reports have also suggested an association between residual B-cell function and stable glycemic control.[74,43,44]

Considerable effort has been given to methods of preserving B-cell function in newly-diagnosed IDD patients. For example, strict glycemic control has been reported to improve B-cell function[45] and to increase the frequency and duration of remissions[48] as compared to conventional treatment. The use of immunosuppressive therapy such as cyclosporine at time of diagnosis may also increase the frequency of remissions in IDDM,[63] but such data are very preliminary and use of these agents must be considered experimental.[16] No specific therapy has yet been demonstrated to prevent ultimate development of IDDM.

In summary, patients with long-standing IDDM have a near-complete loss of insulin secretion in response to all known stimuli. Patients with newly-diagnosed IDDM and those in a remission phase often possess partial responses to meals or to nonglucose stimuli. (The partial preservation of insulin responses to nonglucose stimuli in mild IDDM is reminiscent of NIDDM). At present, there is no proven method for preventing permanent IDDM in individuals with newly-diagnosed disease.

ACKNOWLEDGEMENTS

We gratefully acknowledge the assistance of Patricia Jenkins, Maxine Cormier and Louise Parry in preparation of the manuscript. This work was supported by National Institutes of Health grants AM 17047, AM 12829 and AM 00738, and the Veterans Administration. Dr. Beard was a fellow of the Juvenile Diabetes Foundation.

REFERENCES

1.   C.M. Asplin, T. L. Paquette, and J.P. Palmer, In vivo inhibi-
     tion of glucagon secretion by paracrine beta cell activity in
     man, J Clin Invest 68:314–318 (1981).
2.   J.D. Bagdade, E.L. Bierman, and D. Porte, Jr., The significance
     of basal insulin in the evaluation of the insulin response to
     glucose in diabetic and non-diabetic subjects, J Clin Invest
     46:1549–1557 (1967).
3.   J.C. Beard, J.D. Best, M.A. Pfeifer, J.B. Halter, and D. Porte,
     Jr., Corticosteroids alter B-cell sensitivity to hyperglycemia
     in man, Clin Res 30:522A (1982).
4.   J.C. Beard, C. Weinberg, M.A. Pfeifer, J.D. Best, J.B. Halter,
     and D. Porte, Jr., Interaction of glucose and epinephrine in
     the regulation of insulin secretion, Diabetes 31:802–807 (1982).
5.   J.R. Brooks, Operative approach to pancreative carcinoma,
     Seminars in Oncology 6:357–367 (1979).
6.   J.D. Brunzell, R.P. Robertson, R.L. Lerner, M.R. Hazzard, J.W.
     Ensinck, E.L. Bierman, and D. Porte, Jr., Relationships between
     fasting plasma glucose levels and insulin secretion during
     intravenous glucose tolerance tests, J Clin Endocrinol Metab
     42:222–229 (1976).
7.   E. Cerasi, Potentiation of insulin release by glucose in man.
     I. Quantitative analysis of the enchancement of glucose-
     induced insulin secretion by pretreatment with glucose in
     normal subjects, Acta Endocrinol 79:483–501 (1975).
8.   E. Cerasi, R. Luft, and S. Efendic, Decreased sensitivity of
     the pancreatic beta cells to glucose in prediabetic subjects,
     Diabetes 21:224–234 (1972).
9.   M. Chen, D. Porte, Jr., The effect of rate and dose of glucose
     infusion on the acute insulin response in man, J Clin
     Endocrinol Metab 42:1168–1175 (1976).
10. E.W. Chideckel, J. Palmer, D.J. Koerker, J. Ensinck, M.B.
     Davidson, and C.J. Goodner, Somatostatin blockade of acute and
     chronic stimuli of the endocrine pancreas and the consequences
     of this blockade on glucose homeostasis, J Clin Invest
     55:754–762 (1975)
11. D.L. Curry, L.L. Bennett, and G.M. Grodsky, Dynamics of insulin
     secretion by the perfused rat pancreas, Endocrinolgy 83:572–578
     (1968).
12. R.A. DeFronzo, J.D. Tobin, and R. Andres, Glucose clamp tech-
     nique: a method for quantifying insulin secretion and resis-
     tance, AM J Physiol 237(3):E214–E223 (1979).
13. A. Drash, J.B. Field, L.Y. Garces, F.M. Kenny, D. Mintz, and
     A.M. Vazquez, Endogenous insulin and growth hormone response in
     children with newly-diagnosed diabetes mellitus, Pediat Res
     2:94–102 (1968).
14. D. Drucker and B. Zinman, Pathophysiology of beta-cell failure
     after prolonged remission in insulin-dependent diabetes
     mellitus, Diabetes Care 1:83–87 (1984).

15. J. Dupre, J.D. Curtis, R.H. Unger, R.W. Waddell, and J.C. Beck, Effects of secretin, pancreozymin, or gastrin on the response of the endocrine pancreas to administration of glucose or arginine in man, J Clin Invest 48:745-757 (1969).

16. G.S. Eisenbarth, Immunotherapy of type 1 diabetes (editorial), Diabetes Care 6:521-523 (1983).

17. H. Elrick, Plasma insulin responses to oral and intravenous glucose administration, J Clin Endocrinol 24:1076-1082 (1964).

18. O.K. Faber, and C. Binder, B-cell function and blood glucose control in insulin-dependent diabetics within the first month of insulin treatment, Diabetologia 13:263-268 (1977).

19. O.K. Faber, and C. Binder, C-peptide response to glucagon. A test for the residual B-cell function in diabetes mellitus, Diabetes 26:604-610 (1977).

20. S.S. Fajans, J.C. Floyd, R.F. Knopf, and J.W. Conn, A comparison of leucine-and acetoacetate-induced hypoglycemia in man, J Clin Invest 43:2003-2008 (1964).

21. P. Felig, E.B. Marliss, and G.F. Cahill Jr., Metabolic response to human growth hormone during prolonged starvation, J Clin Invest 50:411-421 (1971).

22. P. Felig, J. Wahren and R. Hendler, Influence of maturity-onset diabetes on splanchnic glucose balance after oral glucose ingestion, Diabetes 27:121-131 (1978).

23. J.D. Fitz, E.M. Sperling and H.G. Fein, A hypocaloric high-protein diet as primary therapy for adults with obesity-related diabetes, Diabetes Care 6:328-333 (1983).

24. J.C. Floyd, Jr., S.S. Fajans, J.W. Conn, R.F. Knopf, and J. Rull, Stimulation of insulin secretion by amino acids, J Clin Invest 45:1487-1502 (1966).

25. W. Gepts and P.M. Lecompte, The pancreatic islets in diabetes, Amer J Med 70:105-114 (1981).

26. D. Giugliano, A. Ceriello, P. DiPinto, Impaired insulin secretion in human diabetes mellitus: the effect of naloxone-induced opiate receptor blockade, Diabetes 31:367-370 (1982).

27. C.J. Goodner, M.J. Conway and J. H. Werrbach, Control of insulin secretion during fasting hyperglycemia in adult diabetics and in nondiabetic subjects during infusion of glucose, J Clin Invest 48:1878-1889 (1969).

28. C.J. Goodner and D. Porte, Jr., Determinants of basal islet secretion in man. in: "Handbook of Physiology; Endocrinology; Endocrine Pancreas, Chapter 38," Steiner DF, Freinkel N (eds), Washington DC, Am Physiol Soc, (1972) pp 597-609.

29. G.M. Grodsky and L. L. Bennett, Multiphasic aspects of insulin release after glucose and glucagon, in: "Diabetes," J. Ostman, ed., Proc Sixth Cong Int Diabetes Fed, (1969), pp 462-469, Excerpta Medica Foundation, Amsterdam.

30. J.B. Halter, R.J. Graf and D. Porte, Jr., Potentiation of insulin secretory responses by plasma glucose levels in man: Evidence that hyperglycemia in diabetes compensates for impaired glucose potentiation, J Clin Endocrinol Metab 48:946–954 (1979).

31. J.B. Halter and D. Porte, Jr., Mechanisms of impaired acute insulin release in adult onset diabetes: Studies with isoproterenol and secretin, J Clin Endocrinol Metab 46:952–960 (1978).

32. E. Heinze, W. Beisher, L. Keller, G. Winkler, W.M. Teller, and E.F. Pfeiffer, C-peptide secretion during the remission phase of juvenile diabetes, Diabetes 27:670–676 (1978).

33. C. Hendriksen, O.K. Faber, J. Drejer, and C. Binder, Prevalence of residual B-Cell function in insulin-treated diabetics evaluated by the plasma C-peptide response to intravenous glucagon, Diabetologia 13:615–619 (1977).

34. C.B. Hollebneck, Y-D.I. Chen, and G.M. Reaven, A Comparison of the relative effects of obesity and noninsulin dependent diabetes mellitus on in vivo insulin stimulated glucoase utilization, Diabetes 33:622–626 (1984).

35. R.R. Holman and R.C. Turner, Maintenance of basal plasma glucose and insulin concentrations in maturity-onset diabetes, Diabetes 28:227–230 (1979).

36. H. Kajinuma, A. Kaneto, T. Kuzuya, and K. Nakao, Effects of methacholine on insulin secretion in man, J Clin Invest 28:1384–1388 (1968).

37. S.C. Kalhan and P.A.J. Adam, Inhibitory effect of prednisone on insulin secretion in man: model for duplication of blood glucose concentration, J Clin Endocrinol Metab 41:600–610 (1975).

38. J.H. Karam, G.M. Grodsky, K.N. Ching, Staircase glucose stimulation of insulin secretion in obesity, Diabetes 23:763–770 (1974).

39. J.L. Leahy, S. Bonner-Weir, and G. Weir, Abnormal glucose regulation of insulin secretion in models of reduced B-cell mass, Diabetes 33:667–673 (1984).

40. R.J. Lerner and D. Porte, Jr., Studies of secretin-stimulated insulin responses in man, J Clin Invest 51:2205–2209 (1972).

41. R.J. Lerner and D. Porte, Jr., Acute and steady-state insulin responses to glucose in nonobese diabetic subjects, J Clin Invest 51:1624–1631 (1972).

42. S.R. Levin, J.H. Karam, S. Kane, G.M. Grodsky, and P.H. Forsham, Enhancement of arginine-induced insulin secretion in man by prior administration of glucose, Diabetes 20:171–176 (1971).

43. J. Ludvigsson and L.G. Heding, C-peptide in diabetic children after stimulation with glucagon compared with fasting C-peptide levels in non-diabetic children, Act Endocrinologica 85:364–371 (1977).

44. J.A. Lutterman, T.J. Benraad, and A. Vantlaar, The relationship between residual insulin secretion and metabolic stability in Type 1 diabetes, Diabetologia 21:99–103 (1981).

45. S. Madsbad, T. Krarup, O.K. Faber, C. Binder, and L. Regeur, The transient effect of strict glycemic control on B-cell function in newly-diagnosed type 1 diabetic patients, Diabetologia 22:16–20 (1982).

46. J.R. McRae, S.A. Metz, and R.P. Robertson, A role for endogenous prostaglandins in defective glucose potentiation of nonglucose insulin secretagogues in diabetics, Metabolism 30:1065–1075 (1981).

47. S.A. Metz, J.B. Halter, and R.P. Robertson, Paradoxical inhibition of insulin secretion by glucose in human diabetes mellitus, J Clin Endocrinol Metab 48:827–835 (1979).

48. J. Mirouze, J.L. Selam, T.C. Pham, E. Mendoza, and A. Orsetti, Sustained insulin-induced remissions of juvenile diabetes by means of an external pancreas, Diabetologia 14:223–227 (1978).

49. R.L. Parker, R.S. Pildes, K.L. Chao, M. Cornblath, and D.M. Kipnis, Juvenile diabetes mellitus, a deficiency in insulin, Diabetes 17:27–35 (1968).

50. M.J. Perley and D.M. Kipnis, Plasma insulin responses to oral and intravenous glucose: Studies in normal and diabetic subjects, J Clin Invest 46:1954–1962 (1967).

51. M.A. Pfeifer, J.B. Halter, and D. Porte, Jr., Insulin secretion in diabetes mellitus, Am J Med 70:579–588 (1981).

52. D. Porte Jr. and A.A. Pupo, Insulin responses to glucose: evidence for a two-pool system in man, J Clin Invest 48:2309–2319 (1969).

53. D. Porte Jr., and R.H. Williams, Inhibition of insulin release by norepinephrine in man, Science 152:1248–1250 (1966).

54. G.M. Reaven, E. Bernstein, B. Davis, and J. M. Olefsky, Nonketotic diabetes mellitus: insulin deficiency or insulin resistance? Am J Med 68:80–86 (1976).

55. J.F. Rehfield and F. Stadil, The effect of gastrin on basal and glucose-stimulated insulin secretion in man, J. Clin Invest 52:1415–1426 (1973).

56. R.P. Robertson and M. Chen, A role for prostaglandin E (PGE) in defective insulin secretion and carbohydrate intolerance in diabetes mellitus, J Clin Invest 60:747–753 (1977).

57. R.P. Robertson, J.B. Halter, and D. Porte, Jr., A role for alpha-adrenergic receptors in abnormal insulin secretion in diabetes mellitus, J Clin Invest 57:791–795 (1976).

58. K. Saito, N. Yaginuma, and T. Takahashi, Differential volumetry of A,B, and D cells in the pancreatic islets of diabetic and nondiabetic subjects, Tohoku J Exp med 129:273–283 (1979).

59. E. Samols, G. Marri, and V. Marks, Promotion of insulin secretion by glucagon, Lancet 2:415–416 (1965).

60. M. Schebalin, S.I. Said and G.M. Makhlouf, Stimulation of insulin and glucagon secretion by vasoactive intestinal peptide, Am J Physiol 232:E197–E200 (1977).

61. K. Shima, R. Tanaka, S. Morishita, Studies on the etiology of brittle diabetes: relationship between diabetic instability and insulinogenic reserve, Diabetes 26:717-725 (1977).

62. S. Srikanta, O.P. Ganda, R. A. Jackson, R.E. Gleason, A. Kaldany, M.R. Garavoy, E.L. Milford, C.B. Carpenter, J.S. Soeldner, and G.S. Eisenbarth, Type 1 diabetes mellitus in monozygotic twins: chronic progressive beta cell dysfunction, Annals Int Med 99:320-326 (1983).

63. C.R. Stiller, J. Dupre, M. Gent, Effect of cyclosporine in type 1 diabetes: clinical course and immune response, Diabetes 33(Suppl 1):13A (1984).

64. R.C. Turner, R.R. Holman, D. Matthews, T.D.R. Hockaday, and J. Peto, Insulin deficiency and insulin resistance interaction in diabetes: estimation of their relative contribution by feedback analysis from basal plasma insulin and glucose concentrations, Metabolism 28:1086-1096 (1979).

65. R.C. Turner, S.T. McCarthy, R.R. Holman, and E. Harris, Beta-cell function improved by supplementary basal insulin secretion in mild diabetes, Brit Med Jl:1252-1254 (1976).

66. C.A. Verdonk, R.A. Rizza, R.L. Nelson, V.L.W. Go, J.E. Gerich, and F.J. Service, Interaction of fat-stimulated gastric inhibitory polypeptide on pancreatic alpha and beta-cell function, J Clin Invest 66:1119-1125 (1980).

67. W.K. Ward, J.C. Beard, J.B. Halter, M. A. Pfeifer and D. Porte, Jr., Pathophysiology of insulin secretion in noninsulin dependent diabetes mellitus, Diabetes Care 7:491-502 (1984).

68. W.K. Ward, D.C. Bolgiano, B. McKnight, J.B. Halter, and D. Porte, Jr., Diminished B-cell secretory capacity in patients with noninsulin dependent diabetes mellitus, J Clin Invest 74:1318-1328 (1984).

69. W.K. Ward, J.B. Halter, J.D. Best, J.C. Beard, and D. Porte, Jr., Hyperglycemia and B-cell adaptation during prolonged somatostatin infusion in man, Diabetes 32:943-947 (1983).

70. W.K. Ward, J.B. Halter, J.C. Beard, and D. Porte, Jr., Adaptation of B and A-cell function during prolonged glucose infusion in human subjects, Am J Physiol 246 (Endocrinol Metab) E405-E411 (1984).

71. K.W. Warren, J.W. Braasch, and C.W. Thurn, Diagnosis and surgical treatment of carcinoma of the pancreas, Curr Probl Surg 132:3-70 (1968).

72. T.A. Welborn, P. Garcia-Webb, and A.M. Bonser, Basal C-peptide in the discrimination of Type I from Type II diabetes, Diabetes Care 4:616-619 (1981).

73. P. Westermark and E. Wilander, The influence of amyloid deposits on the islet volume in maturity-onset diabetes mellitus, Diabetologia 15:417-421 (1978).

74. D.K. Yue, R.C. Baxter, and J. R. Turtle, C-peptide secretion and insulin antibodies as determinants of stability in diabetes, Metabolism 27:35-44 (1978).

INTERNALIZATION OF INSULIN:

STRUCTURES INVOLVED AND SIGNIFICANCE

Barry I. Posner[1], Masood N. Kahn[1] and John J.M. Bergeron[2]

Departments of Medicine[1] and Anatomy[2]
The Royal Victoria Hospital and
McGill University
Montreal, Canada

ABSTRACT

The binding of insulin to its receptor is followed by aggregation of hormone-receptor complexes and their internalization into the cell. Internalized hormone is concentrated in Golgi-enriched not lysosomal endocytotic structures which, in rat liver, contain lipoprotein particles and can be resolved by centrifugation techniques into three different entities. Recent work has shown that the bulk of endocytotic structures can be resolved from biochemically defined (i.e., galactosyltransferase-containing) Golgi elements. The endosomal apparatus or endosomes appear to function as a sorting center wherein internalized hormone-receptor complexes are concentrated and dissociated prior to directing hormone to lysosomes and receptor back to the cell surface for reutilization. Endosomes are heterogeneous and different functions might be subserved by different endosomal structures. Since an insulin stimulable receptor kinase activity can be identified in endosomes certain aspects of insulin action might be initiated herein.

INTERNALIZATION OF INSULIN AND OTHER PEPTIDE HORMONES[1]:
STRUCTURES INVOLVED AND SIGNIFICANCE

I. INTRODUCTION

It is generally accepted that tissue resistance to the action of insulin plays a role in the pathogenesis of Type II Diabetes Mellitus.[41] Though there is considerable controversy as to the site(s) of this resistance and its exact nature,[10] the fact of its

existence has given clinical relevance to investigating the mechanism of insulin's action on target tissues. One approach to the
study of hormone action is to analyze the nature of the interaction
between hormone and target cell. The initial site of interaction
between insulin and its target tissue is the cell surface receptor.
However, such an interaction appears to be only the beginning of a
journey into the cell interior.

II. Structures Involved in Internalization of Insulin

A. Cell Surface

The fluid mosaic model of membrane structure derives from the
recognition that membrane proteins are distributed in a substantially random manner and are able to undergo translational motion in
the plane of the cell membrane.[44] The application of this model
to peptide hormone receptors was swift and supported by observations
of receptor mobility.[11,24] The binding of peptide hormones to
their receptors appears, at physiologic temperatures, to be followed
by aggregation.[43] In cultured fibroblasts hormone–receptor complexes appear to aggregate in coated pits, a process especially well
worked out for LDL.[6] Though coated pits are widely found in
mammalian cell membranes, the extent to which they play a role
wherever found as sites of hormone–receptor aggregation remains to
be determined.

B. Golgi and Lysosomal Elements

A number of studies using morphologic and biochemical approaches
have shown that, subsequent to hormone–receptor complex formation at
the cell surface, the hormone is rapidly internalized in a
receptor-dependent manner.[38] The internalized hormone is rapidly
concentrated in structures whose nature has been debated for several
years.[20] Our early studies, employing both electron microscope
radioautography and subcellular fractionation, demonstrated uptake
of ^{125}I–insulin into Golgi-enriched subcellular fractions of rat
liver.[38] Golgi vesicular elements in rat liver were identified by
two criteria: the morphological one of intraluminal lipoprotein
particles and the biochemical marker of galactosyltransferase.[3,14]
We interpreted our data to indicate uptake into bonafide Golgi
elements since by electron microscope radioautography, the radiolabeled hormone was in lipoprotein-containing structures and by
subcellular fractionation ^{125}I–insulin was found in elements
cosedimenting with galactosyltransferase.[38] Figure 1 illustrates
the rapid accumulation of ^{125}I–insulin into the Golgi heavy
fraction prior to its accumulation into a combined Golgi light and
intermediate fraction. The Golgi heavy fraction is heterogeneous
and contains many small vesicles with which a major fraction of
internalized radiolabel was associated. These are probably endocytotic vesicles into which hormone was first internalized prior to

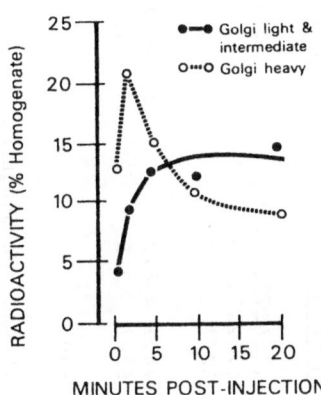

Fig. 1   Time course of association of radiolabel with Golgi
          fractions after injection of ^{125}I–insulin. The figure
          is modified from Posner et al.[39]

its transfer to other structures.[38]

   Since some studies purported to show concentration of
internalized hormone in lysosomes, we compared the uptake of
[125]I–insulin into highly purified Golgi and lysosomal fractions.[40] Table 1 illustrates the characteristically high galactosyltransferase and low acid phosphatase concentration of Golgi
fractions which is the obverse of the enzyme activities in lysosomal
fractions. It is evident that ^{125}I–insulin was concentrated in
Golgi fractions to a much greater degree (at least 5 to 20 fold)
than in lysosomal fractions and that chloroquine, though concentrated to a greater extent in lysosomes, did not influence the relative extent of ^{125}I–insulin accumulation in Golgi and lysosomal
fractions. Furthermore, virtually all radiolabel in the latter was
located over lipoprotein–containing vesicles [i.e., "unique"
vesicles[27,40]] and was never seen over secondary lysosomes.[40]

   Though the structures involved in the early phase of peptide
hormone internalization are not lysosomes, there is evidence for
ultimate degradation of peptide hormones in lysosomes. For example,
studies of gold and ferritin labeled ligands have shown ultimate
accumulation of these particles in lysosomes.[13,35] The extent to
which this is the exclusive fate of internalized protein ligands has
not been established and other routes of cellular clearance are
possible.

Table 1.   Enzyme activity, chloroquine concentration and its effect on ^{125}I-insulin accumulation in Golgi and lysosomal fractions

Cell Fraction	Relative Specific Activity		^{125}I-insulin (cpm/mg protein)[a]		Chloroquine Concentration (Fractions)[b] (Homogenate)
	AP	GT	Control	+Chloroquine	
Golgi light	2.9±0.3	37.3±1.8	18,035±5,321	104,154±22,416	1.9±0.3
intermediate	4.0±0.1	33.4±1.5	32,387±3,615	209,712±39,332	3.2±0.5
heavy	2.1±0.1	17.7±1.4	8,580±1,237	24,586± 2,252	2.5±0.3
Lysosomal L$_2$	24.1±2.8	0.7±0.3	1,804± 490	10,767± 4,672	18.0±0.7
Fractions L$_3$	18.2±2.0	0.3±0.1	577± 97	3,637± 315	7.9±0.2

AP, Acid Phosphatase.   GT, galactosyltransferase.

a   Each animal received 12 x 10^6 cpm of ^{125}I-insulin 20 min before sacrifice. Chloroquine treatment was 10mg/100 body wt. 2 hrs and 1 hr respectively before ^{125}I-insulin injection. All values are mean ± SE of four fractionations. Consult Posner et al.40 for details of cell fractionation and enzyme assays.

b   Subcellular fractions, prepared 60 min after chloroquine, were extracted and measured as described elsewhere (40). Each value is the mean ± SE of three fractionations.

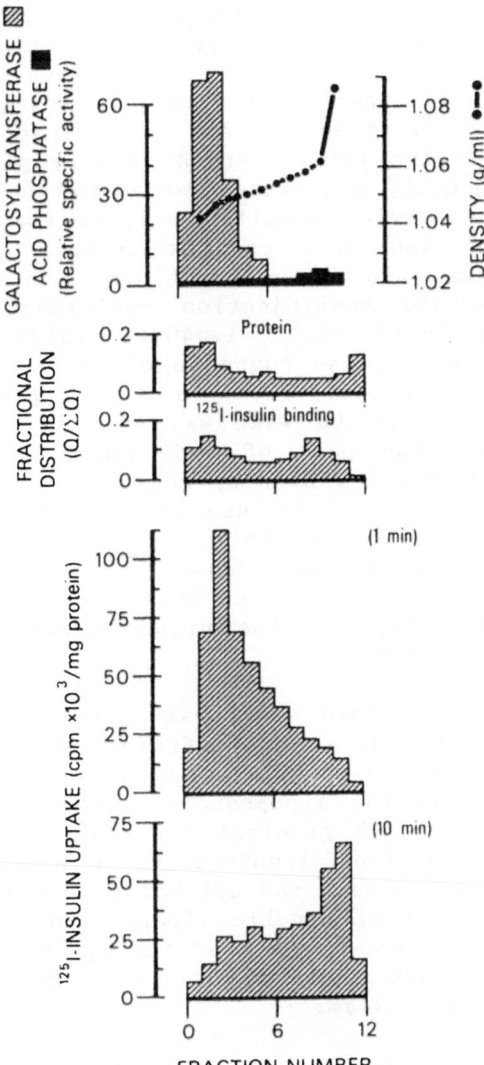

Fig. 2   Distribution of marker enzymes, protein, ^{125}I-Insulin binding and radioactivity following ^{125}I-insulin administration in Golgi intermediate subfractions generated by Percoll gradient centrifugation. Animals received 12 x 10[6] cpm of ^{125}I-insulin and were studied at 1 and 10 minutes after radiolabel injection. Galactosyltransferase, acid phosphatase, ^{125}I-insulin binding and protein were assayed as described by Khan et al.[28] wherein further details may be obtained.

C. The Endosomal Apparatus

The discovery of "unique" vesicles cosedimenting in lysosomal fractions[27] was rapidly followed by the demonstration that the lipoprotein-containing vesicles in Golgi fractions were heterogeneous. Thus, it was shown using Percoll gradient centrifugation, that in both Golgi intermediate and heavy but not Golgi light fractions there were two receptor-rich vesicle populations (Figure 2) — the lighter density structures cosedimenting with galactosyltransferase and the heavier density vesicles containing some acid phosphatase.[28] This led to a re-examination of the internalization of ^{125}I-insulin into these fractions. In Figure 2, it is seen that at 1 minute postinjection radiolabel was largely in elements of low density (density = 1.040 to 1.049) but by 10 minutes the majority of radiolabel was found in elements of higher density. Subsequently, the radioactivity in all gradient fractions diminished.[28] In contrast to what was seen in Golgi intermediate and heavy fractions, the peak of radiolabel in the Golgi light fraction remained in the low density region.[28] It is important to note that the integrity of ^{125}I-insulin was substantially retained across the gradient and, on morphological analysis, was exclusively over lipoprotein-containing structures.[28] We interpreted these data to indicate initial uptake into Golgi vesicles with subsequent transfer to "unique" vesicles (the higher density elements) which cosedimented in Golgi fractions.

More recent data raised the possibility of the independent uptake of peptide hormones, at two different rates, into these two populations of lipoprotein-containing vesicles.[4] In addition, it was not clear that all the lipoprotein-containing vesicles in the light region of the Percoll gradient (see Figure 2) were the same; perhaps there was one pool involved in a biogenetic route and another engaged in endocytosis and catabolism. The possibility that a substantial proportion of hepatic lipoprotein may be derived via endocytosis has been given strong credence by the appreciation that the liver in most animals probably accounts for the bulk of low density lipoprotein catabolism.[1,7]

The advent of a powerful new technique for resolving endocytotic structures has permitted us to examine critically the extent to which internalized ^{125}I-insulin cosedimenting with galactosyltransferase (Figure 2) is actually located in the same structures containing this enzyme. The technique is based upon the polymerization of diaminobenzidine (DAB) to a dense complex by horseradish peroxidase in the presence of H_2O_2. Courtoy and his colleauges coupled horseradish peroxidase to galactosylated bovine serum albumin and allowed this ligand for the asialoglycoprotein receptor to be internalized by rat liver. Following this, they prepared cell fractions containing the ligand and showed that on adding DAB and H_2O_2, the endocytotic structures were shifted to

a higher density on subsequent centrifugation.[8] This density
technique has been applied by us to study ^{125}I-insulin uptake, and
it has become clear that the bulk of endocytotic elements containing
[125]I-insulin are devoid of galactosyltransferase.[26]

The structures involved in concentrating internalized substances within the cell have been described in a variety of ways
(Table 2). It would now appear that these structures can not only
be distinguished from plasma membrane [38] and lysosomes[39] but, in
major part, from Golgi elements themselves.[26] We favor referring
to this distinctive intracellular system as the endosomal apparatus
or endosomes.[22]

It is clear from the above considerations that endosomes are
heterogeneous and consist of at least 3 types of structures. Those
cosedimenting with Golgi heavy elements are probably involved in the
early phase of endocytosis. The other two endosomal elements can be
resolved on Percoll gradient centrifugation of Golgi intermediate
and heavy fractions. The heavier density endosomes or "unique"
vesicles are likely very similar or identical to the endosomal elements cosedimenting with lysosomes. In recent studies we have found
that chloroquine concentrates significantly in the heavier endosomes
and virtually negligibly in the lighter endosomes.[30] This
provides a further distinction between these two endosome
populations and, additionally, indicates that the heavier endosomes
contain acidic interiors.[42,47]

III. Recycling of Receptors - A Role for Endosomes

The above discussion has emphasized the internalization of
insulin and other peptide hormones but it is now quite clear that it
is hormone-receptor complexes which are internalized. This was
suggested by early observations that ligand uptake is receptor-
mediated and that internalized ligand concentrates in receptor-rich

Table 2.   Terminology for Structures Involved in Internalization

---

Lysosomes (20)
Golgi Fractions (elements) (38)
Ligandosomes (45)
Compartment for Uncoupling Receptor and Ligand (CURL) (18)
Receptosomes (50)
Multivesicular Bodies (35, 49)
Tubular Vesicles (48)
Lipoprotein-containing vesicles (38,39)
'Unique' vesicles (27, 39)
Endosomes (22)

---

cell fractions.[38] This view is further supported by the recognition that ligands are metabolized by cells far more rapidly than
their receptors. Thus, insulin is metabolized rapidly (t 1/2 ≃ 30
minutes) and the insulin receptor much more slowly (t 1/2 ≃ 10
hours) by target cells.[32]

Using photoaffinity labeling techniques Fehlman et al. have
provided strong evidence for insulin-receptor internalization and
recycling. Thus, photoaffinity-labeled insulin receptors of
cultured hepatocytes become trypsin-insensitive on incubation at
37°C[16] but, on more extended incubation (up to 6 hours) become
partially sensitive to trypsin indicating an initial loss from and
subsequent return to enzyme accessibility at the cell surface.[17]
Similar studies of rat adipocytes confirmed the internalization of
photolabeled receptors.[5]

These studies can be criticized on the basis that an unnatural
linkage between receptor and ligand was formed. Nevertheless, they
are supported by a range of observations. Thus, exposing chick
liver cells to insulin resulted in a loss (down-regulation) of cell
surface receptors with a corresponding increase in intracellular
receptor content.[32] The injection of insulin has been shown to
effect a loss of insulin receptors from liver cell plasma membranes[12,37] along with a corresponding increase in endosomal
receptors.[12] Comparable observations have been made by exposing
isolated adipocytes to insulin.[21]

The use of antibodies prepared against various receptors has
contributed greatly to defining more precisely the fate of the
receptor. Thus, several groups using antibody to the LDL receptor,[5] the transferrin receptor[15] and the Fc receptor on macrophages[36] have shown that receptor is internalized along with
ligand. In elegant studies Geuze, Schwartz and their colleagues
have used double-label immunoelectron microscopy to colocalize an
asialoglycoprotein and its receptor.[18] They showed that ligand
and receptor were closely associated at the plasma membrane and in
clathrin-coated vesicles close to the surface. However, an endosomal compartment was identified wherein they could demonstrate the
dissociation of ligand from receptor, with the former found in the
lumen of vesicles and the latter concentrated in tubular elements
free of ligand. They interpreted these observations to indicate the
existence of a cell compartment which they called CURL (see Table 2)
in which ligand-receptor complexes dissociated.[18] An important
question is the extent to which CURL corresponds to the heavier
endosomes which are apparently acidic (vide supra).

Other studies have shown that there are different routes for
the handling of ligands depending, presumably at least in part, on
the ease with which they are dissociated from receptor. Thus,
Hopkins, using transferrin-peroxidase to mark ligand and a

transferrin receptor specific antibody, has shown the existence of both a peripheral endosomal system and a juxtanuclear area involved in the handling of ligand-receptor complexes.[23] He suggests that each compartment plays a specific role in directing internalized receptors to particular cellular domains. In a study comparing the uptake of the asialoglycoprotein (ASGP) receptor with that for polymeric IgA (membrane secretory component) Geuze, Schwartz and colleauges showed that the intracellular routes for these 2 receptors corresponded at an early stage but subsequently diverged with each entering distinctive endosomal regions.[19] The IgA receptor and its ligand were directed to the bile canalicular surface and secreted into the bile.[33]

The above noted studies attest to the complexity of the endosomal apparatus but especially the role of this system in directing the flow of ligand-receptor complexes and the dissociated species as well. Figure 3 attempts to schematize the major intracellular routes traversed by hormones and their receptors. The endosomal apparatus (EN) is depicted as playing a major role in directing traffic to Golgi and lysosomes. A key question is how receptor is recycled to the plasma membrane. In this scheme, receptor is visualized as recycling from endosomes and/or via the Golgi apparatus and secretory granules (Sg). The demonstration that ^{125}I-insulin is internalized into secretory granules of the pancreas[9] as well as the appearance of peptide hormones in secretions from various cells is consistent with such a role for this route.

In concluding this section, it is worthwhile noting that the endosomal apparatus plays a role in facilitating the entry of agents such as enveloped viruses and bacterial toxins into the cytosol.[22] Here low pH appears to play a key role in the process by which the agent penetrates endosomal membranes. In summary, the endosomal apparatus appears to be a distinctive entity engaged in sorting intracellular traffic of hormones and their receptors and other penetrating agents as well. In the next few years, the exact composition of this apparatus should become clearer as receptor antibodies, ultrathin cryoelectron microscopy and the DAB density shift procedure, among other new techniques, are applied to its study.

IV. Significance of Internalization

Since the original observations of Terris and Steiner identifying insulin degradation by hepatocytes as a receptor-mediated phenomenon[46] it has been broadly accepted that an important consequence of the internalization of peptide hormones is their degradation within the cell. As noted above the dissociation of hormone from receptor within the endosomal apparatus would appear to be an essential prior step. It is also clear that receptor down

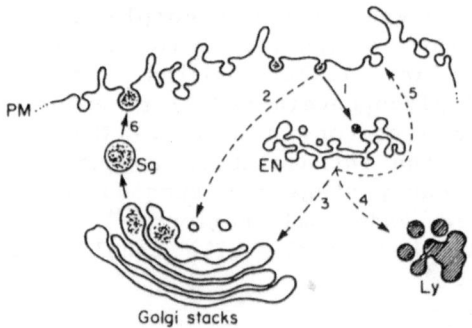

Fig. 3   Scheme of possible intracellular routes traversed by
           hormone-receptor complexes and individual hormone and
           receptor.   1, internalization to endosomal apparatus
           (EN); 2, possible limited internalization to Golgi; 3, 4,
           dissociation of hormone-receptor complex with sorting and
           distribution of hormone to lysosomes (Ly) and hormone
           receptor to Golgi; 5, 6, recycling of receptors directly
           from EN (5) or via the secretory pathway and secretory
           granules (Sg).

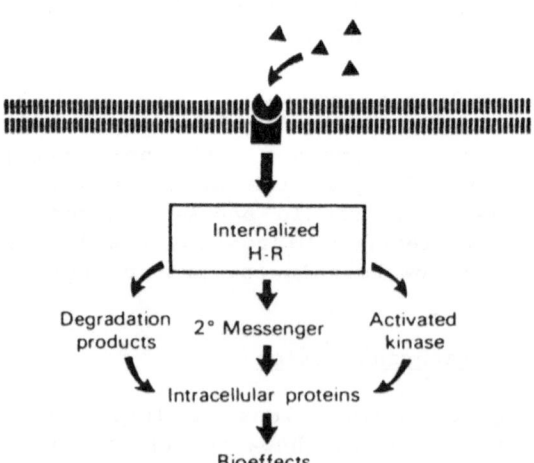

Fig. 4   A model of insulin action following internalization of
           the hormone-receptor complex. For discussion see text.

regulation is a consequence, at least in part, of receptor internalization (vide supra).

An interesting and important issue is the role of insulin-
receptor complex internalization in insulin action. Figure 4 depicts
several possible ways in which the internalization of hormone-
receptor complexes might lead to hormone action. Insulin degradation
products may play a role in augmenting insulin action.[31] Though a
second messenger, mediating insulin action, has been suggested to
derive from plasma membranes[34] such molecules might derive from
intracellular membranes as well. Most recently it has been shown
that the β-subunit of the insulin receptor is a protein kinase,[25]
and it has been suggested that this kinase effects insulin action by
phosphorylating key intracellular proteins. It is possible that the
activated receptor kinase with or without associated insulin is
internalized and brought into contact with key substrates. Our
observation that the endosomal insulin receptor can function as an
insulin-stimulable kinase[29] is compatible with this possibility.

ACKNOWLEDGEMENTS

These studies have been supported by grants from the Medical
Research Council of Canada and the U.S. Public Health Service.

REFERENCES

1. A.D. Attie, R.C. Pittman, and D. Steinberg, Hepatic catabolism
   of low density lipoprotein: mechanisms and metabolic consequences, Hepatology, 2:269-281 (1982).
2. S.K. Basu, J.K. Goldstein, R.G.W. Anderson, and M.S. Brown,
   Monensin interrupts the recycling of low density lipoprotein
   receptors in human fibroblasts, Cell, 24:493-502 (1981).
3. J.J.M. Bergeron, J.H. Ehrenreich, P. Siekevitz, and
   G.E. Palade, Golgi fractions prepared from rat liver homogenates: isolation procedure and morphological characterization, J. Cell Biol, 59:73-88 (1973).
4. J.J.M. Bergeron, L. Resch, R. Rachubinski, B. Patel, and B.I.
   Posner, Effect of colchicine on internalization of prolactin in
   female rat liver: an in vivo radioautographic study, J. Cell
   Biol, 96:875-886 (1983).
5. P. Bernahu, J.M. Olefsky, P. Tsai, P. Thamm, D. Saunders, and
   D. Brandenburg, Internalization and molecular processing of
   insulin receptors in isolated rat adipocytes, Proc Natl. Acad.
   Sci. U.S.A. 79:4069-4073 (1982).
6. M.S. Brown, and J.L. Goldstein, Receptor-mediated endocytosis:
   insights from the lipoprotein receptor system, Proc. Natl.
   Acad. Sci. U.S.A. 76:3330-3337 (1979).

7. Y. S. Chao, A.L. Jones, G.T. Hradek, E.E.T. Windler, and R.J. Havel, Autoradiographic localization of the sites of uptake, cellular transport, and catobolism of low density lipoproteins in the liver of normal and estrogen-treated rats, Proc. Natl. Acad. Sci. U.S.A. 78: 597-601 (1981).

8. P.J. Courtoy, J. Quintart, and P. Baudhuin, Shift of equilibrium density induced by 3, 3-diaminobenzidine cytochemistry: a new procedure for the analysis and purification of peroxidase-containing organelles, J. Cell Biol, 98:870-876 (1984).

9. J. Cruz, B.I. Posner, and J.J.M. Bergeron, Receptor-mediated endocytosis of ^{125}I-Insulin into pancreatic acinar cells in vivo, Endocrinology 115:1996-2008 (1984).

10. R.A. Defronzo, and E. Ferrannini, The pathogenesis of non-insulin-dependent diabetes: an update, Medicine, 61:125-140 (1982).

11. C. de Haen, The non-stoichiometric floating receptor model for hormone-sensitive adenylyl cyclase, J. Theor. Biol. 58:383-400 (1976).

12. B. Desbuquois, S. Lopez, and H. Burlet, Ligand-induced translocation of insulin receptors in intact rat liver, J. Biol. Chem. 257:10852-10860 (1982).

13. R.B. Dickson, M.C. Willingham, and I. Pastan, α_2-Macroglobulin adsorbed to colloidal gold: a new probe in the study of receptor-mediated endocytosis, J. Cell Biol, 89:29-34 (1981).

14. J.H. Ehrenreich, J.J.M. Bergeron, P. Siekevitz, and G.E. Palade, Golgi fractions prepared from rat liver homogenates: isolation procedure and morphological characterization, J. Cell Biol. 59:45-72 (1973).

15. C.A. Enns, J.W. Larrick, H. Suomalainen, J. Schroder, and H.H. Sussman, Co-migration and internalization of transferrin and its receptor on K562 cells, J. Cell Biol. 97:579-585 (1983).

16. M. Fehlmann, J.-L. Carpentier, A. Le Cam, P. Thamm, D. Saunders, D. Brandenburg, L. Orci, and P. Freychet, Biochemical and morphological evidence that the insulin receptor is internalized with insulin in hepatocytes, J. Cell Biol. 93:82-87 (1982).

17. M. Fehlmann, J.L. Carpentier, E. Van Obberghen, P. Freychet, P. Thamm, D. Saunders, D. Brandenburg, and L. Orci, Internalized insulin receptors are recycled to the cell surface in rat hepatocytes, Proc. Natl. Acad. Sci. USA, 79:5921-5925 (1982).

18. H.J. Geuze, J.W. Slot, G.J.A.M. Strous, H.F. Lodish, and A.L. Schwartz, Intracellular site of asialoglycoprotein receptor-ligand uncoupling: double-label immunoelectron microscopy during receptor-mediated endocytosis, Cell 32:277-287 (1983).

19. J.J. Geuze, J.W. Slot, G.J.A.M. Strous, J. Peppard, K. von Figura, A. Hasilik, and A.L. Schwartz, Intracellular receptor sorting during endocytosis: comparative immunoelectron microscopy of multiple receptors in rat liver, Cell, 37:195-204 (1984).

20. P. Gorden, J.-L. Carpentier, P. Freychet, and L. Orci, Internal-
     ization of polypeptide hormones: mechanism, intracellular
     localization and significance, Diabetologia, 18:263-274 (1980).
21. A. Green, and J.M. Olefsky, Evidence for insulin-induced
     internalization and degradation of insulin receptors in rat
     adipocytes, Proc. Natl. Acad. Sci. USA, 79:427-431 (1982).
22. A. Helenius, J. Mellman, D. Wall, and A. Hubbard, Endosomes,
     Trends Biochem. Sci. 7:245-250 (1983).
23. C.R. Hopkins, Intracellular routing of transferrin and trans-
     ferrin receptors in epidermoid carcinoma A431 cells, Cell,
     32:321-330 (1983).
24. S. Jacobs, and P. Cuatrecasas, The mobile receptor hypothesis
     and cooperativity of hormone binding: application to insulin,
     Biochim. Biophys. Acta, 433:482-495 (1976).
25. M. Kasuga, Y. Fujita-Yamaguchi, D.L. Blithe, M.F. White, and
     C.R. Kahn, Characterization of the insulin receptor kinase
     purified from human placental membranes, J. Biol. Chem.
     258:10973-10980 (1983).
26. D.G. Kay, M.N. Khan, B.I. Posner, and J.J.M. Bergeron,
     ^{125}I-insulin in hepatic Golgi fractions: application of the
     diaminobenzidine (DAB)-shift protocol, Biochem. Biophys. Res.
     Commun. 123:1144-1148 (1984).
27. M.N. Khan, B.I. Posner, A.K. Verma, R.J. Khan, and J.J.M.
     Bergeron, Intracellular hormone receptors: evidence for
     insulin and lactogen receptors in a unique vesicle sedimenting
     in lysosome fractions of rat liver, Proc. Natl. Acad. Sci. USA,
     78:4980-4984 (1981).
28. M.N. Khan, B.I. Posner, R.J. Khan, and J.J.M. Bergeron, Intern-
     alization of insulin into rat liver Golgi elements: evidence
     for vesicle heterogeneity and the path of intracellular pro-
     cessing, J. Biol. Chem. 257:5969-5976 (1982).
29. M.N. Khan, S. Savoie, J.J.M. Bergeron, and B.I. Posner,
     Endosomes of rat liver: preparation and characterization,
     Abstract, Amer. Soc. Cell Biol. Meeting (1984).
30. R.J. Khan, M.N. Khan, J.J.M. Bergeron, and B.I. Posner,
     Prolactin internalization into rat liver Golgi fractions:
     differential effects of chloroquine. Biochim. Biophys. Acta.
     (in press).
31. K. Kikuchi, J. Larner, R. J. Freer, and A. R. Day, Effect of
     insulin fragments on biological activity of insulin and
     desoctapeptide insulin, I. Potentiation of biological activi-
     ties, J. Biol. Chem. 256:9441-9444 (1981).
32. M. Krupp, and M.D. Lane, On the mechanism of ligand-induced
     down-regulation of insulin receptor level in the liver cell, J.
     Biol. Chem. 256:1689-1694 (1981).
33. L.C. Kuhn and J.P. Kraehenbuhl, The sacrificial receptor-
     translocation of polymeric IgA across epithelia, Trends Biochem
     Sci. 7:299-302 (1982).

34. J. Larner, G. Galasko, K. Cheng, A.A. Depaoli-Roach, L. Huang, P. Daggy and J. Kellogg, Generation by insulin of a chemical mediator that controls protein phosphorylation and dephosphorylation, Science 206:1408-1410 (1979).

35. J.A. McKanna, H.T. Haigler, and S. Cohen, Hormone receptor topology and dynamics: morphological analysis using ferritin-labeled epidermal growth factor, Proc. Natl. Acad. Sci. USA 76:5689-5693 (1979).

36. I.S. Mellman, H. Plutner, R.M. Steinman, J.C. Unkeless and Z.A. Cohn, J. Cell Biol. 96:887-895 (1983).

37. V. Pezzino, R. Vigneri, N.B. Pliam, and I.D. Goldfine, Rapid regulation of plasma membrane insulin receptors, Diabetologia 19:211-215 (1980).

38. B.I. Posner, J.J.M. Bergeron, Z. Josefsberg, M.N. Khan, R.J. Khan, B.A. Patel, R.A. Sikstrom, A.K. Verma, Polypeptide hormones: intracellular receptors and internalization, Recent Prog. Horm. Res. 37:539-582 (1981).

39. B.I. Posner, M.N. Khan and J.J.M. Bergeron, Endocytosis of peptide hormones and other ligands, Endocr. Revs. 3: 280-298 (1982).

40. B.I. Posner, B. Patel, M.N. Khan, J.J.M. Bergeron, Effect of chloroquine on the internalization of ^{125}I-insulin into subcellular fractions of rat liver: evidence for an effect of chloroquine on Golgi elements, J. Biol. Chem. 257:5789-5799 (1982).

41. G.M. Reaven, Insulin resistance in noninsulin-dependent diabetes mellitus. Does it exist and can it be measured? Amer J. Med 74 (No. 1A): 3-17 (1983)

42. D.-J. Reijngoud, and J.M. Tager, Chloroquine accumulation in isolated rat liver lysosomes, FEBS Lett 64:231-235 (1976).

43. Y. Schecter, J. Schlessinger, S. Jacobs, K-J Chang, and P. Cuatrecasas. Fluorescent labeling of hormone receptors in viable cells: preparation and properties of highly fluorescent derivatives of epidermal growth factor and insulin, Proc. Natl. Acad. Sci. USA 75:2135-2139 (1978).

44. S.J. Singer, and G.L. Nicolson, The fluid mosaic model of the structure of cell membranes, Science 175: 720-731 (1972).

45. G.D. Smith and T.J. Peters, The localization in rat liver of alkaline phosphodiesterase to a discrete organelle implicated in ligand internalization, Biochim. Biophys. Acta 716: 24-30 (1982).

46. S. Terris, and D.F. Steiner, Binding and degradation of ^{125}I-insulin by rat hepatocytes, J. Biol. Chem. 250:8389-8398 (1975).

47. B. Tycko and F.R. Maxfield, Rapid acidification of endocytic vesicles containing α_2 - macroglobulin, Cell 28:643-651 (1982).

48. D.A. Wall, G. Wilson, and A. Hubbard, The galactose specific recognition system of mammalian liver: the route of ligand internalization in rat hepatocytes, Cell, 21:79-93 (1980).

49. R.J. Walsh, B.I. Posner, and B. Patel, Binding and uptake of ^{125}I-iodoprolactin by epithelial cells of rat choroid plexus: an in vivo autoradiographic analysis, Endocrinology, 114:1496-1505 (1984).

50. M.C. Willingham, and I. Pastan, The receptosome: an intermediate organelle of receptor-mediated endocytosis in cultured fibroblasts, Cell 21:67-77 (1980).

INSULIN RESISTANCE IN NON-INSULIN DEPENDENT (TYPE II)

AND INSULIN DEPENDENT (TYPE I) DIABETES MELLITUS

Jerrold M. Olefsky, Robert R Revers, Mel Prince, Robert R. Henry, William T. Garvey, John A. Scarlett, and Orville G. Kolterman

University of California
San Diego
Department of Medicine/Endocrinology M-023E
La Jolla, California, U.S.A   92093

ABSTRACT

Insulin resistance is a characteristic feature of non-insulin dependent diabetes mellitus (NIDDM) due to target tissue defects in insulin action. Abnormalities of cellular insulin action can be divided into receptor and post-receptor defects. Patients with impaired glucose tolerance are insulin resistant due to decreased insulin receptors resulting in decreased insulin sensitivity and rightward shifted in vivo dose response curves. Patients with NIDDM are insulin resistant due to a combination of receptor and post-receptor defects. The greater the severity of the diabetes (greater fasting hyperglycemia) the greater the post-receptor defect, and in those patients with more significant fasting hyperglycemia the post-receptor defect is the predominant abnormality leading to the insulin resistant state. At least one of the abnormalities underlying this post-receptor defect involves a decrease in glucose transport system activity in freshly isolated adipocytes. This defect in glucose transport, is not expressed in cultured fibro-blasts, indicating that the abnormality in glucose disposal seen in vivo and in glucose transport seen in freshly isolated cells is an acquired phenomenon. Consistent with this, the post-receptor defect is partially reversible by insulin therapy, which leads to a 50-70% reversal of the reduced rates of in vivo glucose disposal and in vitro glucose transport. Insulin resistance also exists in poorly controlled IDDM patients, due to a postreceptor defect in insulin action. This insulin resistance is not present in well controlled IDDM patients,

and is completely reversible when poorly controlled patients are
treated with intensive insulin therapy.

Insulin is produced in the pancreatic beta cell as the primary
biosynthetic product preproinsulin. This peptide is rapidly
converted to proinsulin (MW ~ 9000). Proinsulin is converted to
insulin (MW ~ 6000) plus C-peptide in the secretory granule with a
small amount (~ 5 percent) of the proinsulin remaining uncon-
verted. After a brief time in the peripheral circulation (half-life
six to 10 minutes), insulin interacts with target tissues to exert
its biologic effects. One of insulin's major biologic effects is
the promotion of overall glucose metabolism, and abnormalities of
this aspect of insulin action can lead to a number of important
clinical and pathophysiologic states including Type II diabetes,
also known as non-insulin-dependent diabetes mellitus
(NIDDM).[35,38-40] Since insulin travels from the beta cell through
the circulation to the target tissues, abnormalities at any of these
loci can influence the ultimate action of the hormone.[38] These
abnormalities, all of which lead to decreased insulin effect, are
referred to as insulin-resistant states.

CAUSES OF INSULIN RESISTANCE

Mutation in the Structural Gene for Insulin Leading to a
Biologically Defective Insulin Molecule

For many years it has been postulated that diabetes may be due
to the secretion of a structurally abnormal insulin molecule in some
patients. However, such a case has not been described until quite
recently despite extensive research.[14,37,49] A patient who dis-
played fasting hyperglycemia (~ 200 mg/dl) and fasting hyperinsulinemia (~ 100 μU/ml) but who exhibited normal sensitivity
to exogenously administered insulin has now been studied. Detailed
chemical studies revealed that the patient's insulin contained
leucine instead of phenylalanine in the biologic active site of the
insulin molecule at position 24 of the insulin B chain.[49] This
mutated insulin species had greatly reduced binding and biologic
potency which accounted for the diabetic syndrome. It is likely
that more patients with this abnormality will be discovered and the
key clinical finding leading to suspicion of this syndrome is the
presence of endogenous hyperinsulinemia in a patient who responds
normally to exogenous insulin.

Incomplete Conversion of Proinsulin to Insulin

Proinsulin is normally converted to insulin by proteolytic action
within the beta-cell secretory granule. In control subjects only
about 5 percent of the beta-cell secretory product consists of

proinsulin, and its conversion to insulin is usually almost complete. When the conversion of proinsulin to insulin is incomplete, excessive amounts of proinsulin are secreted into the circulation. To maintain glucose homeostasis, beta-cell secretory activity is increased because proinsulin has reduced biologic activity, and thus circulating proinsulin levels are elevated. Since proinsulin crossreacts with insulin (in radioimmunoassay in vitro), an apparent hyperinsulinemic state exists.[12,24]

Circulating Insulin Antagonists

Circulating antagonists can generally be grouped into hormonal and nonhormonal categories. Hormonal antagonists include all of the known counter-regulatory hormones such as cortisol, growth hormone, glucagon, and catecholamines. Well known clinical syndromes such as Cushing's disease and acromegaly exist in which elevated levels of these hormones can induce an insulin-resistant diabetic state. However, excessive levels of counter-regulatory hormones are not an important contributory factor to insulin resistance in the usual case of obesity or NIDDM.[38]

Nonhormonal antagonists include free fatty acids, anti-insulin antibodies, and anti-receptor antibodies. Several years ago Randle et al.[43] hypothesized that elevated circulating levels of free fatty acids could impair peripheral glucose utilization. The proposed mechanism underlying this effect is the uptake of fatty acids by cells and the oxidation of these fatty acids intracellularly. As a result of the elevated cellular rates of fatty acid oxidation, glycolysis, and glucose uptake are inhibited and this inhibition leads to antagonism of insulin action. A derivative of this hypothesis is the assumption that any situation which leads to elevated rates of fatty acid oxidation (even without increased circulating free fatty acids levels) could lead to reduced rates of glucose uptake.[43]

Anti-insulin antibodies develop in essentially all patients treated chronically with exogenous insulin.[22] These antibodies can alter the usual time course of exogenous insulin action by binding and releasing insulin within the plasma compartment. However, these antibodies prove to be clinically significant in causing a true insulin-resistant state in only unusual cases. A few patients have been described who spontaneously develop anti-insulin antibodies in the absence of exogenous insulin therapy.[22] These antibodies can interfere with the insulin radioimmunoassay in vitro and thus lead to apparent hyperinsulinemia, but the antibodies do not cause insulin resistance.

In recent years a fascinating syndrome has been described in which patients develop antibodies directed against the insulin receptor.[11,18,19] This condition is quite rare, and is associated

with acanthosis nigricans, severe insulin resistance, and diabetes
mellitus. The circulating antibodies apparently bind to the insulin
recptor in vivo, thus making the receptor inaccessible to insulin
which results in an insulin resistant state.

Insulin Receptor and Post-Receptor Defects

Insulin exerts its biologic effects by initially binding to its
specific cell-surface receptor.[17,36,41,46] After this binding
event, the insulin-receptor complex is formed and one or more signals
of insulin action are generated. The signal, or "second messenger"
may involve the generation of a chemical mediator, a conformational
change within the plasma membrane, phosphorylation, alterations in
ion flux, or other information transfers.[7,8] Regardless of its
precise physicochemical nature, this signal (or signals) interacts
with a variety of effector units which mediate the entire host of
biologic actions attributable to insulin. In many instances, the
effector unit consists of a series of steps such as a sequentially-
linked enzyme system (specifically, activation of glycogen phosphorylase) or a series of enzymes involved in the degradation of a
particular substrate (glucose). Clearly, insulin action involves a
cascade of events, and abnormalities anywhere along this sequence
can lead to insulin resistance. For convenience, tissue abnormalities in insulin action can be categorized under the headings of
receptor and post-receptor or post-binding defects.

Decreased cellular insulin receptors have now been described in
a variety of pathophysiologic situations. The most common of these
are obesity[2,16,32,46] and NIDDM.[4,9,30,32] Decreased insulin
receptors have also been described in acromegaly,[29] following glu-
cocorticoid therapy[21,31] or after oral contraceptive therapy,[6]
and in several other less common conditions.[3,42] Since the first
step in insulin action involves binding to the receptor, it is
apparent that a decrease in cellular insulin receptors could lead to
insulin resistance. However, this potential relationship is not as
clear as it would seem since the normal relationship between insulin
receptors and insulin action is not straightforward because of the
fact that cells possess spare receptors.[15,28]

The spare receptor concept is based on the observation that a
maximal insulin effect is achieved at a concentration of insulin at
which less than the total number of cellular receptors are occupied.
For example, it has been shown that in isolated adipocytes, maximal
insulin stimulation of glucose transport occurs when only 10 percent
of the adipocyte insulin receptors are occupied.[28,33] Thus, 90
percent of the normal complement of receptors are "spare". All of
these spare receptors are potentially fully functional, but which
receptors are occupied at any given point is purely a random event;
any group of occupied receptors amounting to 10 percent of the total
would lead to the same metabolic response. Therefore, the cellular

response to increasing insulin concentration is a continuous increase in receptor occupancy and biologic action until the critical number of occupied receptors needed to generate a maximal response is reached. Further increases in the prevailing insulin concentration beyond this point lead to a continued increase in receptor occupancy with no further increase in biologic response since a step or steps distal to the receptor are now the rate-limiting event.

Given this relationship between insulin binding and insulin action, the predicted functional consequence of a decrease in the number of receptors would be a rightward shift in the dose-response curve for insulin action, that is, insulin's effect would be decreased at lower insulin concentrations while a normal maximal response would be elicited at higher insulin concentrations.[20,32] As shown in Figure 1, a decrease in the number of receptors results in a rightward shift in the insulin-biologic function dose-response curve with decreased responses at all submaximal insulin concentrations and normal insulin action at maximally effective hormone concentrations. As receptor loss becomes more pronounced, the insulin-biologic function dose-response curve shifts further to the right and the degree of rightward shift is proportional to the decrease in the number of receptors. The only time a decrease in the number of insulin receptors can lead to a decrease in maximal insulin action is when less than 10 percent of the original receptor complement is present (Figure 1). Of course, the precise proportion of spare receptors varies according to cell type and is also dependent upon which particular insulin action is measured. The role of a decrease in the number of insulin receptors in the insulin resistance of NIDDM will be discussed later.

It is apparent that the overall scheme of insulin action represents a multistep sequence in which the binding of insulin to receptors is only the initial event. A defect in any of the effector systems distal to receptor binding can also lead to impaired insulin action and insulin resistance. These defects can involve abnormal coupling between insulin-receptor complexes and the glucose transport system, decreased activity of the glucose transport system per se, or a variety of intracellular enzymatic defects located in various pathways of glucose metabolism. In this context the term "post-receptor defect" refers to any abnormality in the insulin action sequence following the initial insulin-receptor binding step. This defect could theoretically include an abnormality of the insulin receptor which does not affect insulin binding, but does affect insulin action. The role of post-receptor defects in NIDDM will be discussed later. While the biochemical mechanisms underlying postreceptor defects are generally poorly understood, the functional sequelae of this type of abnormality can be predicted. In this situation one sees a proportionate decrease in insulin action at all insulin concentrations, including maximally effective hormone levels.[7,32,38] Thus, a decrease in the capacity of a rate-limiting

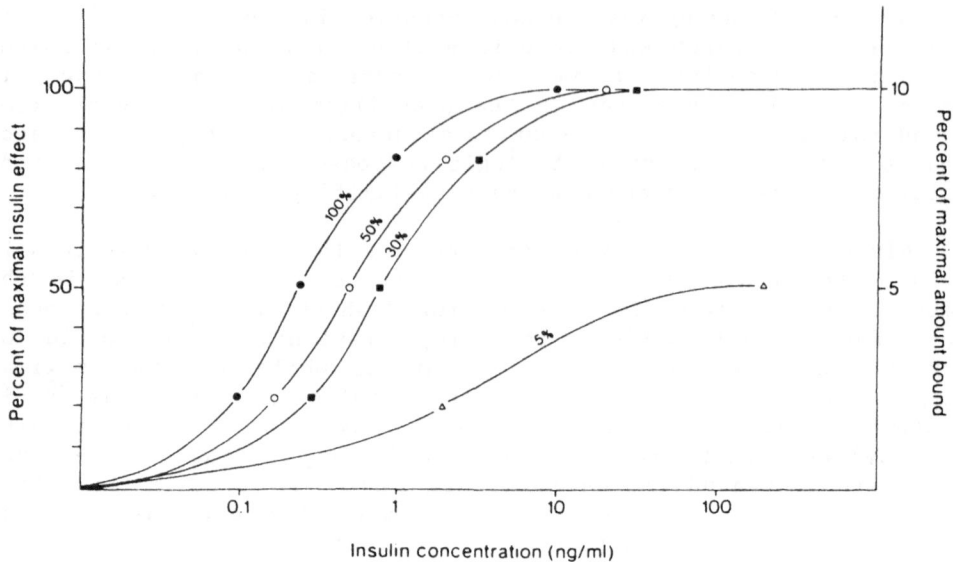

Fig. 1   This figure illustrates the predicted functional con-
            sequence of a progressive loss of insulin receptors on
            the insulin biologic function dose-response curve.
            Results represent theoretical dose-response curves in
            which the percent of the maximal insulin effect (left
            axis) and the percent of the normal maximal amount bound
            (right axis) are plotted as a function of the insulin
            concentration. With progressive receptor loss, the dose-
            response curves are increasingly shifted to the right
            with no change in maximal insulin action, although more
            insulin is necessary to elicit the maximal insulin
            reponse. If enough receptors are lost (greater than 90%)
            so that 10% of the original receptor complement are not
            present, then a rightward shift in the dose-response
            curve as well as a decrease in maximal insulin response
            will occur(Δ).

step in the insulin action-glucose metabolism scheme leads to a
reduction in the maximal absolute insulin effect, and this defect
cannot be overcome by the addition of more and more insulin.

     From the foregoing discussion, it is apparent that abnormal
beta-cell secretory products or circulating insulin antagonists are
unusual causes of insulin resistance and can be etiologically implicated in NIDDM only rarely. Consequently, the available evidence
points to a target tissue defect in insulin action as the cause of
the insulin resistance in this condition. Therefore, the following
sections will be devoted to a discussion of the mechanisms of
insulin resistance in non-insulin-dependent diabetes mellitus with

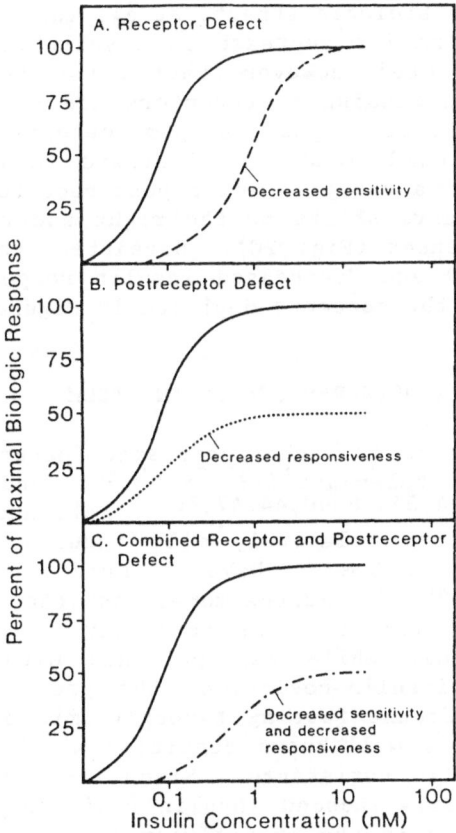

Fig. 2   The curves in this figure represent theoretical insulin
          biologic action dose–response curves depicting the
          results of an isolated receptor defect (A), an isolated
          post–receptor defect (B) and a combined receptor and
          post–receptor defect (C).

particular emphasis on the relative roles of receptor versus
post–receptor defects.

On the basis of our understanding of normal insulin action, the
effects of receptor versus post–receptor defects on the in vivo
insulin–biologic function dose–response curve can be predicted, and
by studying the insulin dose–response curve in insulin–resistant
states the following distinctions which are summarized in Figures 2A
to 2C can be made: (1) An isolated decrease in the number of insulin
receptors leads to a rightward shift in the insulin dose–response
curve with no change in maximal insulin action, and this receptor
defect is termed a decrease in insulin sensitivity (Fig. 2A). (2)
A pure post–receptor defect in insulin action leads to a propor–

tionate reduction in biologic effects at all insulin concentrations. This normally is termed a decrease in insulin responsiveness (Fig. 2B). It should be noted, however, that since the biochemical steps which follow insulin binding to receptors are not known, it is possible that certain kinds of post-receptor defects involving the coupling mechanisms could lead to rightward shifted dose-response curves. (3) If both a receptor and a post-receptor defect co-exist, the dose-response curve shifts to the right and the maximal insulin responsiveness decreases (Fig. 2C). Hereafter, the terms "decreased insulin sensitivity" and "decreased insulin responsiveness" will be used in relation to the concepts depicted in Figures 2A to 2C.[20]

CHARACTERISTICS OF INSULIN RESISTANCE IN NIDDM

Insulin resistance is a characteristic feature of patients with impaired glucose tolerance[34,35,38-40,44] and patients with NIDDM.[1,5,13,23,27,34,35,38-40,44,47,50] Patients with impaired glucose tolerance have relatively mild insulin resistance whereas patients with NIDDM have more severe insulin resistance.[34,35,38-40,44] Furthermore, as the degree of carbohydrate intolerance worsens, the frequency of insulin resistance increases.[34,44] Thus, while all patients with impaired glucose tolerance are not insulin-resistant, the great majority of NIDDM patients with significant fasting hyperglycemia display this abnormality. Obesity is a well-known condition which also leads to the development of insulin resistance. Since most adult NIDDM patients are overweight, obesity-induced insulin resistance is thought to be a contributing factor in the hyperglycemia of these patients. However, obesity cannot account for all of the insulin resistance in this type of diabetic patient since the insulin resistance is greater than that which can be accounted for on the basis of the obesity alone. Furthermore, many non-obese patients with NIDDM are also insulin-resistant. This subject has been reviewed several times in recent years.[27,35,38-41,47]

In Vivo Studies

We have used the euglycemic glucose clamp technique to provide direct quantitative evidence for insulin resistance in patients with impaired glucose tolerance (chemical diabetes) and patients with overt NIDDM. Fasting serum glucose levels were consistently less than 115 mg/dl in the patients with impaired glucose tolerance but their oral glucose tolerance tests were abnormal. Fasting hyperglycemia greater than 140 mg/dl was found in the NIDDM patients and the mean fasting glucose level in this group of patients was 225 mg/dl. They were divided into two groups consisting of 13 non-obese patients (relative weight less than 1.10, mean 0.96) and 10 obese patients (relative weight greater than 1.15, mean 1.31). Figures 3A and 3B present the mean steady-state plasma insulin levels and

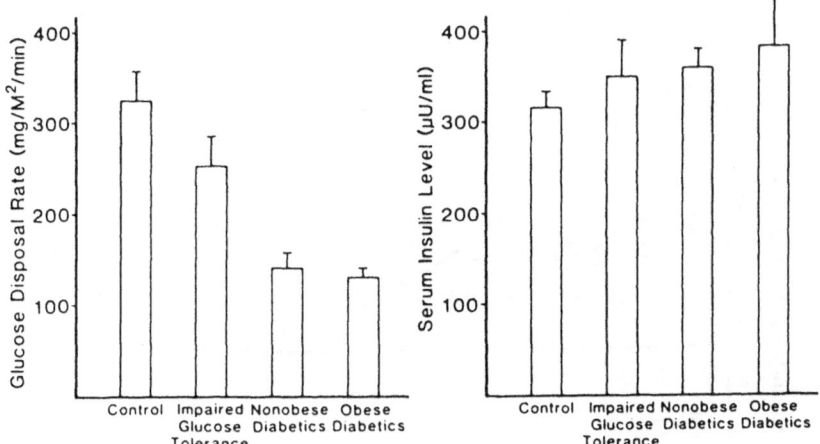

Fig. 3   The graphs depict the mean steady-state glucose disposal
          rates (A), and serum insulin levels (B) for control
          subjects, patients with impaired glucose tolerance, and
          nonobese and obese NIDDM patients during euglycemic
          glucose clamp studies performed at an insulin infusion
          rate of 120 mU/M^2/min. Results are plotted as the mean
          ± SE.

peripheral glucose disposal rates in these patients during
euglycemic glucose clamp studies in which an insulin infusion rate
of 120 mU/M^2/min was used. As can be seen, steady-state insulin
levels were comparable in all patients, but the glucose disposal
rates were decreased in the diabetic groups and the magnitude of
this defect was greatest in the patients with the most carbohydrate
intolerance. Thus, the mean glucose disposal rate was reduced by 24
percent in the patients with impaired glucose tolerance and by 56
percent and 60 percent in the non-obese and obese NIDDM groups.[27]

Abnormal beta-cell secretory products or circulating insulin
antagonists can lead to insulin resistance in NIDDM patients only in
rare circumstances.[35,38-40] Consequently, the cause of this
insulin resistance must reside at the level of the target tissues.
To help elucidate this abnormality, studies of insulin binding to
receptors have been performed. Figure 4A summarizes measurements of
insulin binding to receptors on circulating monocytes from control
subjects and NIDDM patients with fasting hyperglycemia. It is
obvious that the ability of cells from the diabetic patients to bind
insulin is greatly reduced and this reduction is due to a reduced
number of cellular insulin receptors. When similar studies were
performed in a group of patients with impaired glucose tolerance,
analogous results were obtained (Figure 4B). Thus, taken as a

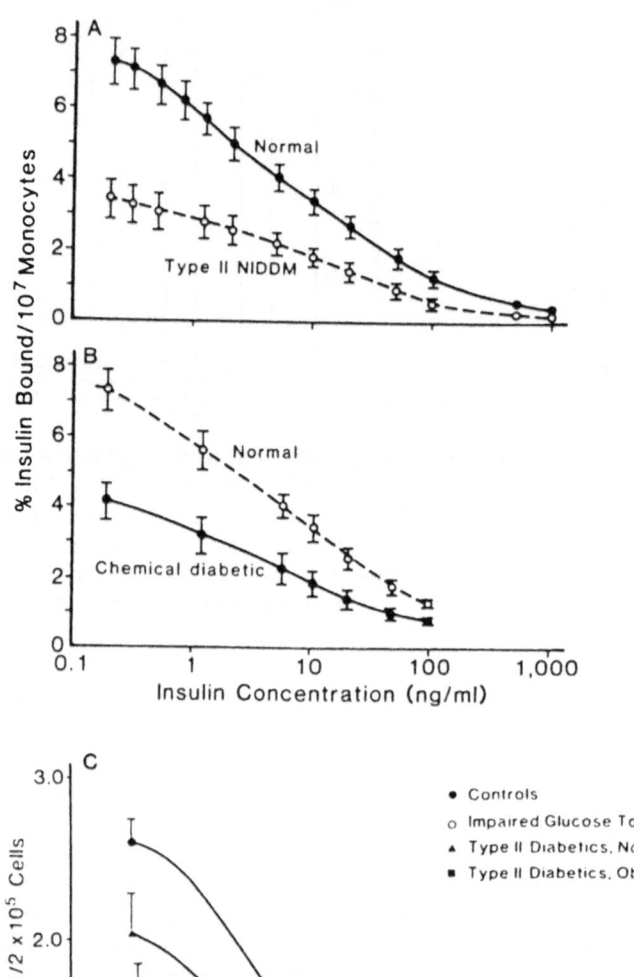

Figure 4

Fig. 4   A. Comparison of [^{125}I]insulin binding to isolated
           monocytes obtained from 31 NIDDM patients (O) and 40
           control subjects (normal)(●).   B.   Comparison of
           ^{125}I-insulin binding to isolated monocytes obtained
           from 24 control subjects (normal) (O) and 14 patients
           with impaired glucose tolerance (●).   C.   Insulin binding
           by isolated adipocytes from control subjects (●) is
           compared with patients with impaired glucose tolerance
           (O), and nonobese (▲) and obese (■) NIDDM patients.

group, insulin binding to circulating monocytes is reduced in these
patients and the overall magnitude of this decrease in insulin binding is about the same for both diabetic groups.   Since circulating
monocytes are not a primary target tissue for insulin, similar studies were performed using a known target tissue; specifically, isolated adipocytes.   Figure 4C demonstrates that results analogous to
those observed in monocytes were found in this cell type.   Scatchard
analysis and average affinity profile analysis revealed that the
decreases in insulin binding seen in Figures 4A, 4B, and 4C are due
to decreases in receptor number with no change in binding affinity.

As discussed earlier, the simple demonstration of decreased
insulin receptors in the setting of insulin resistance does not
necessarily imply cause and effect.   To clarify the role of this
cellular abnormality in the pathogenesis of the in vivo insulin
resistance of diabetes, the in vivo dose-response relationship was
examined by performing additional euglycemic glucose clamp studies
at insulin infusion rates of 40, 240, 1200, or 1800 mU/M^2/min.[27]

As can be seen in Figure 5A, the curve for the patients with
impaired glucose tolerance lies to the right of the curve for the
control subjects.   Thus, the mean glucose disposal rates at insulin
levels of 100, 300, and 1000 µU/ml are significantly less (p <
0.01) when compared to controls.   However, the patients with impaired
glucose tolerance achieve a maximal rate of glucose disposal which
is not significantly different from that of the control subjects.
Therefore, the insulin-resistant state associated with impaired glucose tolerance appears to result solely from a decrease in cellular
insulin receptors with no evidence of a post-receptor defect in
insulin action.

The NIDDM patients exhibit both a rightward shift in their
dose-response curve and a marked decrease in the maximal rate of
glucose disposal.   There is a tendency for these changes to be more
pronounced in the obese diabetic patients with the greatest difference between the two groups appearing at the highest insulin concentration.   The differences in the glucose disposal rates for the
obese and the non-obese NIDDM patients are not significant at the
two lower insulin levels, but do reach statistical significance

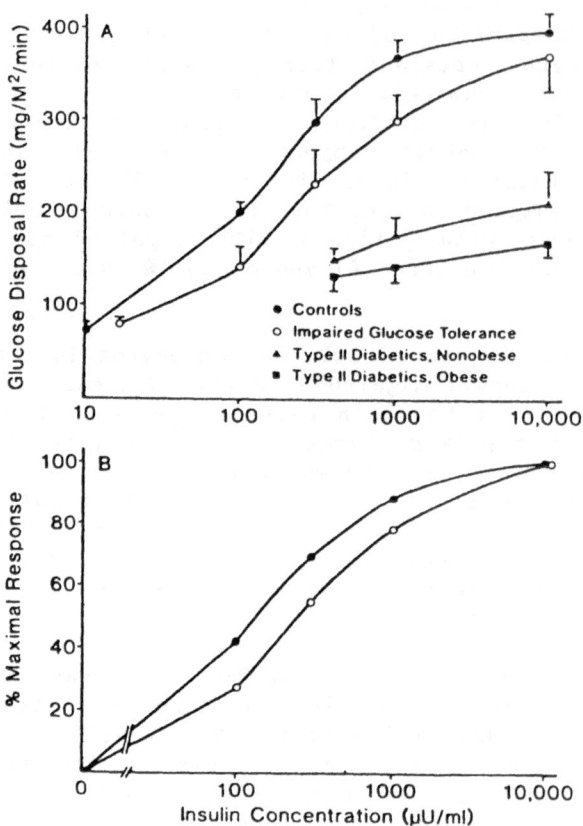

Fig. 5   A.   Mean dose-response curves for control subjects (●)
            are compared with patients with impaired glucose toler-
            ance (O), and nonobese (▲) and obese (■) NIDDM
            patients. B. Mean dose-response curves for the control
            subjects (●) and patients with impaired glucose tolerance
            (O) plotted as the percent of maximal response.

(p < 0.05) at the highest insulin level. Clearly the predominant
lesion responsible for the insulin-resistant state in the patients
with fasting hyperglycemia appears to be a post-receptor defect in
insulin action leading to a marked decrease in maximal insulin
responsiveness. The abnormality is present in both non-obese and
obese NIDDM patients, which suggests that this post-receptor defect
in insulin action is not caused by obesity. This demonstrates that
in impaired glucose tolerance the insulin resistance is due to
decreased insulin receptors which lead to decreased insulin
sensitivity.   In   the   patients   with   significant   fasting
hyperglycemia, decreased insulin receptors and a post-receptor
defect in insulin action exist, which lead to both decreased insulin
sensitivity and decreased insulin responsiveness.

The functional form of the dose—response curves for the control subjects and the patients with impaired glucose tolerance can be better appreciated by plotting the data as a percent of the maximal insulin effect (Fig. 5B).[26,27,33,48] This analysis could not be done accurately for the NIDDM patients because their dose-response curves were so flat. The results show that the half—maximally effective insulin level is 135 μU/ml for the control subjects compared to 240 μU/ml for the patients with impaired glucose tolerance (note the log scale on the abscissa). Therefore, this form of analysis quantitates the rightward shift in the dose-response curve for the patients with impaired glucose tolerance.

Decreased cellular insulin receptors should lead to a shift to the right of the insulin dose—response curve, and this was observed in the patients with impaired glucose tolerance. Implicit in this observation is a relationship between cellular insulin binding and in vivo insulin action. The half—maximally effective insulin level is largely determined by the degree of insulin binding and, therefore, this value was plotted as a function of insulin binding for individual control subjects and patients with impaired glucose tolerance (Figure 6).

As can be seen, a significant inverse relationship exists ($r = -0.53$, $p < 0.02$), indicating that patients with higher levels of insulin binding require lower insulin concentrations to elicit a half—maximal response.

To provide further evidence that the alterations in in vivo insulin action seen in the patients with impaired glucose tolerance were due to decreased cellular insulin binding, the glucose disposal rate was plotted as a function of the amount of cellular bound insulin as shown in Figure 7. The amount of insulin bound at each of the insulin concentrations shown in Figure 5 was determined from the adipocyte binding data plotted in Figure 4C. This assumes that insulin binding to adipocytes accurately reflects insulin binding to other target tissues in vivo. As can be seen in Figure 7, when the glucose disposal rate is examined as a function of insulin binding, the same biologic effect is elicited in both groups of patients by a given amount of bound insulin. This indicates that when one accounts for the decreased ability of tissues from patients with impaired glucose tolerance to bind insulin, no defect in the steps of insulin action distal to the binding event can be detected.

Inspection of the individual data in the NIDDM patients showed that the patients with the lower fasting glucose levels were less insulin—resistant and had the smallest reductions in maximal glucose disposal rates, which suggested that the degree of post—receptor defect is greater as the severity of the diabetic state increases. This relationship is shown directly in Figure 8 where the fasting serum glucose level is plotted as a function of the maximal glucose

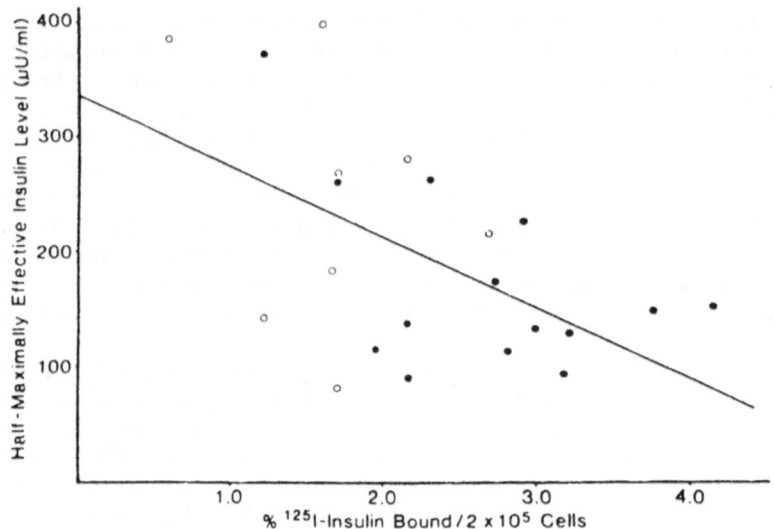

Fig. 6   This figure shows the relationship between the insulin
              concentration that produced half-maximal stimulation of
              glucose   disposal   (from   the   individual   dose-response
              curves)   and   the   percent ^{125}I-insulin   bound   (at   0.2
              ng/ml) in individual control subjects (O) and patients
              with impaired glucose tolerance (0).   Since the half-
              maximally   effective   insulin   concentration   cannot   be
              accurately   assessed   in   NIDDM   patients   (because   of   the
              flat curves) they were not included in this analysis.

disposal rate in the patients with impaired glucose tolerance and
NIDDM (the decrease in maximal glucose disposal is a measure of the
magnitude of the post-receptor defect).   When patients in this group
were examined, a highly significant inverse linear relationship was
found (r - -0.72, p < 0.001) indicating that as the maximal glucose
disposal rate falls, the fasting glucose level rises.   In the
patients with mild impairment of glucose tolerance (normal fasting
glucose levels), maximal insulin-stimulated glucose disposal rates
are normal and no post-receptor defect exists.   In these patients
the insulin resistance is characterized only by decreased insulin
sensitivity due to decreased cellular insulin receptors.   As the
diabetic state worsens and fasting hyperglycemia develops, a post-
receptor defect emerges, and this becomes the primary cause of the
insulin resistance in the patients with the most severe fasting
hyperglycemia.   Thus, the greater the post-receptor defect, the more
severe the fasting hyperglycemia.

In Vitro Studies

        The biochemical nature of the post-receptor defect in the

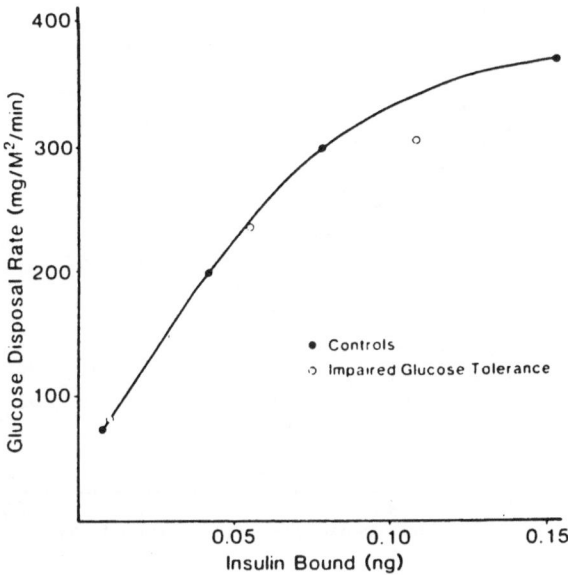

Fig. 7   Shown here are the mean glucose disposal rates for the
         control subjects (●) and patients with impaired glucose
         tolerance (O) plotted as a function of the amount of
         insulin bound. The amount of insulin bound was cal-
         culated by multiplying the insulin concentrations plotted
         in Figure 5 by the percent insulin bound at that concen-
         tration (as calculated from the competition curves in
         Figure 4C).

patients with significant fasting hyperglycemia remains to be elucidated. However, since no post-receptor defect exists in insulin's
ability to inhibit hepatic glucose production or in insulin's anti-
lipolytic effect,[13] it seems likely that the post-receptor abnormality is specific for one or more aspects of cellular glucose
uptake and metabolism. Studies of in vitro 3-0-methyl glucose
transport are consistent with this formulation (Figures 9A and 9B).
Thus, in patients with impaired glucose tolerance, the in vitro glucose transport dose-response curves are shifted to the right with
normal maximal insulin action; this finding is consistent with
decreased insulin sensitivity due to decreased insulin receptors
only. In the patients with NIDDM, not only were the dose-response
curves shifted to the right, but there was also a marked decrease in
maximal insulin-stimulated glucose transport; these findings are
consistent with decreased insulin sensitivity plus decreased insulin
responsiveness due to a combined receptor and post-receptor defect
in insulin action. Clearly these in vitro results are remarkably
well-correlated to the in vivo results obtained using the multiple
euglycemic clamp approach which leads us to conclude that the post-

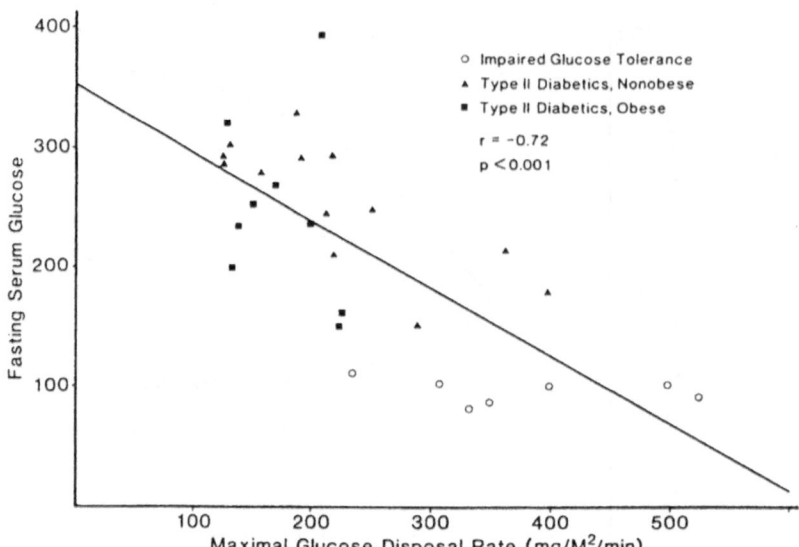

Fig. 8   The relationship between the fasting serum glucose level
           and the maximal glucose disposal rate in individual
           patients with impaired glucose tolerance (O), nonobese
           patients with NIDDM (▲) and obese patients with NIDDM
           (■). The inverse linear relationship seen in the
           figure indicates that as the maximal glucose disposal
           rate falls the fasting glucose level rises.

receptor defect demonstrated in patients with NIDDM is due to a
defect in the activity of the plasma membrane glucose transport
carrier.

     The pathogenesis of the carbohydrate intolerance seems rela-
tively straightforward in those patients with impaired glucose tolerance who are insulin-resistant and relatively hyperinsulinemic.
Thus, it seems reasonable to postulate that the decreased insulin
receptors lead to decreased insulin sensitivity in these patients,
and if adequate hyperinsulinemia cannot be generated to overcome
this defect in insulin action, carbohydrate intolerance develops.

     The relationship between insulin resistance and the diabetic
state in NIDDM patients with fasting hyperglycemia is more complex.
Essentially all patients with severe fasting hyperglycemia are
insulin-resistant and the degree of this resistance is much greater
than that found in patients with impaired glucose tolerance. The
available evidence indicates that the insulin resistance is largely
related to a post-receptor defect in insulin action, and it is possible that this post-receptor defect may be secondary and progres-

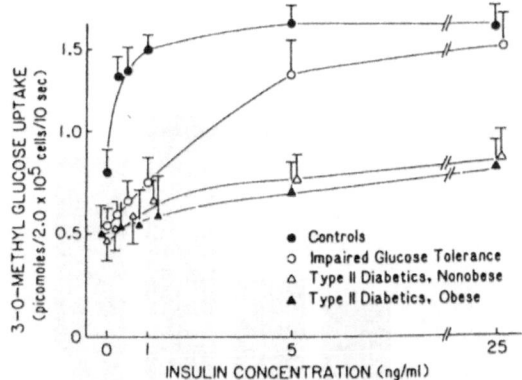

Fig. 9   Dose-response   curves   for   insulin   action   on
          3-0-methylglucose transport in adipocytes from normals
          (●), subjects with impaired glucose tolerance (O), lean
          subjects and NIDDM (Δ), and obese subjects with NIDDM
          (▲).

sive with the severity of the chronic diabetic state. Although
patients wth fasting hyperglycemia can have normal or elevated basal
insulin levels, they are uniformly hypoinsulinemic in response to a
glucose challenge. This could indicate that the insulin resistance
in these patients is secondary to the insulin deficiency. A possible corollary of this idea is that a large part of the insulin
resistance of diabetic patients with severe hyperglycemia could be
reversed if the diabetic state were corrected with insulin therapy.

Hepatic Glucose Production

    It should not be implied that abnormalities of peripheral glu-
cose uptake are the only target tissue defects leading to hyperglycemia in NIDDM, since overproduction of glucose by the liver is
also a major contributing abnormality. As seen in Figure 10, the
rates of basal hepatic glucose output (HGO) are increased in NIDDM,
whether patients are obese or not, whereas HGO is normal in subjects
with impaired glucose tolerance. The importance of this abnormality
is best depicted by examining the relationship between HGO and FBS
in individual subjects. Figure 11 demonstrates a very close correlation between these variables indicating that it is the rate of
glucose production by the liver which most directly modulates the
level of fasting hyperglycemia in NIDDM.

    Our current view is that the peripheral insulin resistance (due
primarily to a post-receptor defect) provides the foundation for
hyperglycemia. In the face of severe peripheral insulin resistance,
NIDDM patients have little ability to compensate for increases in
glucose entry into the circulation regardless of whether this extra
glucose comes from endogenous sources (the liver) or from ingested

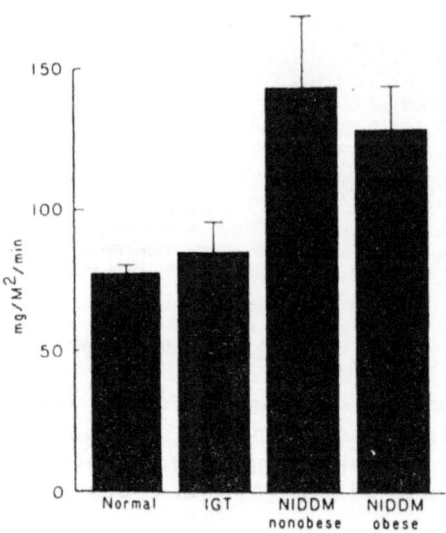

Fig. 10   Basal hepatic glucose production rates in normals, patients with impaired glucose tolerance (IGT) and Type II diabetics (NIDDM non-obese and obese).

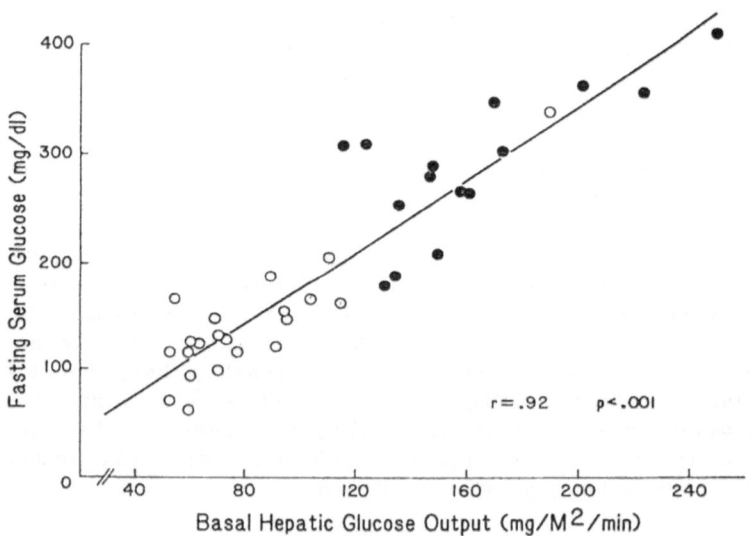

Fig. 11   Relationship between fasting serum glucose level and basal hepatic glucose production rate in NIDDM patients.

food. Thus, while normal subjects compensate for an increase in glucose influx by increasing glucose disposal, NIDDM patients cannot. Because of this, every incremental increase in basal HGO leads to a corresponding increase in the fasting glucose level. This formulation would also account for the marked elevations of postprandial glucose levels in NIDDM following increased glucose entry into the peripheral circulation from ingested food.

Reversibility of Insulin Resistance in NIDDM

One way to determine whether the insulin resistance of NIDDM is acquired is to conduct studies in cultured fibroblasts. These cells can be studied in tissue culture several generations removed from the in vivo milieu. Presumably abnormalities which persist in culture are primary or genetic, whereas those which disappear are secondary or acquired. As seen in Figure 12A and B, insulin binding and glucose transport are perfectly normal in fibroblasts cultured from patients with NIDDM. These results are in marked contrast to the findings in freshly isolated cells (Figures 4 and 10) and indicate that the cellular insulin resistance in NIDDM is acquired and therefore potentially reversible.

In this regard, recent evidence indicates that when NIDDM patients are treated with frequent insulin injections so as to achieve near normalization of the blood glucose level, the post-receptor defect can be substantially reversed.[48] This is seen in Figure 13 which compares the in vivo dose response curves in six patients before and after a two-week period of intensive insulin treatment (the dose-response curves of control subjects are also shown for comparison).

This period of intensive insulin treatment, which markedly improved glycemic control, did not change insulin binding to cells from these patients, this demonstrated that the treatment-induced increase in glucose disposal rates seen in Figure 13 is due to amelioration of a post-receptor defect in insulin action. Consistent with these in vivo results, studies of glucose transport on isolated adipocytes in these same patients before and after insulin treatment also reveal a marked reversal of the decreased maximal glucose transport rates (Figure 14). The pattern of improvement in vitro glucose transport corresponds closely to the in vivo improvement in overall glucose disposal further supporting the conclusion that it is the defect in glucose transport which is largely responsible for the post-receptor defect in NIDDM. From these results one can conclude that the post-receptor defect in NIDDM is acquired and at least partially reversible and, therefore, is secondary to some aspect of the chronic diabetic state, possibly the insulin deficiency.

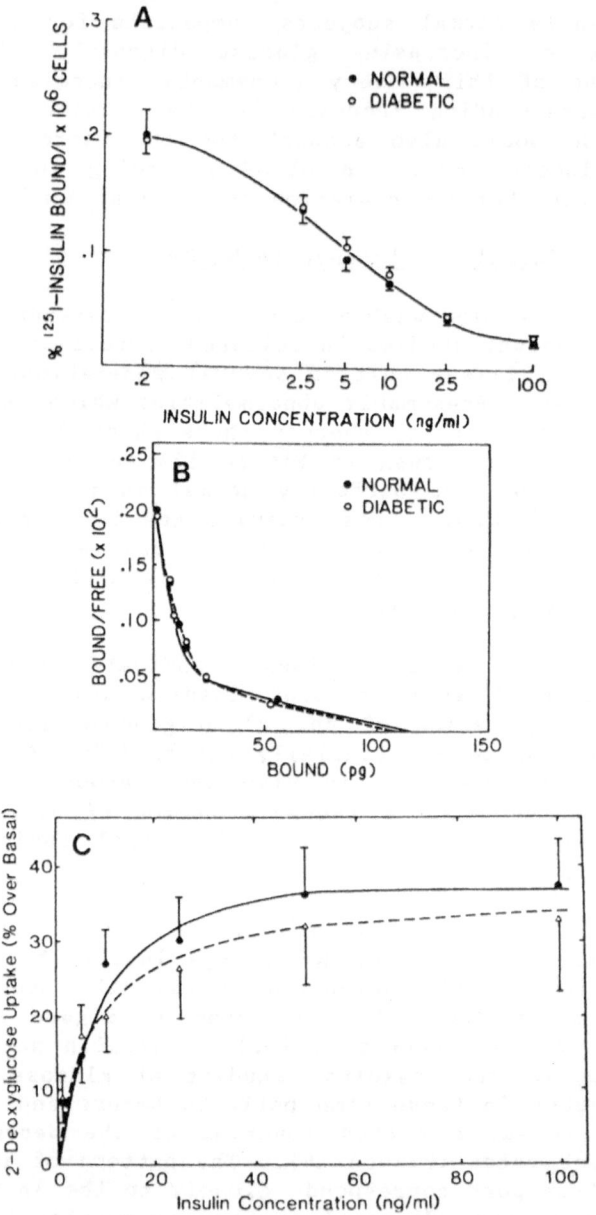

Fig. 12   A Comparison of ^{125}I-insulin binding in fibroblasts
from control and NIDDM subjects. Fibroblasts monolayers
from 8 control (●) and 8 NIDDM diabetic patients (O) were
incubated in the presence of ^{125}I-insulin (0.2 ng/ml)
plus various concentrations of unlabeled insulin for 3 h

(Continued on the next page)

at 16°C. Each point represents the mean ± SEM, and data are corrected for nonspecific binding. The data are expressed as % specific ^{125}I-insulin bound/10^6 cells. B. Scatchard analysis of ^{125}I-insulin binding to fibroblasts from control and NIDDM subjects. C. Effect of insulin concentration of 2-deoxy-D-glucose transport in fibroblasts from control and NIDDM subjects. Fibroblast monolayers from six control (●) and six NIDDM (Δ) subjects were incubated for 60 min at 37°C with the indicated concentrations of insulin. $[^3H]2$-deoxy-d-glucose transport (final concentration, 0.1mM) was then measured in triplicate over a 3 min period. The insulin-stimulated 2-deoxy-d-glucose uptake data are expressed as a percentage over basal (noninsulin-exposed) update values. Each point represents the mean ± SEM.

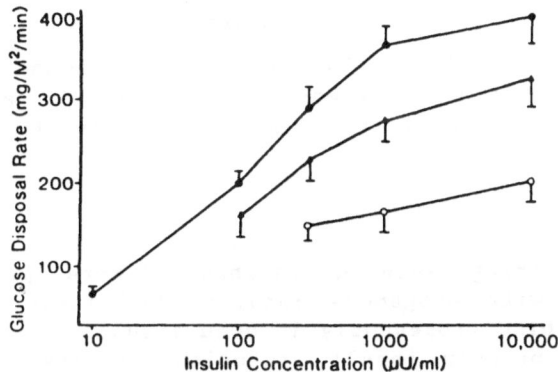

Fig. 13   Mean in vivo insulin dose-response curves for Type II diabetic subjects before (O) and after (▲) insulin treatment and for control subjects (●).

Insulin Resistance in IDDM

We have recently examined the issue of whether insulin resistance exists in IDDM and if so, whether it is related to the degree of control and is reversible. Some of the clinical and metabolic features of the study group are seen in Table 1. Subjects 1-5 all participated in home glucose monitoring two to four times daily, with frequent adjustments in insulin dosage. In contrast, subjects 6-10 assessed control by daily measurement of urinary glucose and maintained a relatively fixed insulin dosage. The hemoglobin A_1C levels in the latter group were significantly higher than those in the well controlled group (11.7 ± 0.6 vs 7.2 ± 0.2%; p < 0.001). As seen in Table 1, insulin antibodies were readily detectable in

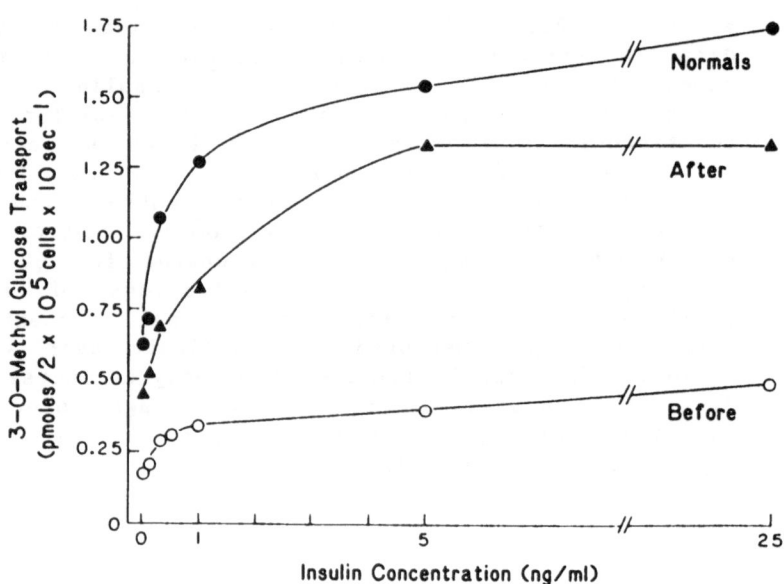

Fig. 14   Mean   in   vitro   insulin   dose-response   curves   for
           3-0-methylglucose transport before (O) and after (▲)
           insulin treatment and in normal subjects (●).

all patients.

     Since circulating insulin antibodies were present in all
patients treated with exogenous insulin (See Table 1), and since
these antibodies bind exogenously infused insulin, we first explored
the relationship between insulin infusion and the time course of
development of steady-state free insulin concentrations.   As can be
seen in Figure 15, steady-state serum insulin concentrations were
achieved within 25 min in normal subjects, whereas in the Type I
diabetic patients it took longer for the exogenous insulin to
equilibrate with the antibody space, and consequently, steady-state
levels of free insulin were not achieved until 90 min.   Therefore,
to compare insulin action in normal subjects and Type I diabetic
patients, it was necessary to carry out the glucose clamp studies
for at least 180 min.   Consequently, all of the glucose clamp
studies performed at each of the exogenous insulin infusion rates
were carried out until circulating free insulin concentrations had
reached a steady state and the effect of this steady state insulin
concentration to promote glucose metabolism had also plateaued.

     Using this approach, we performed 30 separate studies in 10
Type I diabetic patients in which the R_d (rate of glucose disposal) was determined under euglycemic conditions at a variety of
steady state serum insulin levels.   Using the mean values at each

Table 1. Clinical and metabolic characteristics of the diabetic patients studied.

Patient no.	Age (yr)	Sex	Ht (in.)	Wt (kg)	RBW Diabetics	Duration of diabetes (yr)	Glycosylated hemoglobin (%)	Antibody-binding capacity (mU/ml)
Well controlled type I diabetics								
1	39	M	75	205	1.06	1	7.5	259
2	37	M	68	194	1.17	8	7.6	1261
3	30	M	69	143	0.88	2	7.3	894
4	32	M	65	118	0.77	27	7.3	720
5	26	M	70	165	0.99	2	6.4	111
Mean ± SE	33 ± 2				0.97 ± 0.07	8 ± 5	7.2 ± 0.2	649 ± 210
Poorly controlled type I diabetics								
6	36	M	69	150	0.88	20	13.8	179
7	28	F	62	110	0.88	9	11.9	3726
8	22	F	64	116	0.90	1	11.5	439
9	31	M	67	160	0.99	6	9.9	1206
10	33	F	63	132	0.98	9	11.4	
Mean ± SE	30 ± 2				0.93 ± 0.02	9 ± 3	11.7 ± 0.6	1387 ± 810
Normal subjects	31 ± 1	9M 12F			0.96 ± 0.02		5.5 – 7.0	

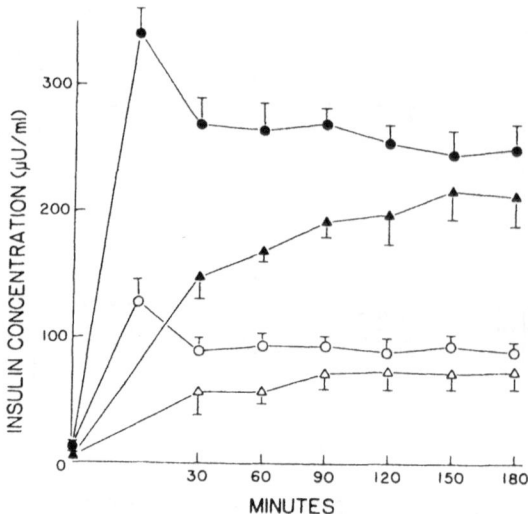

Fig. 15   Mean ± SE serum free insulin levels during euglycemic
glucose clamp studies: normal subjects (n = 21) at
insulin infusions at rates of 40 (O) and 120 (●) mU/M^2
· min vs Type I diabetic patients at 40 (Δ) and 120
(▲) mU/M^2 · min (n = 7 and 10, respectively).

insulin infusion rate, the in vivo dose-response curve was con-
structed for the 5 well controlled Type I diabetic patients and the
5 poorly controlled Type I diabetic patients and compared to the
results of similar studies in a group of 21 normal subjects (Figure
16).   The dose-response curve for well controlled diabetic subjects
was comparable to normal, with half-maximally effective insulin
levels of 84 µU/ml compared to 70 µU/ml in normal subjects and
virtually identical maximal R_d values (433 ± 11 vs 411 ± 17
mg/M^2 · min in normal subjects).   On the other hand, R_d values
were significantly reduced in the poorly controlled diabetic
patients at all insulin levels including maximally effective insulin
concentrations.   These data demonstrate that poorly controlled Type
I diabetic subjects are insulin resistant, whereas well controlled
Type I diabetic subjects are not insulin resistant, at least insofar
as insulin's ability to stimulate glucose uptake is concerned.

Basal hepatic glucose production was higher in the Type I diabetic patients than in normal subjects (132 ± 7, 101 ± 16, and
76 ± 7 mg/M^2 · min in the poorly controlled diabetic patients,
well controlled diabetic patients, and normal subjects,
respectively).   However, the suppressive effects of insulin were
quite comparable among all three groups, and hepatic glucose production was virtually 100% suppressed in all subjects at each infusion rate.   It should be noted that studies at low physiological

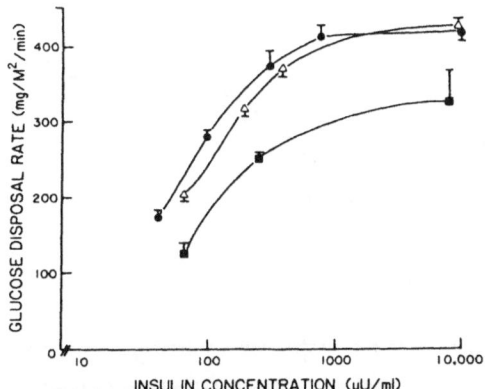

Fig. 16   Dose-response curve for insulin's ability to stimulate
           glucose disposal (milligrams per M^2 · min) in normal
           subjects (●), five well controlled Type I diabetic
           patients (Δ), and five poorly controlled Type I
           diabetic patients (■). Data represent the mean ± SE
           at each point.

insulin levels were not performed in the Type I diabetic patients,
and therefore, it is always possible that differences might have
been noted under these conditions.

Before and After Studies

     The above data indicated that in vivo insulin action was normal
in well controlled Type I diabetic patients, whereas poorly controlled patients were insulin resistant. Consistent with this, previous studies have indicated that insulin deficient dogs[45] and
rats[25] are insulin resistant. Therefore, to further assess the
effect of diabetic control on insulin resistance, we studied one
Type I diabetic patient at a time when he was in poor control and
then subsequently after good control was established with multiple
daily insulin injections.

     The results of glucose clamp studies conducted before and after
6 weeks of control achieved by insulin therapy are shown in Figure
17. At both insulin infusion rates employed, R_d values were
markedly reduced compared to those in normal subjects before insulin
therapy. After the 6-week period of insulin treatment, overall R_d
values increased to normal levels at all three insulin infusion
rates.

     These studies show that in vivo insulin action on glucose dis-
posal and suppression of hepatic glucose production was normal in
well controlled Type I diabetic patients. It should be noted, how-

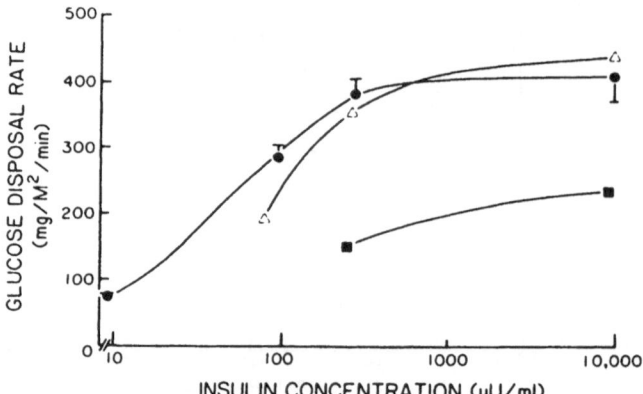

Fig. 17   Dose-response curve for insulin's ability to stimulate
glucose disposal (milligrams per M^2 · min) in normal
subjects (●) and in a poorly controlled Type I diabetic
patient before therapy (■) and after 6 weeks of
intensive insulin management (Δ).

ever, that while the ultimate steady state effect of insulin was
normal, the kinetics of the development of insulin's effect on glucose disposal were delayed in the Type I diabetic patients. The
reason for the delay is most likely due to the presence of circulating insulin antibodies, which prolong the time it takes for any
given rate of insulin infusion to produce a steady-state level of
free insulin. For this reason, R_d values did not reach their
maximal value until after 2-3 h of insulin infusion in the diabetic
patients.

The lack of inherent insulin resistance in well controlled Type
I diabetic patients is an important observation, in view of current
efforts to achieve tighter euglycemic control in these patients.
These results also raise the possibility that it may be useful to
take into account differences in the kinetics of insulin action due
to circulating insulin antibodies in designing the algorithms for
insulin administration. Although one patient was using a sc insulin
infusion system, none of our patients were maintained at euglycemic
conditions by their usual insulin regimens. Therefore, it is
unlikely that peripheral hyperinsulinemia was achieved, whereas this
phenomenon has been reported in Type I diabetic patients who were
kept at near-euglycemic levels with sc insulin delivery systems.[10]
In this latter situation, it is still possible that the peripheral
hyperinsulinemia would lead to an insulin-resistant state, either by
down-regulating cellular insulin receptors or causing desensitization
of insulin action at a post-receptor site.

These studies do not elucidate what aspect of this abnormal

metabolic environment causes the insulin resistance; however, they do suggest that the site of the insulin resistance may be located at a post-receptor locus. Thus, while under poor glycemic control, the IDDM subjects demonstrated markedly reduced R_d values at maximally effective insulin concentrations. Since these very high circulating insulin concentrations (10,000 μU/ml) would occupy enough receptors to elicit a maximal insulin response, the observed decrease in maximal glucose disposal most likely reflects a reversible abnormality distal to the initial insulin-binding step.

SUMMARY

The insulin resistance associated with NIDDM appears to be caused by decreased insulin binding in conjunction with a significant post-receptor defect in insulin action. In the untreated state, the post-receptor defect appears to be the predominant lesion and the magnitude of this post-receptor defect appears to correlate directly with the degree of fasting hyperglycemia in individual patients. In vitro studies using isolated adipocytes suggest that the post-receptor defect in insulin action resides at the level of the glucose transport system. Insulin treatment partially ameliorates the post-receptor defect in insulin action which suggests that it is an acquired defect secondary to some aspect of the altered metabolic state. In IDDM, insulin resistance due to a post-receptor defect exists in poorly controlled patients. However, this defect is entirely dependent upon the degree of glycemic control and is reversible with aggressive insulin therapy.

ACKNOWLEDGEMENT

This work was supported by funds from the Medical Research Service of the Veterans Administration, grant AM 33649 from the NIAMDD, NIH, and grant RR 00827 from the General Clinical Research Branch, NIH. The authors would like to thank Elizabeth Martinez for her secretarial assistance in preparing this manuscript.

REFERENCES

1. F.P. Alford, F.I. Martin, and M.J. Pearson, The significance and interpretation of mildly abnormal oral glucose tolerance, Diabetologia, 7:173-180 (1971).
2. R.S. Bar, P. Gordon, J. Roth, C.R. Kahn, and P. De Meyts, Fluctuations in the affinity and concentration of insulin receptors on circulating monocytes of obese patients: Effects of starvation, refeeding and dieting, J. Clin. Invest., 58:1123-1135 (1976).

3. R.S. Bar, W.R. Levis, M.M. Rechler, et al., Extreme insulin
    resistance in ataxia telangiectasis. Defect in affinity of
    insulin receptors, N. Engl. J. Med., 298:1165-1171 (1978).

4. H. Beck-Nielsen, The pathogeneic role of an insulin-receptor
    defect in diabetes mellitus of the obese, Diabetes,
    27:1175-1181 (1978).

5. H. Beck-Nielsen, O. Pedersen, and H.O. Lindskov, Increased
    insulin sensitivity and cellular insulin binding in obese dia-
    betics following treatment with glibenclamide, Acta
    Endocrinol., 90:451-462 (1979).

6. A. Bertoli, R. De Pirro, A. Fusco, et al., Differences in
    insulin receptors between men and menstruating women and
    influence of sex hormones on insulin binding during the
    menstrual cycle, J. Clin. Endocrinol. Metab., 50:246-250 (1980).

7. M.P. Czech, Molecular basis of insulin action, Annu. Rev.
    Biochem., 46:359-384 (1977).

8. M.P. Czech, Insulin action and the regulation of hexose
    transport, Diabetes, 29:399-409 (1980).

9. R. De Fronzo, D. Deibert, R. Hendler, P. Felig, and V. Soman,
    Insulin sensitivity and insulin binding to monocytes in
    maturity-onset diabetes, J. Clin. Invest., 63:939-946 (1979).

10. P. Felig, and M. Bergman, Intensive ambulatory treatment of
    insulin-dependent diabetes, Ann. Int. Med., 97:225-230 (1982).

11. J.S. Flier, C.R. Kahn, J. Roth, and R.S. Bar, Antibodies that
    impair insulin-receptor binding in an unusual diabetic syndrome
    with severe insulin resistance, Science, 190:63-65 (1975).

12. K.H. Gabbay, K. De Luca, J.N. Fisher Jr., M.E. Mako, and A.H.
    Rubenstein, Familial hyperproinsulinemia: an autosomal
    dominant defect, N. Engl. J. Med., 294:911-915 (1976).

13. H. Ginsberg, G. Kimmerling, J.M. Olefsky, and G.M. Reaven,
    Demonstration of insulin resistance in maturity-onset diabetic
    patients with fasting hyperglycemia, J. Clin Invest., 55:454-460
    (1975).

14. B.D. Given, M.E. Mako, H.S. Tager, et al., Diabetes due to sec-
    retion of an abnormal insulin, N. Engl. J. Med., 302:129-135
    (1980..

15. J. Gliemann, S. Gammeltoft, and J. Vinten, Time course of
    insulin-receptor binding and insulin-induced lipogenesis in
    isolated rat fat cells, J. Biol. Chem. 250:3368-3374 (1975).

16. C.R. Kahn, D.M. Neville Jr., and J. Roth, Insulin-receptor
    interaction in the obese-hyperglycemic mouse. A model of
    insulin resistance, J. Bio. Chem., 248:244-250 (1973).

17. C.R. Kahn, Membrane receptors for hormones and neuro-
    transmitters, J. Cell. Biol., 70:261-286 (1976).

18. C.R. Kahn, J.S. Flier, R.S. Bar, et al., The syndromes of
    insulin rsistance and acanthosis nigricans. Insulin-receptor
    disorders in man, N. Engl. J. Med., 294:739-745 (1976).

19. C.R. Kahn, K.L. Baird, J.S. Flier, and D.B. Jarrett, Effects of autoantibodies to the insulin receptor on isolated adipocytes: studies of insulin binding and insulin action, J. Clin. Invest., 60:1094-1166 (1977).

20. C.R. Kahn, Insulin resistance, insulin insensitivity, and insulin unresponsiveness: a necessary distinction, Metabolism, 27:1893-1902 (1978).

21. C.R. Kahn, I.D. Goldfine, D.M. Neville Jr., and P. De Meyts, Alterations in insulin binding induced by changes in vivo in the levels of glucocorticoids and growth hormone, Endocrinology, 103:1054-1066 (1978).

22. C.R. Kahn, and A.S. Rosenthal, Immunologic reactions to insulin: Insulin allergy, insulin resistance, and the autoimmune insulin syndome, Diabetes Care, 2:283-295 (1979).

23. H. Kalant, T.R. Csorba, and N. Heller, Effect of insulin on glucose production and utilization in diabetes, Metabolism, 12:1100-1111 (1963).

24. Y. Kanazawa, M. Hayashi, M. Kieuchi, K. Hirmatsu, and K. Kosaka, Familial proinsulinemia: a possible cause of abnormal glucose tolerance, Eur. J. Clin. Invest., 8:327 (1978) (Abstract).

25. M. Kobayashi, and J.M. Olefsky, Effects of streptozotocin-induced diabetes on insulin binding, glucose transport, and intracellular glucose metabolism in isolated rat adipocytes, Diabetes, 28:87-95 (1979).

26. O.G. Kolterman, J. Insel, M. Saekow, and J.M. Olefsky, Mechanisms of insulin resistance in human obesity - evidence for receptor and post-receptor defects, J. Clin. Invest., 65:1273-1284 (1980).

27. O.G. Kolterman, R.S. Gray, J. Griffin, et al., Receptor and post-receptor defects contribute to the insulin resistance in noninsulin dependent diabetes mellitus, J. Clin. Invest., 68:957-969 (1981).

28. T. Kono, and F.W. Barham, The relationship between the insulin-binding capacity of fat cells and the cellular response to insulin: Studies with intact and trypsin-treated fat cells, J. Biol. Chem., 246:6210-6216 (1971).

29. M. Muggeo, R.S. Bar, J. Roth, C.R. Kahn, and P. Gordon, The insulin resistance of acromegaly: evidence for two alterations in the insulin receptor on circulating monocytes, J. Clin. Endocrinol. Metab., 48:17-25 (1977).

30. J.M. Olefsky, and G.M. Reaven, Decreased insulin binding to lymphocytes from diabetic patients, J. Clin. Invest., 54:1323-1328 (1974).

31. J.M. Olefsky, J. Johnson, F. Liu, P. Jen, and G.M. Reaven, The effects of acute and chronic dexamethasone administration on insulin binding to isolated rat hepatocytes and adipocytes, Metabolism, 24:517-527 (1975).

32. J.M. Olefsky, The insulin receptor: Its role in insulin
     resistance in obesity and diabetes, Diabetes, 25:1154-1165
     (1976).

33. J.M. Olefsky, Effects of fasting on insulin binding, glucose
     transport, and glucose oxidation in isolated rat adipocytes:
     Relationships between insulin receptors and insulin action, J.
     Clin. Invest., 58:1450-1460 (1976).

34. J.M. Olefsky, and G.M. Reaven, Insulin binding in diabetes:
     Relationships with plasma insulin levels and insulin sensi-
     tivity, Diabetes, 26:6806-88 (1977).

35. J.M. Olefsky, Insulin antagonists and resistance, in "Diabetes
     Mellitus: Theory and Practice", Ed. 3, H. Rifkin, M. Ellenberg
     (eds)., Medical Examination Publishing Co., Inc., New York.

36   J.M. Olefsky, The insulin receptor: Physiology and patho-
     physiology, in: "Current Concepts," The Upjohn Company,
     Kalamazoo (1980), pp 1-47.

37. J.M. Olefsky, M. Saekow, H. Tager, and A.H. Rubenstein, Char-
     acterization of a mutant human insulin species, J. Biol. Chem.,
     255:6098-6105 (1980).

38. J.M. Olefsky, Insulin resistance and insulin action: an in
     vitro and in vivo perspective, Diabetes, 20:148-162 (1981).

39. J.M. Olefsky, and O.G. Kolterman, Mechanisms of insulin resis-
     tance in obesity and noninsulin-dependent (Type II) diabetes,
     Am. J. Med., 70:151-168 (1981).

40. J.M. Olefsky, and T.P. Ciaraldi, The insulin receptor: Basic
     characteristics and its role in insulin resistant state, in
     "Diabetes Mellitus," Vo. 2, M. Brownlee, ed., Garland STPM
     Press, New York (1981)

41. J.M. Olefsky, Extrapancreatic factors: Insulin resistance in
     obesity and diabetes mellitus, in "Diabetes Mellitus: A Patho-
     physiologic Approach to Clinical Practice," E. Marliss, ed.,
     John Wiley and Sons, New York (in press).

42. S. Oseid, H. Beck-Nielsen, and O. Pedersen, Decreased binding
     of insulin to its receptor in patients with congenital general-
     ized lipodystrophy, N. Engl. J. Med., 296:245-248 (1977).

43. P.J. Randle, C.N. Hales, P.B. Garland, and E.A. Newsholme, The
     glucose fatty-acid cycle. Its role in insulin sensitivity and
     the metabolic disturbances of diabetes mellitus, Lancet,
     1:785-789 (1963).

44. G.M. Reaven, R. Bernstein, B. Davis, and J.M. Olefsky, Non-
     ketotic diabetes mellitus: Insulin deficiency or insulin
     resistance? Am. J. Med., 60:80-88 (1976).

45. G.M. Reaven, W.S. Sageman, and R.S. Swenson, Development of
     insulin resistance in normal dogs following alloxan-induced
     insulin deficiency, Diabetologia, 13:459-462 (1977).

46. J. Roth, C.R. Kahn, M.A. Lesniak, et al., Receptors for
     insulin, NSILA-s and growth hormone: Applications to disease
     states in man, Recent Prog. Horm. Res., 31:95-139 (1975).

47. G.M. Reaven, and J.M. Olefsky, The role of insulin resistance
     in the pathogenesis of diabetes mellitus, <u>Adv. Metab. Disord.</u>,
     9:313-331 (1978).
48. J.A. Scarlett, R.S. Gray, J. Griffin, J.M. Olefsky, and O.G.
     Kolterman, Insulin treatment reverses the insulin resistance of
     Type II diabetes mellitus, <u>Diabetes Care</u>, 5:353-363 (1982).
49. H. Tager, B. Given, D. Baldwin, et al., A structurally abnormal
     insulin causing human diabetes, <u>Nature</u>, 281:122-125 (1979).
50. K.L. Zierler, and D. Rabinowitz, Roles of insulin and growth
     hormone, based on studies of forearm metabolism in man,
     <u>Medicine</u>, 42:385-402 (1963).

INSULIN-MEDIATED AND NON-INSULIN-MEDIATED METABOLIC EFFECTS OF GASTROENTEROPANCREATIC PEPTIDES IN TYPE I AND TYPE II DIABETES

J. Dupre, A. Baer, M. Lee, T.J. McDonald,
J. Radziuk, N.W. Rodger, and S. Sullivan

Department of Medicine
University of Western Ontario
London, Ontario, Canada

INTRODUCTION

The recognition of secretion as a physiological regulator of the exocrine secretions of the pancreas in 1902 led to generalization of the concept of hormonal control of digestive sections,[1] and excited interest in such mechanisms as possible mediators of the functions of the pancreas in control of glycemia.[2] According to the "incretin" hypothesis, hormones released from the gastrointestinal tract in response to ingestion of nutrients serve to activate the glucoregulatory function of the pancreas.[3] With the later identification of insulin as a hormonal effector of these functions, the hypothesis was adapted by suggesting that incretin stimulates insulin secretion. A variety of experiments with crude extracts of gastrointestinal tissues yielded conflicting results[4], and following the recognition of direct effects of glucose on the release of insulin interest in incretin waned. However in the early 1960's it was recognized that the glycemic stimulus to insulin secretion cannot account for differences in blood insulin levels after enteral and parenteral administration of glucose, which are also accompanied by apparent differences in glucose disposal.[5,6] These observations revived the hormonal hypothesis for stimulation of the beta cells by gastrointestinal factors, and a renewed search for candidate peptides that might fill this role was undertaken. Studies of these phenomena have yielded evidence related to the pathophysiology of disorders of intermediary metabolism in diabetes, with indications of differences between Type I and Type II diabetes in this context. However, before discussing the identification of incretins it is necessary to consider the question whether the hypothetical enteroinsular axis is necessary or suffcient to account for differences in glucose homeostasis observed with enteral and parenteral administration of the sugar, and whether mechanisms other than those simply dependent on portal perfusion of the liver and/or the recognized effects of insulin must be invoked.

PHYSIOLOGICAL SIGNIFICANCE OF EFFECTS OF ROUTE OF ADMINISTRATION OF GLUCOSE ON THE GLYCEMIC RESPONSE

Importance of hepatic extraction of glucose

The greater excursion of the concentration of glucose in the blood after parenteral delivery of glucose compared with that after delivery of similar loads into the gastrointestinal tract seemed readily attributable to hepatic extraction of glucose from portal venous blood, which would favour disposal of glucose entering from the gut. This presumption was maintained, in spite of the lack of support from early attempts to validate it based on determinations of hepatic glycogen content after delivery of glucose by the different routes.[7] Later comparisons of the glycemic response to delivery of glucose into systemic or portal veins in anesthetized[8] or conscious experimental animals[9] showed very little difference between glucose tolerance or the insulin responses following delivery of the sugar by the different routes. With the development and validation of tracer techniques for use in the non-steady state it was possible to test this question in man.[10] It transpires that the initial hepatic extraction of glucose entering by way of the gastrointestinal tract and portal venous system is <10% and cannot account for observed differences in oral and intravenous glucose "tolerance".[11] It follows that glucose "tolerance" and the distribution of glucose among tissues competing for its uptake from the systemic pool, a competition in which the liver features as a "peripheral" tissue, must be determined by regulatory factors operating on disposal from this pool.

Uptake of glucose in the limbs

The question whether insulin is a major determinant of the distribution of glucose in physiologic conditions can be studied by examining the uptake of glucose in limb tissues under conditions of intestinal and parenteral delivery of glucose. In such studies in the human forearm it has been shown that the uptake of glucose is greater during intestinal absorption of glucose than during parenteral delivery of glucose, in spite of the higher arterial concentrations of glucose obtained with parenteral delivery.[12] The question whether this difference is simply attributable to the higher arterial concentrations of insulin that prevail with intestinal delivery of the sugar has also been addressed in studies of the forearm uptake of glucose. It was shown that simulation of the concentrations of insulin in arterial blood that are observed during

absorption of glucose from the gut, by means of supplementary infusion of insulin together with parenteral infusion of glucose,
resulted in uptake of glucose in the forearm closely matching that
observed after ingestion of glucose with comparable glycemia.[13]
Thus it appears that enteroinsular potentiation of insulin secretion
is largely responsible for the difference between the rates of
uptake of glucose in the limbs after oral and parenteral administration of glucose.

Non-insulin-dependent actions of intestinal factors in control of glucose disposal

The available evidence increasingly suggests that Type I
diabetes mellitus in the fully developed condition, with virtual
absence of endogenous secretion of insulin, represents a hormone
deficiency state in which optimized treatment with insulin can
largely correct the recognized metabolic disorders. In relation to
attempts to determine whether mechanisms initiated in the intestine
other than those leading to enhancement of insulin secretion are
important in glucose homeostasis, the finding that initial hepatic
extraction of glucose from portal blood is of little quantitative
significance in glucose disposal validates comparisons of the
effects of delivery of glucose by the intestinal and parenteral
routes under conditions of optimal replacement treatment with
insulin. With the development of continuous subcutaneous insulin
infusion programs capable of resulting in longterm near-
normalization of glycemic control, such experiments have become
feasible.[14] We have examined the effect of delivery of identical
infusions of glucose by way of duodenal or superficial vein
catheters in volunteers with C-peptide negative Type I diabetes
mellitus, studied in the course of long term replacement treatment
with insulin by means of continuous subcutaneous insulin infusion.
In these experiments the glucose infusions were given after overnight fast with continuation of the basal infusions of insulin, and
with delivery of supplements of insulin before the administration of
the glucose loads, using the doses determined empirically in control
of prandial glycemia in these subjects. It was found that the blood
glucose levels resulting from delivery of glucose by the different
routes were similar in time course and magnitude. The levels of
free immunoreactive insulin and immunoreactive glucagon in the blood
under these conditions on the two occasions were not significantly
different. It therefore appears that intestinal mechanisms are not
important in glycemic control when similar levels of exogenous
insulin in the systemic blood are imposed. Since the first-pass
extraction of glucose by the liver during absorption of glucose from
the gut in normal subjects is very low,[11] it also seems that the
effects of relative portal hyperglycemia and hyperinsulinemia that
obtain under physiological conditions during absorption of glucose
from the gut do not confer a major advantage on the liver in the
dispoal of glucose entering from the gut. It is therefore suggested

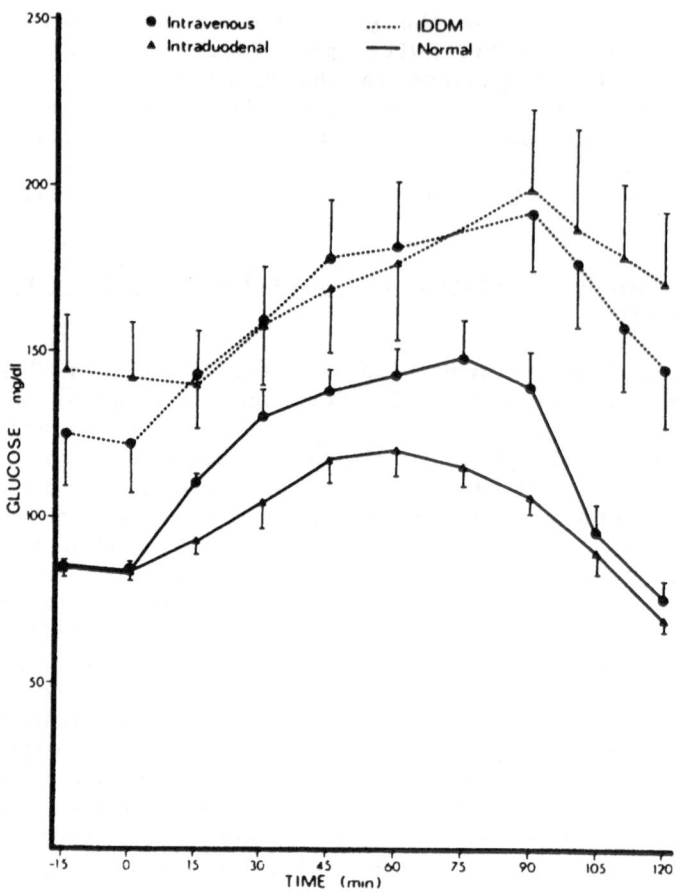

Fig. 1   The figure illustrates mean plasma glucose concentrations
in 6 normal volunteers (solid lines) and 6 subjects with
IDDM rate infusions of glucose (Total 30 gm) in the postabsorptive state at breakfast time.   On one occasion the
infusion was given IV (circle symbols) and on the other it
was given intraduodenally (triangle symbols).   The subjects
with IDDM were receiving continuous subcutaneous infusions
of insulin at rates maintaining the plasma glucose in the
range illustrated and received their usual pre-breakfast
supplementary dose of insulin as a bolus dose at 0 time on
both occasions.   It can be seen in the normal subjects that
the glycemic excursion was significantly reduced when the
infusion was delivered into the duodenum.   In the diabetic
volunteers under the same conditions the mean plasma
glucose curves were not distinguishable on the two occasions.   The plasma levels of free immunoreactive insulin
(not shown) were similar on the two occasions in the volunteers with IDDM, and were significantly higher on the
occasion of intraduodenal infusion in the normal subjects.

that enteroinsular potentiation of insulin secretion is the major determinant of differences between oral and parenteral glucose tolerance in normal man (Fig. 1).

IDENTIFICATION OF INCRETINS

Studies with the identified intestinal peptides believed to serve hormonal functions in control of the exocrine secretions of the gut showed that several of these are pharmacologically capable of stimulating insulin secretion. Thus secretin, gastrin, and cholecystokinin-pancreozymin were shown to potentiate the stimulation of insulin secretion by glucose in various experimental conditions.[15,16]

In assessment of the potential physiologic roles of these peptides, the approach generally taken was that of the so-called copying experiment, in which observed meal-stimulated increments of the peptide in question in the plasma are simulated by parenteral delivery of the purified agent, with examination of its effects on the response to concurrent parenteral delivery of the nutrient. By this approach it appeared that secretin, gastrin and cholecystokinin-pancreozymin are not individually qualified to account for enteroinsular potentiation of the response to glucose in test animals or in man. However, after gastric inhibitory polypeptide was identified in the search for the physiological inhibitor of gastric acid secretion (defined as enterogastrone),[17] examination of its pharmacological properties in animals showed that it is capable of stimulating release of insulin and also glucagon from the pancreas.[18] Furthermore, the copying experiment with highly purified GIP suggested that simulation of the increments of plasma immunoreactive GIP that occur after ingestion of glucose in normal man by means of parenteral infusion of the peptide results in potentiation of insulin secretion.[19] Accordingly this agent appeared to be qualified as a participant in physiologic enteroinsular mechanisms of the hormonal type.

Gastric inhibitory polypeptide as a physiological incretin

The copying experiment is designed to test the question whether the agent selected for study is capable on its own of accounting for the physiologic effect under consideration. The techniques applied to this problem in relation to the role of GIP as a physiological incretin involve two assumptions, the first that endogenous immunoreactive GIP is identical with the exogenous test agent, and the second that the prevailing glycemia is within the physiological range. Recognition of the heterogeneity of immunoreactive GIP in the plasma weakens the first assumption. With respect to the second assumption, recent studies of the interactions of GIP and glucose in man suggest that the potentiation of the response of the beta cell to glucose at concentrations of the sugar within the physiologic range is not sufficient to account for observed physiologic insulin responses.   Such considerations have led to questioning of the suggestion that GIP can account for enteroinsular potentiation of the response to the ingestion of glucose in man.[20]   It is important to note that arguments of this kind cannot exclude a major contribution of the agent in question to the physiologic response. Thus interactions with other hormonal agents or with other mechanisms of potentiation of insulin secretion are probably involved in the system, so complicating interpretation of studies designed to support or reject the role of single agents proposed as mediators.   It is apparent that the role of GIP in regulation of insulin secretion in the normal response to ingestion of carbohydrate or of mixed meals has yet to be fully clarified.

PATHOPHYSIOLOGY OF THE ENTEROINSULAR AXIS IN DIABETES

The enteroinsular axis in diabetes and obesity

Recognition of the enteroinsular axis led to interest in its expression in disorders of carbohydrate metabolism, particularly diabetes mellitus.   It has been shown that apparent enteroinsular potentiation of insulin secretion is preserved in obesity with or without glucose intolerance, and in non-insulin-dependent diabetes with or without obesity.[21]   The net operation of the axis in non-insulin-dependent diabetes with or without obesity was demonstrated in studies of the responses of insulin in the blood when matching glycemic excursions were elicited by oral and parenteral glucose loads.   The greater insulin responses observed when glucose was taken by mouth under these conditions in subjects with normal glucose tolerance, whether obese or non-obese, showed that potentiation of the insulin response to a given glucose stimulus is responsible to a major extent for the exaggerated increase of insulin in the blood in obese subjects.   Thus in non-insulin-dependent diabetics with moderate fasting hyperglycemia (not treated with insulin) the enteroinsular mechanism is clearly operative. Increased insulin responses in obesity are apparent with parenteral delivery of glucose and thus are not simply due to the immediate operation of enteroinsular mechanisms.   It is important to note also that interpretation of the relative doses or oral and parenteral glucose necessary for production of given glycemic excursions in terms of hepatic uptake or distribution of glucose[21] are not warranted in the presence of different blood levels of insulin with the two routes of administration of sugar.

Pathophysiology of GIP in diabetes

With the development of radioimmunoassays for gastric inhibitory polypeptide the functions of this hormone have been examined in studies of the response to ingestion of glucose in non-insulin-dependent diabetes mellitus.

Studies of this kind have yielded evidence of relative hyper-secretion of GIP, inferred from greater increases of immunoreactive GIP in the blood on ingestion of glucose loads.[22,23] Similarly exaggerated responses of GIP have been observed after ingestion of mixed meals in non-insulin-dependent diabetes.[24]. This type of abnormality is also found in obesity with normal glucose toler-ance.[24] These findings appear to be consistent with the hypothetical regulatory interaction between GIP as an incretin, and insulin, so that exaggerated responses of the intestinal "trophic" hormone occur in the presence of relative or absolute deficiency of the response of the beta cell to combined stimulation by glucose and GIP.[25] However, attempts to confirm feed-back inhibition of glucose-stimulated GIP secretion with physiologic doses of insulin in man have not been successful.[26] This failure may be due in part to the hyperinsulinemia that prevailed under the conditions of the experiments, but this question remains to be clarified.[27] Thus the significance of apparent abnormalities of the "suppression" of GIP by insulin in obesity or diabetes is obscure.

Comparison of the responses of GIP to ingestion of meals in Type I and Type II diabetes mellitus

Studies of the responses of plasma immunoreactive GIP to inges-tion of nutrients in diabetes in man have been difficult to inter-pret because of the variability of glycemic control of the subjects before and at the time of study, and because of imprecise charac-terization of the subjects in terms of endogenous insulin secretory capacity and "type" of diabetes. We have compared the responses of plasma immunoreactive GIP after ingestion of standard meals in groups of non-obese diabetics, comparing those with absent or negli-gible endogenous secretion of insulin (absent C-peptide response to IV glucagon), and those with non-ketosis-prone diabetes who retained demonstrable insulin responses to meals (C-peptide responses to IV glucagon also demonstrable).[28] All subjects were maintained with near-normoglycemia by means of longterm continuous subcutaneous insulin infusion with empirically determined supplementary doses of insulin before meals. They were first studied after overnight fast with their basal insulin infusions continuing through the tests, and with administration of the standard supplement before the test meal. The study was repeated in the C-peptide negative volunteers with continuation of the basal infusion but with omission of the pre-meal supplementary dose of insulin. In the other group of subjects (C-peptide positive), in repetition of the study the program of CSII was interrupted for at least 24 hours with no delivery of exogenous insulin before the meal. In the studies in which euglycemia was maintained with the CSII program including the pre-meal supplements in both groups, the responses of plasma immuno-

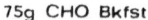

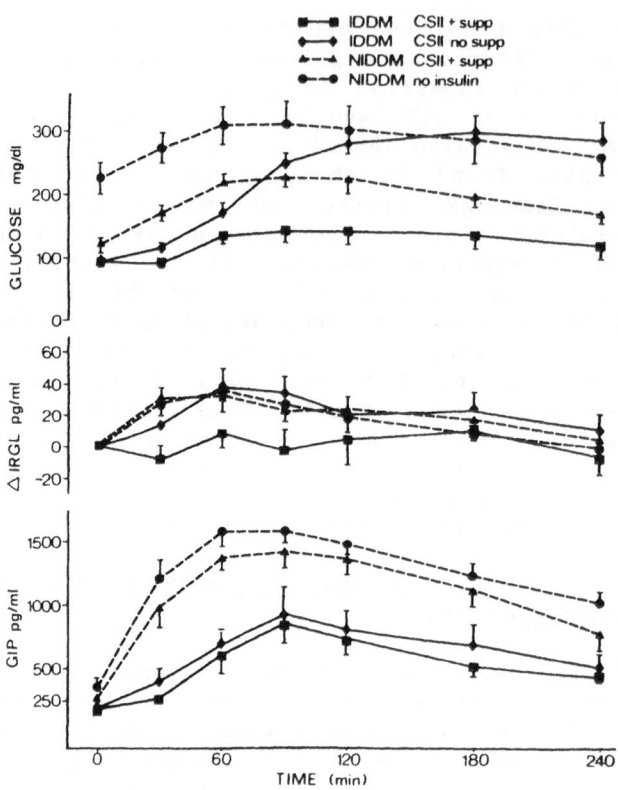

Fig. 2   The volunteers in this study (7 with IDDM and 6 with NIDDM)
          ingested a standard 75 gm carbohydrate breakfast after
          overnight fast, on two occasions, under the following
          conditions, in varied order.   The subjects with IDDM were
          treated   with   longterm   continuous   subcutaneous   insulin
          infusion and with an empirical breakfast-time supplement
          delivered before the meal on one occasion, and omitted on
          the other occasion.   The subjects with NIDDM were in
          similar longterm insulin infusion programs: on one occasion
          they received the continuous infusion together with their
          usual   supplement   and   on   the   other   occasion   insulin
          treatment was withdrawn altogether for 24-48 hours before
          the test meal.   It can be seen that there was good control
          of glycemia in IDDM and NIDDM when the continuous infusion
          was delivered together with the supplement, though it is
          apparent that glycemic control was superior in those with
          IDDM.   When the supplementary dose of insulin was omitted

(continued on next page)

in the subjects with IDDM, the blood glucose rose to abnormally high levels after the breakfast. When insulin treatment was omitted in the subjects with NIDDM, fasting hyperglycemia developed and the peak glycemic levels attained after the breakfast were similar to those in the group of IDDM subjects on the occasion when no insulin supplement was delivered with the meal. It can be seen from the third panel that immunoreactive GIP responses were similar on the two occasions in each group but were significantly lower in the IDDM subjects by comparison with the NIDDM subjects. The centre panel shows the change in immunoreactive glucagon from the 0 time levels which were not significantly different in the two groups or on the two occasions. It can be seen that there was a mean rise in plasma immunoreactive glucagon concentration after the test meal on both occasions in the subjects with NIDDM, as well as in the subjects with IDDM on the occasion when the pre-meal insulin supplement was ommitted. However when the subjects with IDDM received the supplement together with the basal infusion, with optimized control of glycemia, there was no significant deviation of plasma immunoreactive glucagon levels from the 0 time value, as in normal subjects (not shown).

reactive GIP were substantially greater in the C-peptide-positive group than in the C-peptide-negative group. When the supplementary dose of insulin was omitted in C-peptide negative patients there was no significant modification of the response of plasma IRGIP, although there was obvious loss of glycemic control. In the C-peptide-positive subjects the omission of insulin treatment resulted in fasting hyperglycemia and obvious glucose intolerance after the meal, but the response of plasma immunoreactive GIP was again not significantly different from that observed during strict glycemic control. These studies demonstrate a significant difference between the GIP responses of truly insulin deficient diabetics and those with obvious residual insulin secretory capacity. The studies failed to demonstrate an acute effect of exogenous insulin on the responses of GIP to the meal in the two groups. These findings support the suggestion that the secretion of GIP in response to meals differs in Type I and Type II diabetes, and show that this difference is preserved under conditions of equivalent and optimal metabolic control. The prevailing levels of free immunoreactive insulin in the blood in the two groups of subjects during insulin therapy with meal supplements were similar in the postabsorptive and fed states. This, together with the lack of effect of short-term deprival of insulin, suggests that the differences in the GIP responses of the two types of diabetes are not simply dependent on the concentrations of insulin in systemic blood. The pathophysiologic significance of the differences in plasma levels of

GIP in the two conditions is discussed further below (Fig. 2).

NON-INSULIN-MEDIATED METABOLIC EFFECTS OF GIP

Glucagon and the enteroinsular axis

Studies of the pharmacologic effects of GIP in animals demonstrated the capacity of this peptide to stimulate the release of glucagon as well as insulin from the pancreas in vivo and in vitro.[18] It has been suggested that paradoxical increases of immunoreactive glucagon in the blood after meals in diabetic man might be due to the glucagonotropic action of GIP.[29] Such increases in immunoreactive glucagon in the blood are small and difficult to detect with available assays. Studies with infusion of GIP in human volunteers with hyperglucagonemia associated with cirrhosis of the liver have demonstrated that GIP can elicit a rise of immunoreactive glucagon in the blood.[30] This immunoreactive glucagon can be characterized by chromatography and was shown to be similar to pancreatic glucagon. In studies in volunteers with C-peptide negative Type I diabetes mellitus after ingestion of mixed meals we have found no significant increments of plasma immuno- reactive glucagon in subjects maintained in normoglycemia by long- term CSII with administration of insulin supplements before the meals.[31] However, with omission of supplementary insulin, in spite of continuation of the basal insulin infusion these subjects show increases of plasma immunoreactive glucagon after their meals. In subjects with Type I diabetes mellitus, confirmed to be C-peptide negative and receiving conventional once or twice daily depot therapy with insulin, abnormal increases of plasma IRG after mixed meals were also demonstrable. Since similar increases of plasma IRG occur after ingestion of glucose in Type I diabetes mellitus during longterm CSII when supplementary doses of insulin are not given before the meal, and since increases of plasma IRG are not seen after parenteral infusion of glucose under these conditions, it appears that these abnormal responses of immunoreactive glucagon in Type I diabetes may be due to enteroinsular mechanisms, although a contribution from glucagon-like immunoreactants of enteric origin cannot be excluded.

A similar abnormality of plasma IRG has been described in Type II diabetes, and in this condition there is preliminary evidence suggesting that administration of GIP can elicit increases of IRG in the blood.[25] Moreover, while intensive insulin replacement treat- ment by means of CSII in Type I diabetes can suppress the response of plasma IRG after meals, similar regimens failed to produce this effect in preliminary studies of Type II diabetes.[28] Enteroin- sular stimulation of glucagon secretion in Type I and Type II diabetes mellitus under conditions of suboptimal or non-physiologic replacement treatment with insulin may be of pathophysiological importance, especially after ingestion of protein,[32] and the possible role of GIP in this context remains to be clarified.

Gastrointestinal factors in the insulin resistance of diabetes mellitus

The observation that plasma immunoreactive GIP is abnormally elevated after meals in Type II diabetes and in obesity in man led to the suggestion that this agent may contribute to development of insulin resistance as a consequence of excessive stimulation of insulin secretion.[24] Studies of diurnal plasma levels of IRGIP in man with adherence to normal feeding patterns show that concentration of the hormone is elevated above the postabsorptive baseline for most of the 24 hour period. It has therefore been questioned whether high blood levels of GIP maintained through prolonged periods may have effects other than those favouring glucose disposal through its action on the pancreatic beta cell. We have examined the effects of exogenous GIP given by longterm intravenous infusion in rats.[33] In this experiment the rats were fed by constant-rate infusions of weight-maintaining mixtures of amino acids and glucose. The infusions were delivered by way of permanent catheters placed in the duodenum in one group of rats, and in a central vein in two other groups. One of the groups of rats receiving the central vein infusions were administered GIP by the same route in doses resulting in plasma IRGIP levels similar to those dependent on endogenous secretion in the rats receiving duodenal nutrient infusions. The studies were carried out through a period of six days with the animals under minimal restraint in metabolic cages. It was found that parenteral nutrition with concurrent infusion of GIP resulted in development of a hyperglycemic hyperinsulinemic state. The rats receiving the nutrient infusion by way of the intestine maintained similarly elevated levels of GIP throughout the study, but achieved near-normoglycemia with low levels of insulin in the blood. The rats receiving parenteral nutrition without infusion of GIP developed modestly elevated plasma levels of both glucose and insulin. Thus administration of GIP in parenterally fed rats produced a glucose intolerant and apparently insulin resistant state that was not elicited by the other treatments. One conclusion from this experiment, making the assumption that the relative hyperglycemia of the animals receiving this peptide was not attributable to stimulation of glucose production, was that porcine GIP may cause insulin resistance in the rat (see below). The absence of this condition in the intestinally fed rats with similarly elevated levels of endogenous GIP in the blood might be due to differences between the two species of GIP, or to counter-balancing mechanisms elicited by intestinal delivery of food in the enterally fed rats. These findings add plausibility to the hypothesis that hypersecretion of GIP in over-fed subjects, or in Type II diabetes in man, may be a factor in the generation of insulin resistance in these conditions. The lower levels of IRGIP

in the blood in Type I diabetes by comparison with Type II diabetes
under similar degrees of metabolic control, as described above, are
consistent with the lesser degree of insulin resistance generally
found in Type I diabetes by comparison with Type II diabetes in
man. These results suggest that the degrees to which the insulin
resistance of diabetes and of obesity are dependent on enteral as
opposed to parenteral nutrition need to be assessed.

NON-HORMONAL MECHANISMS OF ACTION OF GASTROENTEROPANCREATIC PEPTIDES IN CONTROL OF METABOLISM

The recognition that similar or identical biologically active
peptides may be produced in cells with different modes of delivery
of these agents to the target tissues (Fig. 3) calls for
consideration of the possible interactions among these various
mechanisms under physiological conditions (Fig. 4). Such
interactions may involve aminergic and peptidergic mechanisms in
afferent and efferent limbs linking the gut and the target tissues,
including the endocrine pancreas. Fully satisfactory experimental
approaches to the study of these questions are not available at the
present time. It is nevertheless important to recognize that it is
not reasonable on physiologic grounds to search for a single
mechanism or agent capable of accounting for any given response. In
the context of studies of regulatory functions of gastroenteropancreatic peptides these considerations are futher illustrated by
the recognition of the actions of newly discovered members of this
family of peptides.

Gastrin-releasing polypeptide (GRP)

This peptide was identified as an agent with gastric-acid-
stimulating properties, found in extracts of hog stomach and
duodenum.[34] It is the mammalian analogue of avian bombesin, and
appears to be a neuropeptide, present in the central nervous system
as well as in nervous elements in the gastrointestinal tract and the
pancreas. In relation to the control of pancreatic endocrine
function, pharmacologically it is capable of causing release of
insulin and glucagon from the pancreas, and can stimulate the
release of other endocrine polypeptides, inculding GIP.[35] When
given by intravenous infusion in animals the transient release of
insulin that follows is associated with the expected changes in
glucose turnover, as detected by tracer techniques, and the
potential for participation in the neural control of pancreatic
endocrine function is evident. It is clear that this potential
cannot be assessed by means of simple pharmacologic experiments with
systemic administration of GRP alone. The possible interactions of
this peptide with hormonal and other mechanisms involved in the
glucoregulatory functions of the pancreas remain to be determined.

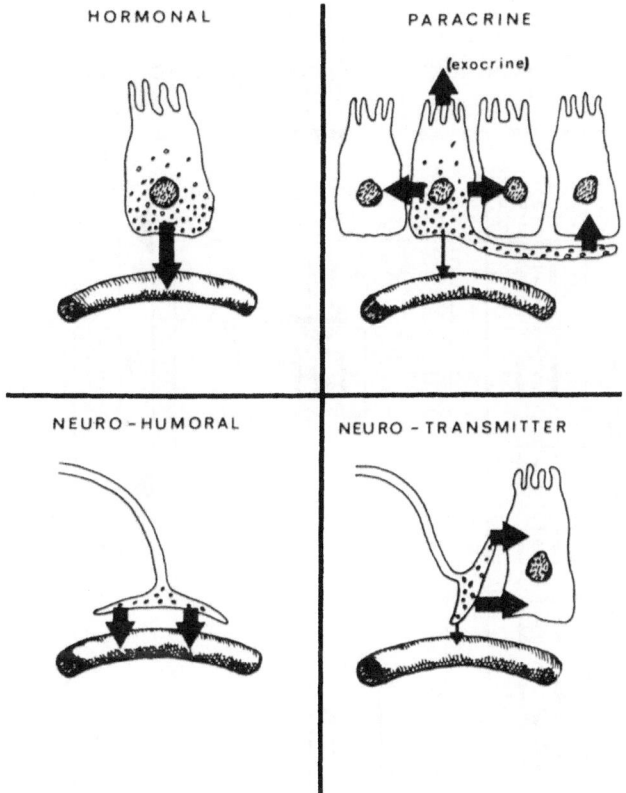

Fig. 3   This figure illustrates the several modes of delivery of
          biologically active regulatory peptides or amines. The
          hormonal, neurohumoral and neurotransmitter modes of action
          are familiar. The scheme illustrating the neurotransmitter
          mode of delivery includes indication of possible "spillage"
          of the neurotransmitter into the venous drainage. The
          illustration of the paracrine mode of action indicates the
          possible exercise of this effect through cell processes,
          and also indicates the possibility of "spillage" into
          venous effluent. This section of the diagram also illus-
          trates the exocrine mode of secretion; the exercise of
          regulatory effects on cells at-a-distance through this
          route has not yet been clearly demonstrated.

Galanin

     In the screening of peptides derived from gastrointestinal
tissues for possible effects in intermediary metabolism a different
type of action has recently been identified. The peptide now known
as "galanin" was isolated in systematic pharmacologic studies of

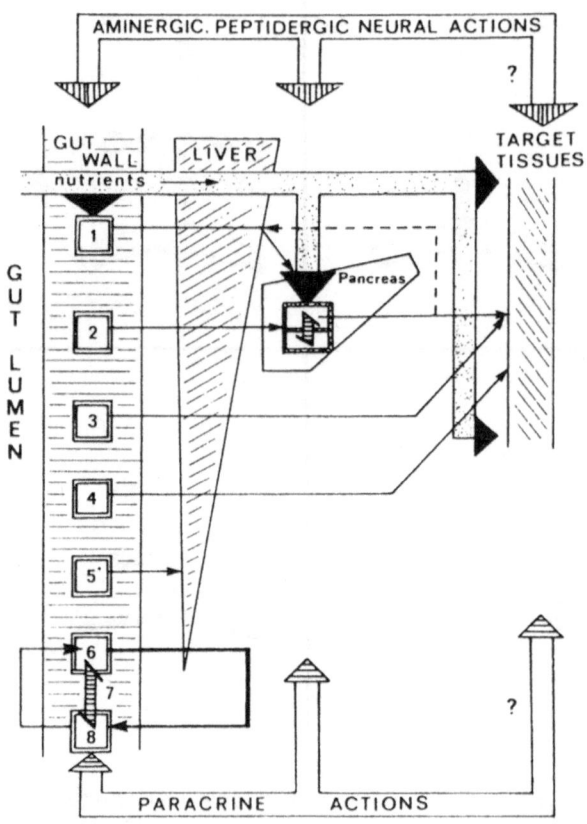

Fig. 4   This scheme illustrates the variety of ways by which
regulatory agents released from specialized sources in the
gut wall may reach the various target tissues, and
indicates a number of possible interactions among these
agents. All of them may interact with the nutrient at the
level of the various target cells. All of them may
interact with aminergic and peptidegic neural control
mechanisms in which the agents are delivered through that
system. It is also indicated that paracine actions and
interactions may take place. In the case of humoral
mechanisms 1-6, the agents have to traverse the liver,
where they may also exert actions. The model of feedback
inhibition of release of humoral agents is illustrated for
mechanism 1, in which a gut hormone acts on an endocrine
target organ to cause release of one of its hormones.
Various interactions at the target level may occur, and are
schematically illustrated for mechanisms 2 and 3.

peptides extractable from the porcine intestinal tract and identified chemically by detection of a C-terminal alpha amide structure.[36] Preliminary evidence suggests that galanin is also a neuropeptide. It has been found to cause hyperglycemia when infused intravenously in experimental animals, and this effect appears to be due to suppression of insulin secretion[37] with reduction of glucose clearance and little or no increase in glucose production. This action differs from that of systemically delivered somatostatin.[38] Galanin also inhibits the rise of plasma insulin concentrations in response to intravenous infusion of glucose in dogs and impairs glucose tolerance.[37] These findings further increase the complexity of a mechanism which may include one or more hormone(s), each capable of interactions with nutrients and metabolites at the level of the target endocrine tissues of the pancreas, with interactions in series or in parallel with peptidergic and aminergic nervous effects, and with paracrine agents, with potentially different polarities in each case.

EXTRAPANCREATIC EFFECTS OF AGENTS OF THE ENTEROINSULAR AXIS

In common with well-recognized endocrine mechanisms in control of exocrine secretions of the gastrointestinal tract, putative hormonal agents of the enteroinsular axis are likely to be capable of effects on targets other than the endocrine pancreas, and may affect intermediary metabolism in these other ways. Pharmacological examples of this potential with gastric inhibitory polypeptide have already come to light. Thus GIP is capable of competitive interactions with glucagon at glucagon receptors in adipocytes.[39] This experimental lead has been followed up with studies of the effects of GIP on liver metabolism, which show that this peptide can stimulate glucose production under certain conditions.[40,41] There is also evidence that GIP can affect the level of lipoprotein lipase activity in isolated cells.[42]

SUMMARY

In this brief review of regulatory function of gastroenteropancreatic peptides in control of intermediary metabolism in normal and diabetic states, with and without mediation by insulin and/or glucagon, a variety of possible mechanisms have been described. It is apparent that the pharmacologic actions of the peptides identified in various locations provide models for multiple routes of delivery and modes of action of effectors in this control system. Examples already exist of each of the hypothetical mechanisms illustrated in the scheme in Figure 4. It is clear that a great deal of study will be necessary in identification of the active agents and assessment of their importance in the physiology of intermediary metabolism. With respect to the possible pathophysio-

logic roles of regulatory peptides of the gastroenteropancreatic
system other than insulin and glucagon, a number of considerations
of Type I and Type II diabetes have been raised. The balance of the
evidence suggests that Type I diabetes may be viewed as an insulin
deficiency syndrome, so that physiological replacement with insulin
may be expected to result in correction of the metabolic abnormalities. Nevertheless, the difficulty of physiologic replacement
treatment, which may call for portal delivery of insulin, is well
recognized, and abnormalities secondary to insulin deficiency even
in "well-treated" Type I diabetes may be compounded by the effects
of gastroenteropancreatic peptides other than insulin, exerted
through the various mechanisms discussed. In Type II diabetes
mellitus, current understanding of the pathophysiology is much less
complete and no convincing description of the etiology exists. The
various metabolic actions of the gastroenteropancreatic peptides,
and their interactions with other endocrine, paracrine and nervous
regulatory mechanisms, represent a dauntingly complex control
system. The elucidation of this system can provide fertile ground
for the development and testing of hypotheses for the pathophysiology of disordered metabolism in Type II diabetes mellitus.

REFERENCES

1. Bayliss, W.M, Starling, E.H., The mechanism of pancreatic
    secretion, J. Physiol. 28:325-353 (1902).
2. Moore, B., Edie, E.S., Abram, J.H., On the treatment of
    diabetes mellitus by acid extract of duodenal mucous membrane,
    Biochem. J. 1:28 (1906).
3. Laughton, N.B., Macallum, A.B., Relation of duodenal mucosa to
    internal secretion of pancreas, Proc. Roy. Soc. Ser. B.
    111:37-46 (1932).
4. Loew, E.R., Gray, J.S., Ivy, A.C., Is duodenal hormone involved
    in carbohydrate metabolism? Am. J. Physiol. 129:659-663 (1940).
5. McIntyre, N., Holdsworth, D.C., New interpretation of oral
    glucose tolerance, Lancet II:20-21 (1964).
6. Dupre, J., Rojas, L., White, J.J., Unger, R.H., Beck, J.C.,
    Effects of secretin on insulin and glucagon in portal and
    peripheral blood in man, Lancet II:26-7 (1966).
7. Scow, R.O., Cornfield, J., Quantitative relations between oral
    and intravenous glucose tolerance curves, Am. J. Physiol.
    179:435-38 (1954).
8. McIntyre, N., Turner, D.S., Holdsworth, D.C., The role of the
    portal circulation in glucose and fructose tolerance,
    Diabetologia, 6:593 (1970).
9. Lickley, H.L.A., Chisholm, D.J. Rabinovitch, A., Wexler, M.
    Dupre, J., Effects of portacaval anastomosis on glucose
    tolerance in the dog: evidence of an interaction between the
    gut and the liver in oral glucose disposal, Metabolism
    24:1157-1168 (1975).

10. Radziuk, J., Norwich, K.H., Vranic, M., Experimental validation of measurements of glucose turnover in non-steady state, Am. J. Physiol. 234:E84-E93 (1978).

11. Radziuk, J., McDonald, T.J., Rubenstein, D., Dupre, J., Initial splanchnic extraction of ingested glucose in normal man, Metabolism 27:657-669 (1978b).

12. Radziuk, J., Inculet, R., Effects of ingested and intravenous glucose on forearm uptake of glucose and glucogenic substrate in normal man, Diabetes 32:977 (1983).

13. Radziuk, J., The effect of additional insulin on intravenous glucose tolerance and the forearm uptake of glucose compared to that following oral glucose, Diabetologia 25:188 (1983).

14. Dupre, J., Champion, M.C., Rodger, N.W., Replacement treatment with insulin, Clinical and Investigative Medicine 5:109 (1982).

15. Unger, R.H., Ketterer, H., Dupre, J., Eisentraut, A.M., The effects of secretin, pancreozymin, and gastric on insulin and glucagon secretion in anesthetized dogs, J. Clin. Invest. 46:630-45 (1967).

16. Dupre, J., Curtis, J.D., Unger, R.H., Waddell, R.W., Beck, J.C., Effects of secretin, pancreozymin, or gastrin on the response of the endocrine pancreas to administration of glucose or arginine in man, J. Clin. Invest. 48:745-57 (1969).

17. Brown, J.C., Dryburgh, J.R., Ross, S.A., Dupre, J., Identification and actions of gastric inhibitory polypeptide, Recent Progress in Hormone Research 31:487-532 (1975).

18. Rabinovitch, A., Dupre, J., Effect of gastric-inhibitory polypeptide present in clear pancreozymin-cholecystokinin on plasma and glucagon in the rat, Endocrinology 94:1139-1144 (1974).

19. Dupre, J., Ross, A.S., Watson, D., Brown, J.C., Stimulation of insulin secretion by gastric-inhibitory polypeptide in man, J. Clin. Endocrinol. and Metab. 37:828 (1973).

20. Sarson, D.L., Wood, S.M., Kansal, P.C., Bloom, S.R., Glucose-dependent insulinotropic polypeptide augmentation of insulin, Diabetes 33:389 (1984).

21. Perley, M.J., Kipnis, D.M., Plasma insulin responses to oral and intravenous glucose on studies in normal and diabetic subjects, J. Clin. Invest. 46:1954-1962 (1967).

22. Ross, S.A., Brown, J.C., Dupre, J., Hypersecretion of gastric inhibitory polypeptide following oral glucose in diabetes mellitus, Diabetes 26:525-529 (1977).

23. Crockett, S.E., Cataland, S., Falko, J., Mazzaferri, E.L., Gastric inhibitory polypeptide: responses to variable doses of glucose in normal subjects and abnormal responses to oral glucose in patients with adult onset diabetes mellitus, Diabetes 24:413 (1975).

24. Creutzfeldt, W., Ebert, R., Wilms, B., Frerichs, H., Brown, J.C., Gastric inhibitory polypeptide (GIP) and insulin in obesity: increased response to stimulation and defective feedback control of serum levels, Diabetologia 14:15-24 (1978).

25. Brown, J.C., Dryburgh, J.R., Ross, S.A., Dupre, J., Identifica-
     tion and actions of gastric inhibitory polypeptide, Recent
     Progress in Hormone Research 31:487-532 (1975).

26. Verdonk, C.A., Rizza, R.A., Nelson, R.L., Go, L.L.W., Gerich,
     J.E., Service, F.J., Interaction of endogenous gastric-
     inhibitory polypeptide with pancreatic alpha and beta cell
     function in man, Diabetes 28:353 (1979).

27. Stockman, F., Ebert, R., Creutzfeldt, W., Preceding hyper-
     insulinemia prevents demonstration of insulin effect on
     fat-induced gastric inhibitory polypeptide (GIP), Diabetes
     33:580 (1984).

28. Dupre, J., Champion, M., Rodger, N.W., Secretion of gastric
     inhibitory polypeptide (GIP) in insulin-dependent (IDDM) and
     non-insulin-dependent (NIDDM) diabetes mellitus, Ref. Program
     64th Annual Meeting of Endocrine Society, p.342 (1982).

29. Ross, S.A., Dupre, J., Effects of ingestion of triglyceride or
     galactose on secretion of gastric inhibitory polypeptide and on
     responses to intravenous glucose in normal and diabetic
     subject, Diabetes 27:327:333 (1978).

30. Dupre, J., Caussignac, Y., Champion, M., Kobric, M., McDonald,
     T.J., Rodger, N.W., Shepherd, G.A.A., VanVliet, S., Gastro-
     intestinal Hormones: the enteroinsular axis and the secretion
     of glucagon, in: "Front of Hormone Res." W. Creutzfeldt, ed.,
     S. Karger, Basel, publisher, Vol. 7:232-245 (1980).

31. Dupre, J., Champion, M., Rodger, N.W., Abnormal response of
     plasma immunoreactive glucagon to meals in insulin-dependent
     diabetes mellitus (IDDM) during treatment by conventional depot
     injection therapy (CSII), Clin & Invest. Med. (2)6:40 (1983).

32. Felig, P., Wahren, J., Sherwin, R., Palaiologos, G., Amino acid
     and protein metabolism in diabetes mellitus, Arch. Intern. Med.
     137:507 (1977).

33. Baer, A., Dupre, J., Prolonged intravenous infusion of gastric
     inhibitory polypeptide with parenteral nutrients elicits
     glucose intolerance and hyperinsulinemia in conscious rats,
     Program 63rd Annual Meeting, The Endocrine Society (1981).

34. McDonald, T.J., Jornvall, H., Nilsson, G., Vagne, M., Ghatei,
     M., Bloom, S.R., Mutt, V., Characterization of gastrin
     releasing peptide from porcine non-antral gastric tissue,
     Biochem. and Biophys. Res. Communications 90:227-233 (1979).

35. McDonald, T.J., Ghatei, M.A., Bloom, S.R., Track, N.S.,
     Radziuk, J., Dupre, J., Mutt, V., A qualitative comparison of
     canine plasma gastroenteropancreatic hormone responses to
     bombesin and the procine gastrin-releasing peptide (GRP),
     Regulatory Peptides 2:193-304 (1981).

36. Tatmoto, K., Rokaeus, A., Jornvall, H., McDonald, T.J., Mutt,
     V., Galanin - a novel biologically active peptide from porcine
     intestine, FEBS Letters 164:124 (1983).

37   (a) McDonald, T.J., Tatemoto, K., Radziuk, J., Dupre, J.,
      Galanin produces hyperglycemia in dogs, Clin. & Invest. Med.
      Vol. 5, No. 3 (1984).
      (b) McDonald, T.J., Dupre, J., Tatemoto, K., Greenburg, J.,
      Radziuk, J., Mutt, V., Galanin inhibits insulin secretion and
      induces hyperglycemia in dogs, Manuscript submitted to Diabetes.
38.   Altzuler, N., Gottlieb, B., Hampshire, J., Interaction of
      somatostatin, glucagon and insulin on hepatic glucose output in
      the normal dog, Diabetes 25:116 (1976).

NEW PROBES TO STUDY INSULIN RESISTANCE IN MEN;

FUTILE CYCLE AND GLUCOSE TURNOVER

Mladen Vranic*, Alexandre Wajngot** and Suad Efendic**

Departments of Physiology and Medicine
University of Toronto*
Toronto, Ontario Canada
Department of Endocrinology
Karolinska Hospital**
Stockholm, Sweden

ABSTRACT

Insulin resistance has been measured in man by nonsteady state tracer methodology. Increase in overall glucose utilization and suppression of glucose production was measured when hyperglycemia was achieved either by infusing glucagon or glucose. With the first method, insulin resistance was assessed in obese man and in lean hypertriglyceridemic patients. With the second method, insulin resistance was assessed in lean mild type II diabetics. These methodologies can only assess deficiences in overall glucose utilization and glucose production, but cannot delineate the defect in glucose uptake by the liver. However, if a given metabolic event is essentially characteristic of only one organ, metabolic abnormalities specific to that organ can be detected in vivo provided there is a probe specific to that metabolic pathway. Therefore, in lean mild type II diabetics the liver glucose futile cycle was assessed by a double tracer method. Previously it was shown that liver glucose futile cycling is increased in diabetic dogs. In healthy control subjects in basal state and during glucose infusion, the futile cycle could not be detected, but it represented a major part of glucose metabolism in liver of type II diabetics. It appears, therefore, that most of the glucose taken up by the liver during the glucose challenge in diabetics reenters the blood stream without being oxidized or polymerized. On the basis of these studies, it was concluded that excessive hyperglycemia in the diabetics during glucose infusion is due to a decrease in irreversible glucose uptake (impaired phosphorylation and futile cycling) and to a decrease in suppression of glucose production. The relative contribution of the liver and periphery to hyperglycemia seems to be almost equivalent. The mechanism behind the increased glucose cycle activity is not clear. It may be due to a relative decrease of glycogen synthase or increase in glucose-6-phosphatase or both. These observations in mild lean type II diabetics may have implications also in some other types of diabetes, since we have observed that futile cycling is even more marked in obese type II diabetics and that it could account in part for the diabetogenic effect of growth hormone in acromegalics.

With respect to metabolic abnormalities in diabetes, we wish to discuss some new probes to study insulin resistance particularly as they relate to developments of tracer methodology and their impact in the understanding of the etiopathology of diabetes. An important factor in the etiopathology of diabetes is decreased insulin sensitivity, which has been more extensively studied in Type II than in Type I diabetics.

Insulin resistance has been measured using a variety of different steady state experimental techniques based on glucose clamp and insulin suppression test. It is also possible to outline whether the abnormality of insulin sensitivity resides primarily at the receptor and/or postreceptor level.[1,2,3,4,5] In order to study insulin release and insulin sensitivity in type 2 diabetics, Cerasi and Luft designed a glucose infusion test (GIT) which led to development of a mathematical model. This made it possible to make quantitative measurements in a large population of diabetics.[6,7] They suggested that impaired insulin release is a primary defect,[8] whereas others felt that it is insulin resistance.[9] The evidence that islet β-cell function is indeed abnormal in NIDDM became very convincing[10] and it is also apparent that not only in NIDDM but also in impaired glucose tolerance there is abnormal insulin secretion and decreased sensitivity to insulin.[11] More recently a new mathematical approach based on minimal modelling has been proposed. This latter approach allows for estimation of the insulin sensitivity index from the dynamic responses of plasma glucose and insulin to a glucose injection. By the use of computer modelling it was possible to sever the feedback loop between plasma insulin and glucose.[12,13] The modelling approaches[6,7,12,13] require only simple experimental design and therefore can be used for wide epidemiological studies to define more precisely the abnormalities of insulin secretion and sensitivity.

The use of radioactive glucose tracers made it possible to assess insulin resistance with respect to glucose production and glucose uptake since this methodology[14] was validated both in and out of steady state.[15,16]

The first attempt to use tracer methodology to define insulin sensitivity in man in nonsteady state conditions used graded glucagon infusions to compare glucoregulatory responses in lean and obsese subjects.[17] The obese were studied first by this approach because they provided a model known to be resistant to insulin. The aim of the studies was to assess not only the effect of insulin but also that of glucagon. Glucoregulation was studied under both steady state and nonsteady state conditions. This was done because we felt that any alteration in glucoregulatory processess would be more pronounced and, therefore, easier to detect when glucose homeostasis was perturbed. To drive glucose out of steady state, we infused stepwise-incremental doses of glucagon in order to compensate for the transient metabolic effect when increments of glucagon concentrations are constant.[18] This hormone stimulates in vivo hepatic glucose production and promotes insulin release from the pancreatic ß-cell. The latter effect was also desirable for the study, because it allowed us to examine the glucoregulatory consequences of insulin delivered into the portal, rather than peripheral circulation. Thus, we used tracer techniques to measure nonsteady and steady state glucose kinetics under the influence of varying concentrations of glucagon and insulin. While an infusion of glucose, combined with tracer, does provide similar information about the peripheral response to insulin, the present approach was chosen because it permitted us to examine not only the response to insulin, but also the response to glucagon and the interaction of these two hormones.

The study compared the glucoregulatory responses in five lean subjects (102 ± 4 percent ideal body weight) to five obese (199 ± 11 percent ideal body weight). Fig. 1 illustrates that a graded infusion of glucagon resulted in more marked hyperglycemic response in the obese than in the lean. The difference occurred for the following reason. In the lean the rate of glucose production exceeded that of glucose utilization only during the first 60 min of infusion, while thereafter both rates became equal, and glucose concentration plateaued. The plateau of glucose concentration was, however, not a consequence of transiency of glucagon effects because both glucose production (Ra) and utilization (Rd) continued to rise. In contrast to the lean, in the obese glucose concentration never plateaued, because glucose production always exceeded glucose utilization, an indication of insulin resistance (as the rates of glucose production and their relation to plasma glucagon concentrations were the same in both groups, these data indicate that the differences are a result of altered sensitivity of glucose utilization to insulin). This difference in insulin sensitivity between the two groups becomes even more evident when insulin concentrations are plotted against glucose utilization, as shown in Fig. 2. In order to explore the effectiveness of insulin partially divorced from the influence of glucose concentration, we examined the relationship between the fractional disappearance of glucose and the plasma insulin concentration (Fig. 3). At basal insulin concentration, the

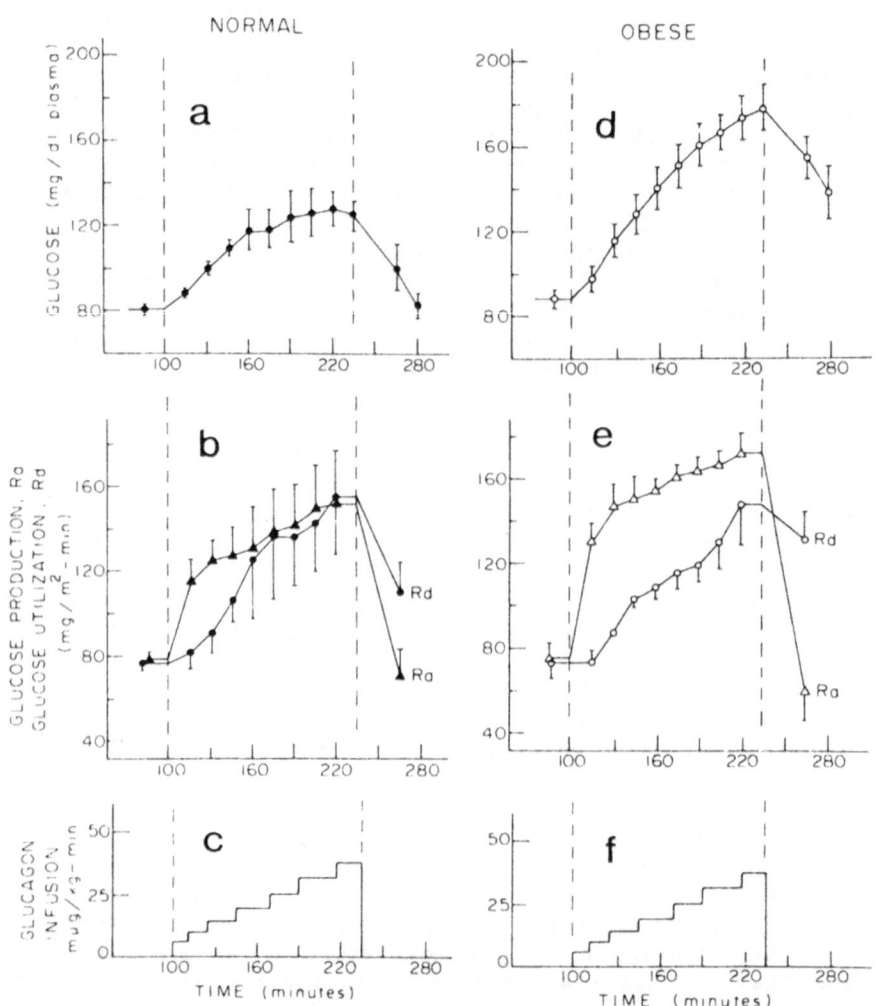

Fig. 1   The effect of a graded glucagon infusion on concentration,
           production and utilization of glucose in five normal (left
           panel) and five grossly obese subjects (right panel). At
           160 min, plasma glucose reached a steady state, whereas
           glucose concentrations in the obese subjects were steadily
           increasing throughout the glucagon infusion period. Glu-
           cose concentrations were significantly higher in the obese
           than in the lean subjects from 180 to 230 min (P<0.05 –
           0.01). Reproduced from ref. 17.

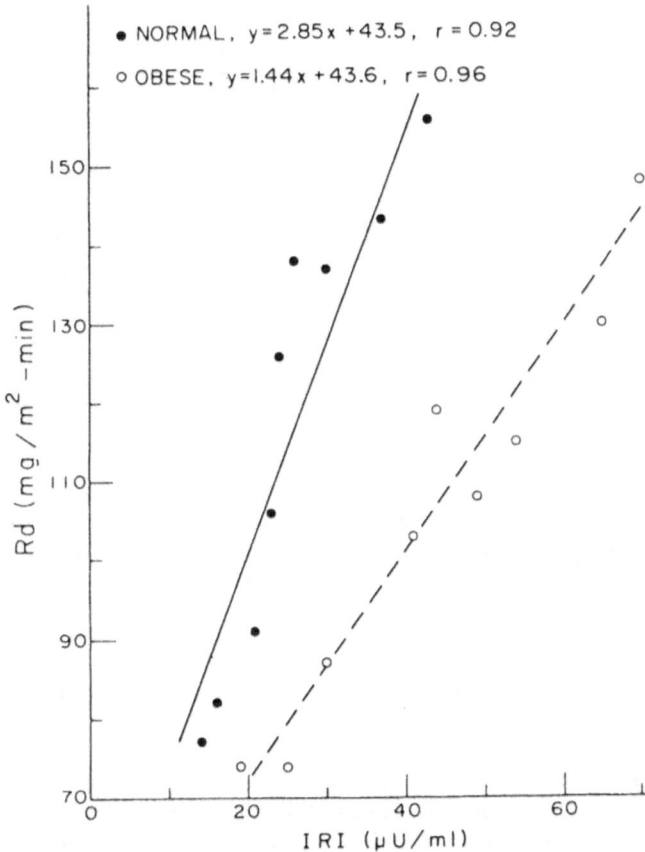

Fig. 2   Correlation between the mean concentrations of immuno-
            reactive insulin (IRI) and the mean rate of glucose
            utilization (Rd) in lean and obese subjects. Reproduced
            from ref. 17.

fractional disappearacne of glucose was much greater in the lean
than in the obese group. With higher concentrations of insulin, the
fractional disappearance rate rose significantly in the lean, but
not in the obese group. Thus, the obese were resistant to the
effect of all observed levels of insulin and the fractional glucose
disappearance did not increase.

    In many obese subjects not only is the sensitivity of glucose
metabolism in various tissue to insulin diminished, but the pancreatic B-cell is also hyperresponsive to glucose. Thus, it is not
clear which of the two changes represents the primary abnormality of
obesity. Interestingly in the obese subjects which we have studied,
the pancreatic B-cells were shown to be normally responsive to

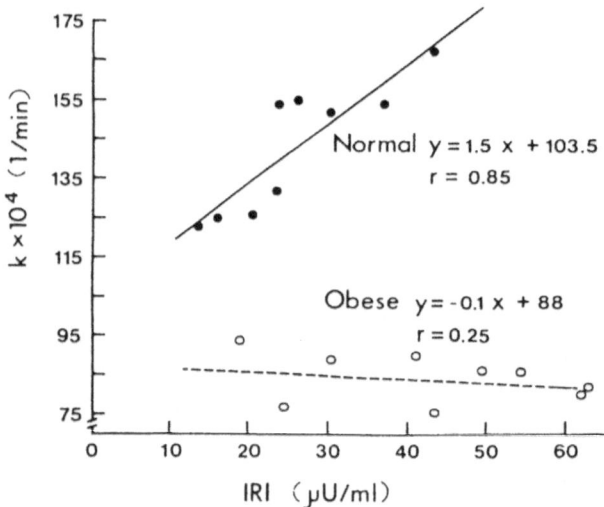

Fig. 3   Correlation between mean concentrations of immunoreactive
          insulin (IRI) and mean fractional disappearance rate of
          glucose (k). A highly significant correlation was found
          in the lean, but no correlation was observed in the obese
          subjects. [Fractional disappearance rate of glucose
          (min^{-1}) = rate of glucose utilization (mg/min) divided
          by glucose mass (mg).] Reproduced from ref. 17.

stimulatory effects of either glucose or glucagon. Hence they did
not release sufficient insulin to overcome the insulin resistance,
and therefore these obese individuals had impaired glucose tolerance.
We suggested that, in the presence of insulin resistance, which may
be the primary event, the responsiveness of B-cells will determine
whether the glucose tolerance will be normal or abnormal in obese
persons (a similar finding of normal B-cell responsiveness associated with insulin resistance was also found in hyperlipemic
patients, which however were lean[19]). On the other hand, when the
B-cells of obese subject are hyperresponsive rather than normally
responsive to a glucose challenge, they will secrete enough insulin
to overcome this resistance. Such a group would then have normal
glucose tolerance.[20]

     To asses insulin resistance we measured the fractional dis-
appearance rate of glucose which is proportional to the rate of
metabolic glucose clearance. These two parameters have been used
extensively to measure insulin resistance because glucose uptake
expressed in these parameters is partially normalized for the prevailing glucose concentration. From the point of view of tracer
methodology metabolic glucose clearance is an equally valid a measurement as glucose production, since both parameters are directly
derived from tracer data. However, both glucose production[21] and

clearance[22],[23] are suppressed by marked hyperglycemia. Therefore, for precise comparison between normal and insulin resistant individuals, glucose levels should not be too divergent or the effect of glycemia should be accounted for.

Insulin resistance was also documented in lean mild type II diabetics using intravenous glucose infusions to induce hyperglycemia.[24] Table 1 depicts clinical data for control subjects and those with mild diabetes. Glucose was infused at 2 mg/kg/min in study A (16 lean healthy subjects), at 4 mg/kg/min in study B (11 lean healthy subjects and at 2 mg/kg/min in study C (9 mild type II diabetics). The studies were closely matched with respect to body weight and age. All diabetics had decreased IV glucose tolerance. As shown in figures 4 and 5 in the basal state, diabetic had normal plasma concentrations of insulin, C-peptide, glucagon and glucose production and utilization. 21% decreased metabolic clearance rate (MCR) ($p<0.001$) at only moderately elevated glucose concentration indicates decreased sensitivity to insulin. During infusion of glucose at 2 mg/kg/min the hyperglycemia attained in the diabetics (170 mg/dl) was higher than in controls (115 mg/dl) but comparable to that of controls exposed to higher glucose load. Insulin response to hyperglycemia was defective in diabetics, because at similar hyperglycemic levels there was a marked increase in insulin and C-peptide concentrations in controls, but not in the diabetics. It is interesting that glucagon response to hyperglycemia was similar in controls and diabetics despite much higher insulin levels attained in controls infused with 4 mg/kg.min. With the lower glucose load metabolic clearance rate decreased more markedly in the diabetics, again suggesting insulin resistance. This was further substantiated by the fact that at the same insulin levels, glucose utilization (irreversible glucose loss) did not increase more in the diabetics than in controls, although the glycemia reached was considerably higher in the diabetics. With the lower glucose load, glucose production was suppressed to the same degree in the controls and diabetics, although the attained glycemia was much more marked in the latter. Since both insulin and hyperglycemia can suppress glucose production some defect in the regulation of glucose production of the diabetics is also indicated.

Another aspect of glucoregulation studied by isotopic methodology addressed the question of whether or not the decreased glucose tolerance of low insulin responders is associated with insulin resistance. In order to answer this question glucose metabolism was studied in eight low insulin responders to glucose and eight controls using a primed-constant tracer infusion technique.[25] The former group demonstrated a lower IVGTT than the controls, although the K-values were well within the normal range. They also attained higher blood glucose levels during IV administration of high and low glucose loads. Glucose turnover studies revealed normal hepatic glucose production, normal total glucose uptake and normal metabolic

Table 1. Clinical Data for the Control Subjects and Those with Mild Diabetes

Group	n	Sex ratio, M/F	Age, yr	Body weight, % of ideal	Fasting plasma glucose mg/dl	mM	OGTT, 1.75 g/kg	IVGTT, K value
A	16	14/2	42.1 ± 2.2	93.1 ± 2.0	<108	<6	Normal	1.97 ± 0.14
B	11	9/2	43.8 ± 2.3	93.2 ± 2.2	<108	<6	Normal	2.48 ± 0.03
C	9	6/3	50.7 ± 2.6	97.8 ± 3.8	108-144	6-8	–	0.72 ± 0.05

Results are expressed as mean ± SEM. OGTT was not done in group C.
Reproduced from 24.

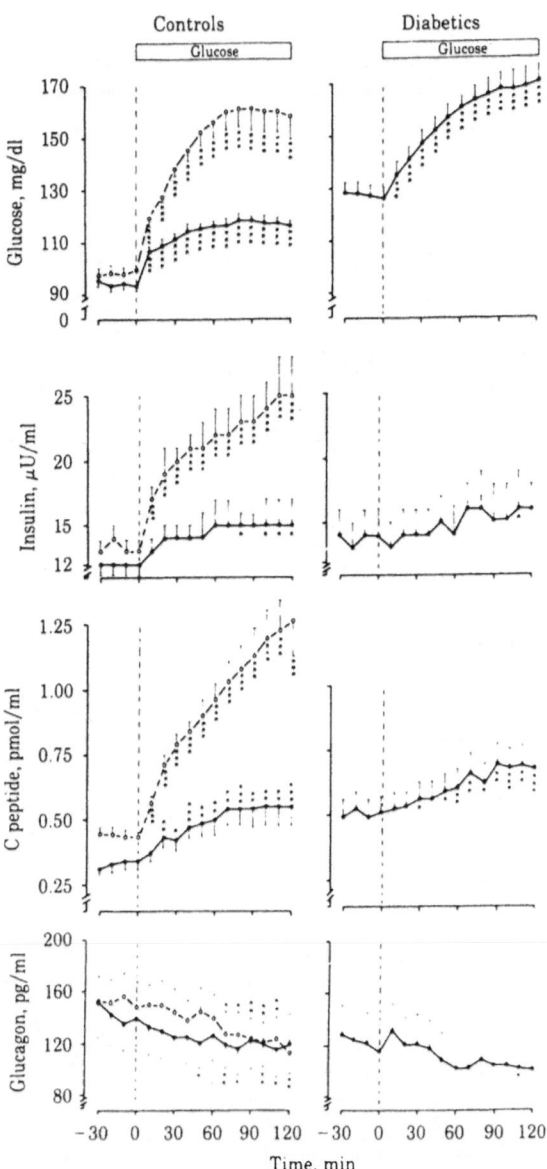

Fig. 4   Effect of glucose infusion on plasma concentration of glucose, insulin, C peptide, and glucagon in controls (left) and subjects with mild type 2 diabetes (right). U, international unit. Glucose was infused at a rate of 4 (o) or 2(●) mg/kg/min. Data are shown as mean ± SEM. Probabilities, compared with basal concentrations for that group: *, P<0.05; **, P<0.001. Reproduced from ref. 24.

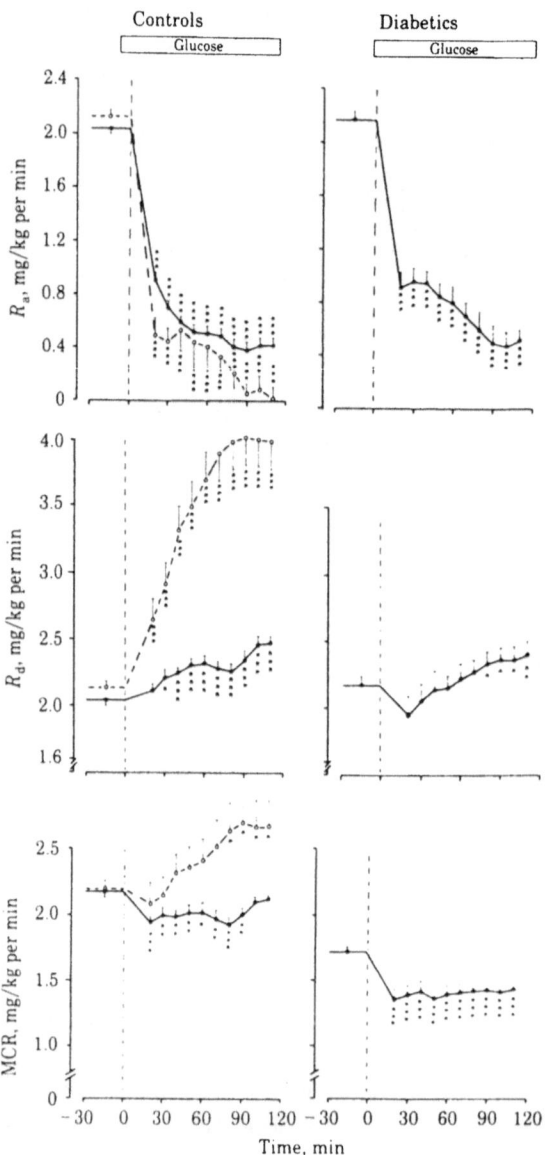

Fig. 5   Effect of glucose infusion on rates of glucose production
            (Ra), utilization (Rd) and metabolic clearance (MCR) in
            controls (left) and subjects with mild type 2 diabetes
            (right). Glucose was infused at a rate of 2 (•) or 4 (o)
            mg/kg/min. Data are shown as mean ± SEM. See legend
            of Fig. 3 for P values. Reproduced from ref. 24.

clearance of glucose in the low responders both in basal state and during a 2 mg/kg/min glucose infusion. These findings suggest normal sensitivity to insulin in these subjects, and imply that the low insulin response is the sole mediator of the observed lowering in IVGTT. However, the low insulin responders seem to be a heterogenous group, because in another study, where computer modelling was used to assess insulin sensitivity in 33 low insulin responders, subgroups with either an enchanced or decreased insulin sensitivity could be identified.[26]

In the assessment of insulin resistance, tracer methodology can be used to assess components of the fuel fluxes. If a given metabolic event is essentially characteristic of only one organ, metabolic abnormalities specific for that organ can be detected in vivo in men and in animals without using any invasive surgical methodology. Most work dealing with insulin resistance dealt with glucose uptake in peripheral tissues and with the overall glucose production by the liver. Glucose uptake by the liver is more difficult to assess in vivo. Balance techniques in man measure total balance across the splanchnic bed and that includes metabolic exchanges occuring in the gut and in the liver. Thus, it is not possible to differentiate between the metabolic events which occur in the two organs. In animals these two events can be differentiated by placing an indewelling catheter also in the portal bed. In man glucose uptake by the liver can be assessed by using a double tracer technique where one glucose tracer is given orally and another is infused intravenously. However, by using this technique[27] it became apparent that during glucose loading the first-pass glucose uptake by the liver is much smaller than was previoulsy thought to be the case. With the error contained in the present double tracer method it may not be possible to detect differences in liver glucose uptake which may exist between normal populations and the different classes of diabetics. These isotopic studies are consistent with the biochemical data, which indicate that at least in the rat, the capacity of the liver to utilize intact glucose for glycogen synthesis is rather limited and the reason for this might reside in the liver's limited capacity to phosphorylate the sugar at physiological concentrations.[28]

A novel way to look at the possible role of liver in overall insulin resistance emerged when futile cycles in the liver were measured by a double tracer methodology. According to the definition of Newsholme and Start, these cycles are created by two nonequilibrium reactions catalyzed by two separate enzymes in opposing directions.[29] It is generally believed that there are three futile cycles in hepatic glucose metabolism causing ATP hydrolysis without any corresponding change in the reactants.[30] These represent three irreversible steps between glucose and pyruvate. First, the glucose cycle (glucose->G6P->glucose); second, the fructose-6-phosphate cycle (F6P->FDP->F6P); and third, the

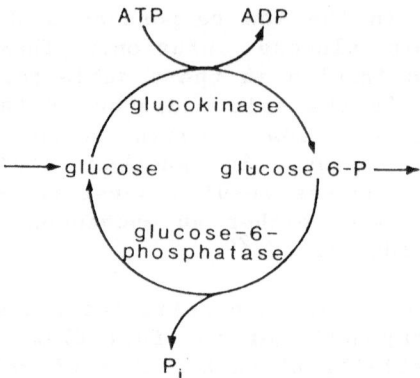

Fig. 6   The glucose cycle fraction of the liver futile cycles.

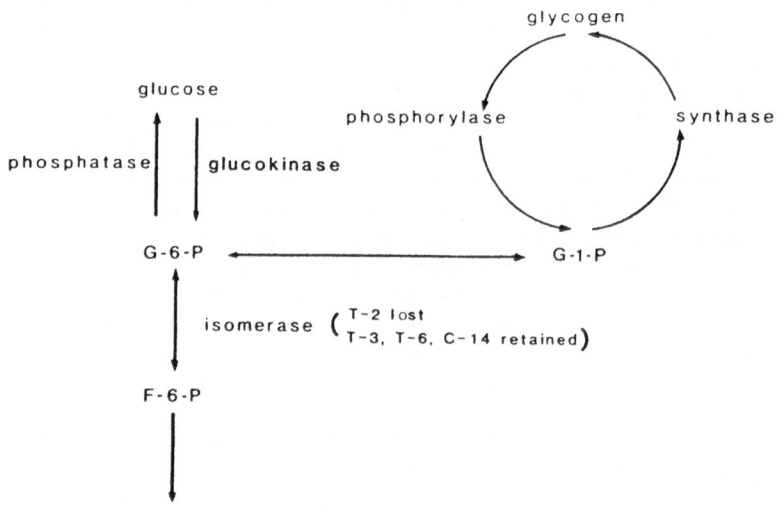

Fig. 7   A schema of a part of the glycolytic and glycogenetic
          pathways illustrating the loss of T-2 label in the
          isomerase reaction.

phosphoenol-pyruvate cycle (pyruvate->PEP->pyruvate). Of the three
cycles, only the first was measured in man (fig. 6) by comparing
total hepatic glucose output (or glucose phosphorylation) (estimated
by 2-T-glucose) with hepatic glucose production (or irreversible
glucose loss) assessed either by 14C glucose (corrected for
recycling) or tritiated glucose labelled at position 3 or 6.[31,32]
When tritiated glucose is labelled in position 2 it loses its tritium
in the hexose isomerase reaction (G6P<--->F6P) which is near its

equilibrium. Therefore, this tracer measures glucose appearance in plasma irrespective of whether it is newly-formed glucose or it originates from the glucose cycle (fig. 7). Glucose cycling fraction of the futile cycle then equals total hepatic glucose output (or glucose phosphorylation) minus the rate of glucose production (or irreversible glucose loss) (fig. 7).

Figure 8 illustrates the values of total glucose output (2-T) and glucose production (3-T) in a) depancreatized dogs in good metabolic control; b) depancreatized dogs in poor metabolic control; and c) in diabetic dogs during maximal stimulation of glucose production by glucagon. In comparison to normal dogs, in which the glucose cycling fraction of total glucose output amounted to 13%,[33] in diabetic dogs it was 48% and 60% in good and poor metabolic control, respectively.[34] Issekutz has shown that in normal dogs, glucose cycling plays an important role whenever glucose production is increased such as during exercise, chronic treatment with methylprednisolone and during infusion of glucagon and mannoheptulose.[35] Glucose infusion per se does not affect glucose cycling in normal animals but it does increase it when glucose production is also elevated.[35]

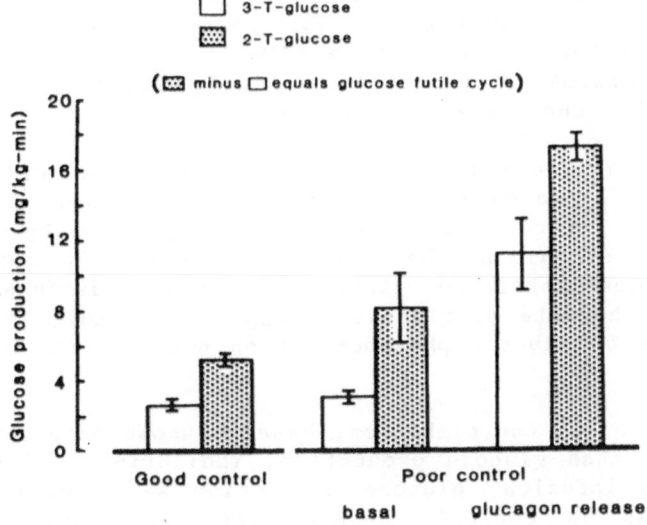

Fig. 8   A comparison of glucose production measured in diabetic dogs using either 2-^{3}H-glucose (striped columns) or 3-^{3}H-glucose (open columns). A Depancreatized dogs in good metabolic control; B. Depancreatized dogs in poor metabolic control; C. During maximal stimulation of glucose production by glucagon release in diabetic dogs. Reproduced from ref. 34.

The aims of our study[36] were to assess in the mild lean type II diabetics: 1) the activity of the glucose cycle part of the hepatic futile cycle in the basal state and during a glucose infusion; and 2) the overall contribution of the glucose cycle and the relative contributions of the liver and the periphery to excessive hyperglycemia during glucose infusion.

In each subject, two experiment were performed in random order in which constant infusions of either 2-T $((2-^3H))$ or 3-T $(3-^3H)$ glucose were given throughout the investigation period. After an equilibrium period of 120 minutes, an infusion of unlabelled glucose was started at 2 mg/kg/min. Seven controls and 7 diabetics were of a similar age (46 $\pm$ 4.8; 52 $\pm$ 4.7) and were near ideal body weight (96 $\pm$4; 103 $\pm$ 4% ideal B.W). The diabetics had marginally increased fasting blood sugar (123 $\pm$ 4 mg%), markedly decreased IVGTT and OGTT, and they were all classified as Type II diabetics. During glucose infusion in normal subjects, plasma glucose plateaued at 130 mg/dl, whereas in diabetics, glycemia of about 160 mg/dl was eventually achieved. C-peptide release was increased in both groups, however, the increase of C-peptide in diabetics did not reflect the much higher glucose concentrations reached during the glucose infusion (figure 9). Figure 4 shows much higher C-peptide levels achieved in normal subjects with hyperglycemia of 160 mg%. Thus, a decreased insulin responsiveness to a glucose challenge was noted in lean, mild NIDDM's. On the other hand, a marginal suppression of glucagon levels by hyperglycemia occurred equally in both groups (figures 4 and 9).

As shown in figure 10 in control subjects with either tracer, rate of glucose appearance (Ra) amounted to 2 mg/kg/min, and during glucose infusion, glucose production was suppressed by 75%. Thus, the glucose cycle could not be detected in either the basal state or during the glucose challenge. There were also no differences in the increments in the rate of glucose disappearance (Rd), implying that the total rate of glucose phosphorylation equalled the irreversible glucose loss.

In contrast, in the diabetics, basal glucose output was significantly larger than glucose production, indicating a glucose cycle. During glucose infusion, glucose production was suppressed to the same extent as in controls despite the fact that glucose and C-peptide levels reached were considerably higher. Thus, a part of the insulin resistance was apparently due to a defect in suppression of glucose production, since it is amply documented that hyperglycemia per se can suppress glucose production.[21] During glucose infusion the difference between total glucose output and glucose production increased and became as high as 0.6 mg/kg/min at 80 min of glucose infusion. Since at the end of glucose infusion, glucose production was about 0.6 mg/kg/min, approximately one-half of the total glucose output was due to glucose released through the glucose

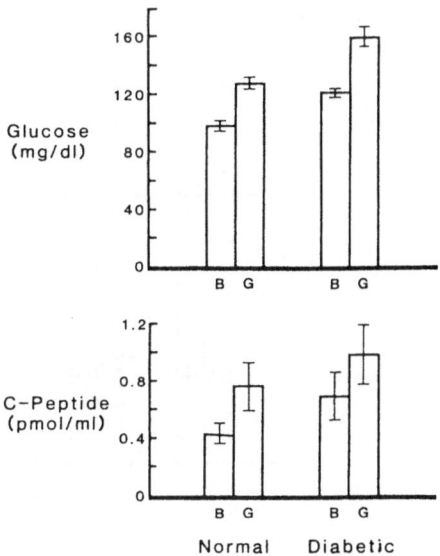

Fig. 9   Mean glucose and C-peptide concentrations before (B) and
at the end of the 2 hr glucose infusion at 2 mg/kg/min
(G) in 7 controls and 8 subjects with mild type 2 diabetes. Paired t-test indicates that increments in all
groups were significant.

cycle. Hyperglycemia in the diabetics resulted in a markedly
increased glucose phosphorylation whereas the irreversible loss of
glucose increased only marginally. With the present methodology, we
could not determine how much glucose is taken by the liver but the
amount of glucose flowing through the futile cycle seems to be quite
significant. Thus, the activity of the glucose cycle is negligible
in healthy subjects under basal conditions as well as during moderate
hyperglycemia. In mild, type II diabetics the activity of the glucose cycle is low after an overnight fast. During glucose infusion
the glucose cycle is considerably increased indicating that a significant amount of glucose taken up by the liver cells reenters the
blood stream without being oxidized or polymerized to glycogen.

    In order to assess the overall contribution of futile cycling
and the relative contributions of liver and periphery to excessive
hyperglycemia in the diabetic glucose-infused patients, we have
compared the rates of glucose disappearance in normal and diabetic
subjects when the same hyperglycemia of 160mg% was reached (Figs. 5
and 10). While in healthy subjects irreversible glucose uptake was
4 mg/kg/min, in diabetics it was only 2.4 mg/kg/min. Thus, in the
diabetics at this level of glycemia (160 mg/dl) irreversible glucose
uptake was decreased by 1.6 mg/kg/min (4-2.4 mg/kg/min). Assuming
that in healthy subjects glucose cycle does not operate at this level

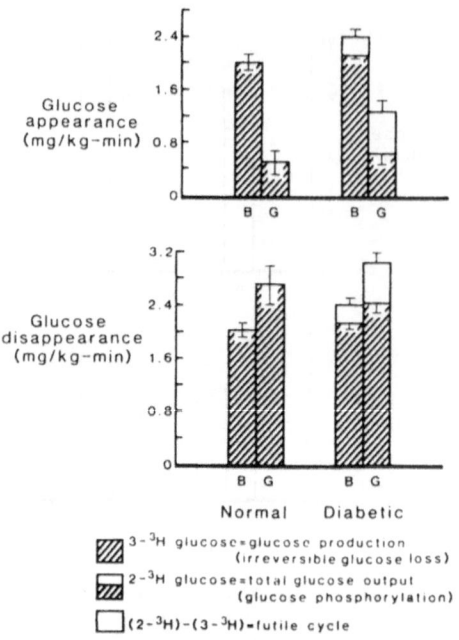

Fig. 10   Mean rates of glucose appearance and disappearance before
           (B) and at the end of the 2 hr glucose infusion at 2
           mg/kg/min (G) in 7 controls and 8 subjects with mild type
           2 diabetes. Futile cycle is not detectable in normals.
           In diabetics, total glucose output is significantly
           larger than glucose production indicating glucose futile
           cycle. The difference was significantly greater at the
           end of glucose infusion.

of glycemia[35], the rate of glucose phosphorylation in healthy subjects would also amount to 4 mg/kg/min (fig. 5) while in diabetics
it was 3 mg/kg/min (fig.10). Thus, in the diabetics at this level
of glycemia glucose phosphorylation was decreased by 1.0/mg/kg/min
(4–3 mg/kg/min). Since futile cycling amounted to 0.6/mg/kg/min, it
appears that the decrease of the irreversible glucose loss in diabetics (1.6 mg/kg.min) was due to defective phosphorylation
(decrease of 1 mg/kg/min) and to futile cycle (0.6/mg/kg.min).
These calculations can also give some indication of the participation
of the liver and the periphery in the deficient rate of irreversible
glucose utilization in the diabetics (1.6/mg/kg/min). Namely, one
could assume that phosphorylation of glucose in the liver is not
rate limiting, so that the main liver defect relates to futile
cycling (0.6 mg/kg/min). On the other hand, since the glucose cycle
does not operate in the periphery, the decrease in the rate of total
phosphorylation would reflect the peripheral deficiency (1
mg/kg/min). Thus, of the total defect of irreversible glucose uptake

in the diabetics, two-thirds would reside in the periphery and one-third in the liver. Furthermore, since at hyperglycemia of 160 mg/dl, glucose production was completely suppressed in the normal subjects (fig. 5) but in the diabetics was maintained at 0.7 mg/kg/min (fig. 5 and 10) it could be that the relative contributions of the liver (glucose production in spite of the hyperglycemia plus glucose cycle) and the periphery (decreased phosphorylation) to hyperglycemia of the diabetics are of similar magnitude.

The reason for the increased futile cycling in diabetes is not yet known. In healthy subjects hyperglycemia inhibits glucose phosphatase and activates glycogen synthase. Hers and colleagues[37] proposed that glucose binds to glycogen phosphorylase a, which in turn initiates the following processes: conversion of phosphorylase a into less active phosphorylase b --> deinhibition of glycogen synthase phosphatase --> conversion of glycogen synthase b into the more active glycogen synthase a --> accelerated glycogen synthesis with concomitant reduction in the tissue concentration of UDP-glucose and G6P. The falling G6P is seen as a main factor responsible for the diminished output of free glucose from the liver (pull hypothesis). An opposite approach was advocated by El-Refai and Bergman,[38] i.e. glucose causes an increase in hepatic G6P by inhibiting glucose-6-phosphatase, which in turn serves to force glucose carbon into glycogen (push hypothesis). Thus, suppression of glucose phosphatase would be the primary event. Finally, it has recently been suggested that glucose initially stimulates glycogen synthase and later on directly inhibits glucose-6-phosphatase.[39] Thus, this unified concept of McGarry and Foster suggests that both the pull and push mechanisms are important, since activation of synthase and inhibition of phosphatase are both primary events. The activity of the glucose cycle depends on the rate of glucose phosphorylation in the liver, its polymerization to glycogen, oxidation and dephosphorylation. Since the hexose isomerase reaction is considered to be non-rate limiting, it could be that the increased glucose cycle could be due to relatively decreased activity of glycogen synthase or to relatively increased activity of glucose-6-phosphatase or to both these defects. In alloxan-diabetic rats an increased activity of glucose-6-phosphatase was found[40,41,42] implying that this enzyme may play a key role in augmentation of glucose cycle also in patients with type II diabetes.

We conclude that glucose intolerance in mild lean type II diabetics is not only due to a decreased peripheral glucose phosphorylation but also to a defect in the liver. As a result of this, a significant part of glucose phosphorylated in the liver cannot be further utilized since it is desphosphorylated through a glucose cycle. In addition, glucose production in the liver is inadequately suppressed by hyperglycemia. We speculate that contributions of liver and periphery to glucose intolerance could be of similar magnitudes. We believe that these observations in mild lean type II diabetics have implications also in some other types of diabetes, since we have demonstrated recently that futile cycling is even more marked in obese type II diabetics and that it could account in part for the diabetogenic effect of growth hormone in the acromegalics.[43]

REFERENCES

1. S. Efendic, R. Luft, and A. Wajngot, Endocrine Review 5:395-410 (1984).
2. S. W. Shen, G.M. Reaven, and J.W. Farquhar, J. Clin. Invest. 49:2151 (1970).
3. R.A. DeFronzo, J.D. Tobin, and R. Andres, Am. J. Physiol. 237:E214 (1979).
4. O.G. Kolterman, L.J. Insel, M. Sackow, and J.M. Olefsky, J. Clin. Invest. 65:1272 (1980).
5. C.R. Kahn, Metabolism 27:1893 (1978).
6. E. Cerasi, and R. Luft, Acta Endocrinol. (Copenh) 55:278-304 (1967).
7. E. Cerasi, Acta Endocrinol (Copenh) 55:163 (1967).
8. E. Cerasi, R. Luft, Diabetes 16:615-627 (1967).
9. G.M. Reaven, and J.M. Olefsky, "Adv. Metab. Disord." R. Levine, and R. Luft, eds., Academic Press, New York, vol. 9, 313-331 (1978).
10. W.K. Ward, J.C. Neard, J.B. Halter, M.A. Pfeifer, D. Porte, Diabetes Care 7:491-504 (1980).
11. S. Efendic, A. Wajngot, E. Cerasi, and R. Luft, Proc. Natl. Acad. Sci. 77:7425-7429 (1980).
12. R.N. Bergman, Y.Z. Ider, C.R. Bowden, and C. Cobelli, Am. J. Physiol. 236:E667 (1979).
13. D.T. Finegood, G. Pacini, and R.N. Bergman, Diabetes 33:362 (1984).
14. R.C. De Bodo, R. Steele, N. Altszuler, A. Dunn, and J.S. Bishop, Recent Prog. Horm. Res. 19:445-488 (1963).
15. J.S. Cowan, and G. Hetenyi, Metabolism 20:360-373.
16. J. Radziuk, K.H. Norwich, and M. Vranic Am. J. Physiol 234:E84-93 (1978).
17. M. Vranic, S. Morita, and G. Steiner, Diabetes 29:169-176 (1980).
18. A.D. Cherrington, M. Vranic, Metabolism 23:729-744 (1974).
19. G. Steiner, S. Morita, and M. Vranic, Diabetes 29:899-905 (1980).
20. M. Perley, D.M. Kipnis, Diabetes 15:867-874 (1966).
21. R.N. Bergman, Federation Proc. 36:265-270 (1977).
22. C.A. Verdonck, R.A. Rizza, J.E. Gerich, Diabetes 30:535-537 (1981).
23. J.D. Best, G.J. Taborsky, J.B. Halter, D. Porte Jr., Diabetes 30:847-850 (1981).

24. R. Wajngot, A. Roovete, M. Vranic, R. Luft, and S. Efendic, Proc. Natl. Acad. Sci. USA 79:4432-4436 (1982).

25. A. Wajngot, R. Luft, M. Vranic, and S. Efendic, Horm. Metab. Res. 14:564-568 (1982).

26. A. Wajngot, R. Luft, and S. Efendic, Acta Endocrinologica 104:1-8 (1983).

27. J. Radziuk, T.J. McDonald, D. Rubenstein, and J. Dupre, Metabolism 28:300-307 (1979).

28. C.B. Newgard, L.J. Hirsh, D.W. Foster, and D. McGarry, J. Biol. Chem. 258:8046-8052 (1983).

29. E.A. Newsholme, C. Start, "Regulation in Metabolism," John Wiley and Sons, London (1973).

30. J. Katz, and R. Rognstadt, Curr. Top Cell. Regul. 64:237-289 (1976).

31. J. Katz, and A. Dunn, Biochemistry 6:1-5 (1967).

32. N. Altszuler, A. Barkai, C. Bjerknes, B. Gottlieb, and R. Steele, Am. J. Physiol. 229:1662-1667 (1975).

33. H.L. Lickley, G.G. Ross, and M. Vranic, Am. J. Physiol. 230:1159-1162 (1979).

34. M. Vranic, H.L. Licley, F.W. Kemmer, G. Perez, G. Hetenyi, T.W. Hatton, and N. Kovacevic, "Etiology and Pathogenesis of Insulin Dependent Diabetes Mellitus," J.M. Martin, R.M. Ehrlich, and F.J. Holland, eds., Raven Press, New York, 153-178 (1981).

35. B. Issekutz, Jr., Metabolism 26:157-170 (1977).

36. S. Efendic, A. Wajngot, and M. Vranic, Proc. Natl. Acad. Sci. USA (1985, in press).

37. H.G. Hers, Ann. Rev. Biochem. 45:167-189 (1976).

38. M. El-Refai, R.N. Bergman, Am. J. Physiol 231:1608-1619 (1976).

39. C.B. Newgard, D.W. Foster, J.D. McGarry, Diabetes 33:192-195 (1984).

40. C.J. Fisher, and M.R. Stetten, Biochim. Biophys. Acta 121:102-109 (1966).

41. S.V. Jakobsson, and G. Dallner, Biochim. Biophys. Acta 198:66-75 (1968).

42. T.L. Hanson, and R.C. Nordlie, Biochim. Biophys. Acta 198:66-75 (1970).

43. S. Karlander, A. Roovete, A. Wajngot, M. Vranic, and S. Efendic, Diabetologia 27:294A. Abstract #260 (1984).

NEW METHODS FOR THE ANALYSIS OF INSULIN KINETICS IN VIVO:

INSULIN SECRETION, DEGRADATION, SYSTEMIC DYNAMICS AND HEPATIC

EXTRACTION

J. Radziuk* and T. Morishima**

*Dept. of Medicine
McGill University
Montreal, Quebec   CANADA

**First Department of Medicine
Osaka University Hospital
Fukushima-Ju
Osaka 553, JAPAN

Glucose is a metabolite which is subject to a high degree of control. It is a principal substrate for the metabolic activity of the central nervous system, but its availability from exogenous sources is sporadic. This has led to the development of hormone systems which titrate the distribution of energy-rich substrates among different tissues in a very precise manner. That these hormone systems are efficient is manifest in the minimal perturbations seen, for example, in plasma glucose concentrations after the ingestion of a carbohydrate containing meal.

Insulin is certainly central in this control of glucose homeostasis. Among the many hormonal feedback loops present in the mammal, the glucose-insulin system represents one of the most tightly coupled stimulus-effector relationships. Small excusions in the blood glucose concentrations are recognized with extreme rapidity and the precise amount of insulin required is delivered to the circulation. The physiological importance of this tight coupling is illustrated by the fact that even minor differences in this loop can result in the deterioration of the glucose tolerance.

The feedback loop just described can be subdivided into three parts:

1.   Insulin secretion and its control by metabolic signals.

2.   Insulin degradation whose regulation is also essential in the
      maintenance of a finely-adjusted insulin concentration.

3.   Insulin action which consists of insulin-membrane interactions,
      as well as intracellular effects.

The final result of these mechanisms is the control of the flux of
metabolites, particularly glucose, into cells as well as of the
rates of a large number of enzyme reactions. It can be seen that
defects in any of the three parts of the insulin-based feedback loop
will lead to various degrees of glucose intolerance and diabetes.
Thus type I diabetes is characterized by a primary deficiency in
insulin secretion (e.g. 1). In type II diabetes, insulinopenia may
be mild or only relative, while insulin resistance may play a more
important part in the generation of hyperglycemia. This insulin
resistance may reflect receptor binding[2-4] or post-membrane
defects.[5] In addition, in some cases hyperinsulinemia with an
attendant insulin resistance has been ascribed to impaired hepatic
uptake of insulin.[6]

     In summary diabetes, as well as other states of impaired
glucose tolerance entail defects in any or all of the above
mechanisms. In order to gain further understanding about their
interplay in the pathophysiology of diabetes, accurate methodology
must be developed to achieve their quantitation in vivo. It must
also be possible to implement these methods in man. Our aim in this
chapter is to describe some of the steps that have been taken in
developing methods for the measurement of insulin secretion,
post-hepatic insulin appearance and hepatic extraction of insulin
continuously in both steady and nonsteady states, and to indicate
applications in the study of diabetes and its development.

1. THE MEASUREMENT OF INSULIN SECRETION - THE USE OF C-PEPTIDE

     The classical determination of insulin in secretion has been
the measurement of the arterial-portal venous gradient of insulin
together with an estimate of hepatic blood flow.[7-10] Portal
sampling of insulin, however, is difficult, primarily because of
inadequate mixing of pancreatic venous blood, or streaming.
Moreover, this method is not generally applicable in human
subjects. The accurate assessment of insulin secretion rates from
systemic insulin levels has been precluded by the large first pass
uptake of newly-secreted insulin by the liver.[11-15] The hepatic
extraction of insulin has frequently been shown to vary - with the
plasma levels of insulin, with the route of nutrient entry or due to
disease state.[16-23] These determinations were made based either
on estimates of global insulin clearance, portal/arterial-hepatic
venous differences in dogs or arterial hepatic vein differences in
man.

With the discovery of proinsulin and its conversion to insulin and C-peptide by Rubenstein and his coworkers[24] an alternative methodology became available. During insulin biosynthesis C-peptide fulfills the important role of assuring proper secondary and tertiary structure of the insulin molecule. C-peptide is then cleaved from the insulin molecule and sequestered in the insulin secretory granule. The result is that, during the process of exocytosis, C-peptide is secreted into the circulation on an equimolar basis with insulin.[24] More recent evidence has demonstrated that the portal molar ration of C-peptide to insulin is close to one in both man[25] and dog.[26] Theoretically, therefore, the determination of C-peptide secretion rates should be equivalent to measuring the rates of insulin delivery. This could be done using peripheral C-peptide concentrations.

The principle assumption on which such a determination would be based is that C-peptide itself is not extracted by the liver or at least extracted at a rate which is low and constant. It has been shown, in this context, that C-peptide almost completely escapes the splanchinic bed in rats[27] and dogs[26] or may undergo a low, constant 12% extraction in pigs.[28] With these observations in mind, plasma concentrations and urinary excretion of C-peptide have been used as indicators of insulin secretion.[29-31] These measurements are necessarily approximate since the clearance of C-peptide may change under different circumstances, for example, in renal disease.

A more accurate determination of insulin secretion was made by Waldhausl et al.[32] in man, based on the assumption that C-peptide was not extracted by the liver. Splanchnic production of C-peptide was estimated by measuring the hepatic venous-arterial concentration difference and multiplying by the hepatic blood flow. This method was also applied in the nonsteady-state situation following an oral glucose load. Subsequent studies demonstrated that in all likelihood human C-peptide is not extracted by the liver since porcine C-peptide escapes the human liver entirely.[33]

The arterial-hepatic venous difference technique is, in general, somehat invasive and an alternative approach to the measurement of C-peptide secretion arises from the consideration of its kinetics. If, in addition to negligible extraction by the liver, C-peptide kinetics are linear, then its concentration will always be proportional to its rate of secretion. Faber et al.[34] demonstrated convincingly that during the infusions of human C-peptide in man, this was the case. These observations were applied to the calculation of C-peptide (and, therefore, insulin) secretion rates by Eaton et al.[35] A two-compartment model was used to describe C-peptide kinetics:

$$\dot{C}(t) = -(K_1+K_3C(t) + K_2Y(t) + S(t) \qquad (1)$$

$$\dot{Y}(t) = K_1C(t) - K_2Y(t) \qquad (2)$$

where $C(t)$ and $Y(t)$ are the amounts of C-peptide in the sampled compartment (includes vascular space) and a more remote compartment respectively; $S(t)$ is the secretion rate of C-peptide; K_3 the fractional extraction of C-peptide from the first compartment and K_1, K_2 are exchange coefficients between the two compartments. K_1, K_2 and K_3 are constant and were estimated from the response to a C-peptide injection given by Faber et al.[34] Equations (1) and (2) were then solved for $S(t)$ which was calculated continuously based on measurements of $C(t)$ smoothed using spline fitting.

A more general approach based on properties of linear systems is to consider the concentrations of C-peptide as the convolution of a unit bolus response and the rate of secretion:

$$C(t) = \int_0^t h(t-\tau)S(\tau)d\tau \qquad (3)$$

where $C(t)$ is now the C-peptide concentration, $S(t)$ the rate of its secretion and $h(t)$ the response in plasma concentration to the injection of a unit bolus of C-peptide. If $h(t)$ is a double exponential then equation (3) is completely equivalent to the description using equation (1) and (2). Whether $h(t)$ is a double exponential or not, however, the equation can be solved for $S(t)$ by deconvolution using an algorithm such as that described by Radziuk.[36]

Since the use of equation (3) presumes linearity, both the linearity of the system and the validity of the calculations can be verified for C-peptide kinetics by first injecting C-peptide, monitoring the response, then infusing it at variable rates. $h(t)$ and $S(t)$ are then known, $C(t)$ is measured at discrete time points t_i, and using $h(t)$ and the $C(t_i)$, the calculated infusion rate, $S_c(t)$ is obtained. By comparing the two quantities $S(t)$ and $S_c(t)$, the degree of accuracy of the calculation can be esti- mated. This was done[37] in dogs. Figure 1 represents a typical decay curve following the injection of a bolus of dog C-peptide. Using this type of response (here fitted by three exponentials) and C-peptide levels shown in Figure 2, the rate of C-peptide appearance is calculated as shown. This compares well to the actual rate of infusion. It can be seen that the decay of C-peptide concentrations occurs slowly, therefore, the errors in assuming that is directly

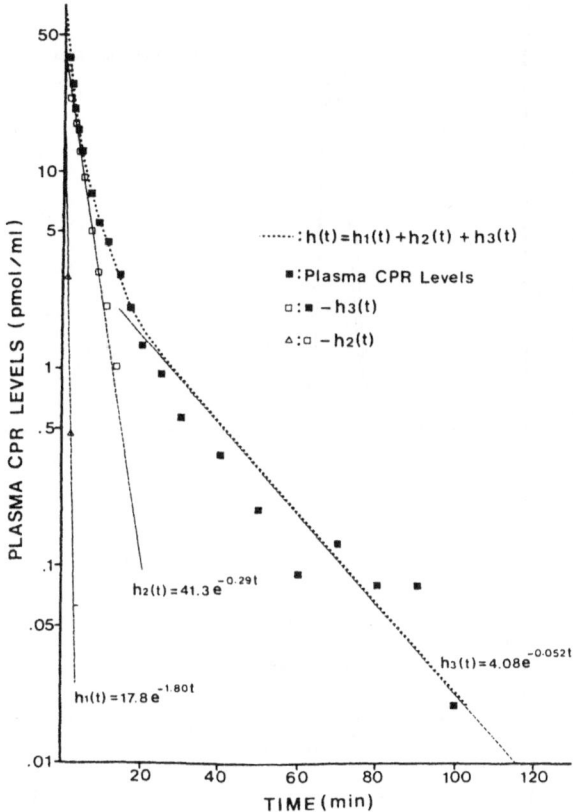

Fig. 1   A typical decay curve following the injection of a bolus
of dog C-peptide.

proportional to the rate of secretion would be minimal. The
extraction of the rates of appearance from the plasma concentrations
using mathematical deconvolution (or an analogous procedure) becomes
more important when the rate of appearance is changing rapidly. It
can be seen in Figure 2 that the plasma concentrations are shifted
relative to the rate of infusion and the peaks not as well resolved
as in the curve obtained after deconvolution. Comparing the areas
under the calculated and infused rates for the five studies reported
94% of the infused C-peptide was accounted for. As an estimate of
the total error (experimental and calculation) the absolute area
between the two sets of curves was found to be 12% of the infused
C-peptide.

The mean metabolic clearance rate of C-peptide in dogs was 10.1
± 1.0 ml/kg/min based on either the response to an infusion or an
injection of C-peptide. This reconfirms the constancy of the
metabolic clearance and, therefore, the linearity of C-peptide

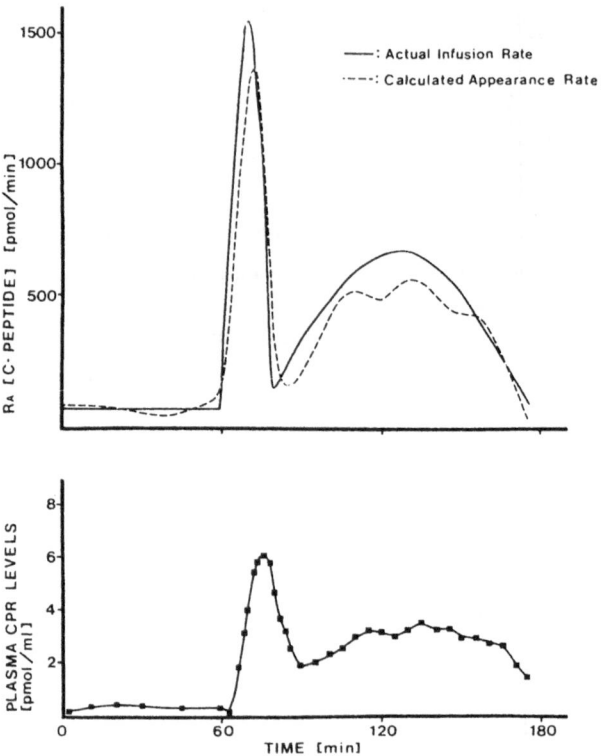

Fig. 2   C-peptide concentrations with the actual and calculated
           infusion rates in a dog.

kinetics is consistent with previous estimates in the dog[23] of
11.5 ± 0.8 ml/kg/min. It is also more than twice the metabolic
clearance rate obtained in man, 4.4 ml/kg/min,[34] and consistent
with a slower decay of concentrations following C-peptide injection.[34,38] Since the equilibration of C-peptide concentrations is
slower in man it, therefore, becomes all the more essential to
extract the rates of secretion mathematically.

AREA UNDER PLASMA C-PEPTIDE RESPONSE AND URINARY C-PEPTIDE AS
INDICATORS OF INSULIN SECRETION.

    A frequent requirement is the comparison of insulin secretion
in the same subject under two sets of physiological circumstances -
for example, following oral and intravenous glucose administration.
It can easily be shown that for an excursion s(t), from basal which
occurs over a finite period of time, a, where C(o) is the basal
C-peptide concentration:

$$\int_0^\infty (C(t)-C(o))dt = \int_0^\infty \int_0^t h(t-\tau)s(\tau)d\tau$$

$$= \int_0^\infty h(t)dt \int_0^a s(t)dt \quad (4)$$

This implies that, if the injection response, h(t), remains the same between two studies, the area under the C-peptide concentration curve is proportional to the area under the secretion curve. This, in turn, confirms the validity of, for example, comparing the C-peptide response following oral and intravenous glucose, in this way.[39] It also explains why urinary C-peptide, which in effect, represents a fraction of the integral of the concentration curve often correlates well to an otherwise determined insulin secretion rate (e.g. (40). One must add that none of the factors which might affect urinary C-peptide excretion should change between two studies which are compared.

It can be concluded, therefore, that peripheral C-peptide concentrations can be accurately used to calculate the rates of insulin secretion by beta cells in a continuous fashion. It requires only the preliminary determination of the concentration response to a bolus C-peptide injection in each individual. Because deconvolution protocols are valid in dogs and human C-peptide kinetics have also been shown to be linear, the calculation is also valid in man.

If only a comparison of the total amount of insulin secreted in response to different metabolic challenges in the same subject is required, only the areas under the plasma concentration curves of C-peptide are required. If renal C-peptide clearance remains constant, then urinary C-peptide is also an accurate reflection of the amount of insulin secreted.

II. POST-HEPATIC INSULIN APPEARANCE - THE USE OF TRACERS

The calculation of the rate of appearance of insulin in the systemic circulation is likely to be more complex than that of C-peptide. Insulin possesses a high degree of bioactivity and, as pointed out above, is a hormone whose concentrations must be tightly controlled. It is bound to receptors, the initiating mechanism by which it exerts its effect, and its concentration is controlled primarily by changes in the rate of secretion, but perhaps also by changes in its rate of removal. Both the volume of distribution and its rate of appearance, therefore, may be subject to changes during the course of an experiment. Both these are components of the metabolic clearance rate of insulin. Changes in this rate imply nonlinearity of the insulin system. The well-established approach to calculating the metabolic clearance rate under these circumstances is the use of exogenous tracers and, under nonsteady state conditions, mathematical modelling to describe insulin kinetics.

A general approach to the tracer—mediated determination of the rate of appearance of a substance in the systemic circulation can be described as follows:

1.   The choice of tracer: The labelled molecule must be (as much as possible) physically and chemically indistinghishable from the native molecule. This ensures identical kinetics for the two substances - e.g., the same binding properties and the same rate of degradation. At the same time the tracer must be administered in miniscule quantities - so as not to perturb the kinetics or action of the endogenous molecule in any way. It is thus a probe and not a perturbation.

2.   The detection of the tracer: The presence of the tracer in minute amounts implies very low concentrations. The identity of kinetics futhermore implies, as much as possible physical identity and, therefore, isotopic labelling. With the introduction of a label into the intact molecule, it follows that some of the degradation products may also be labelled. The separation of the substance in question from labelled metabolic products is, therefore, also a central question.

3.   The mathematical model: The limiting case of steady—state dynamics, although important, is less likely to yield information on how the system responds to challenges or pertubations. It is, therefore, essential to be able to determine the transient response of metabolite or hormone perturbations in the metabolic milieu. These responses obviously generate nonsteady state conditions and., therefore, require some understanding of the dynamics of the system. Traditionally this has been accomplished using compartmental modelling (e.g. 41), but in the context of determining flux rates into and out of the system, more general approaches are possible.[42]

4.   Validation: No method is completely satisfactory unless it can be shown to provide adequate results under circumstances analagous to the endogenous situation. In the case of rates of appearance, this can frequently be tested since endogenous production of the substance in question can often be eliminated or suppressed with the substitution of an exogenous input at a known rate. The calculated and input rates can then be directly compared, validating both the technical and mathematical manipulations involved in obtaining the result. This has already been illustrated with reference to C—peptide kinetics, although in the special case of a linear system.

In the remainder of this section, we will attempt to show how this protocol was applied to the measurement of the post-hepatic rate of insulin appearance.

1. INSULIN TRACER AND THEIR VALIDATION

A variety of insulin tracers have been used for a long time in the assessment of various aspects of insulin kinetics, for example binding or degradation. For insulins nonspecifically labelled with I^{125}, results concerned with both their biological activity and their rates of metabolism have been contradictory.[43-45] In general, the rate of catabolism decreased as the degree of iodination increased.[46-48] It was found, moreover, that the differences between in vivo and in vitro biological effects could be explained by the different rates of metabolism.[49] Because the B1 position of the insulin molecule is distant from the receptor binding site 50 and des-Phe B1-insulin is fully active[51], tracers such as B1-3,5-diiodotyrosine insulin were prepared and exhibited biological behaviour analogous to unlabelled insulin.[52] Alternately mono-iodoinsulin with the I^{125} on the A14 tyrosine was found to have many desirable properties.[53,54] However, either chemical damage during iodination, physical alterations during the decay[54] or the sheer size of iodine atom may affect the behaviour of the insulin molecule. Indeed, analysis of some aspects of behaviour of even the most carefully iodinated insulins reveals some discrepancies.[48, 55]

In contrast to this, tritiated insulin has been prepared by Halban et al.[56] which apart from the isotopic substitution in one amino acid is chemically indistinguishable from the native molecule. It has also been shown to be indistinguishable from native insulin both in its biological and immunological activity, as well as its metabolism.[56, 57]

The validation of this tracer in vivo was performed by infusing it at a constant rate with the concomitant infusion of unlabelled insulin at constant rates of different magnitues. If the tracer is appropriate, then its metabolic clearance rate (MCR) will equal that of the unlabelled insuln. This is because:

$$MCR = \frac{Ra}{C} = \frac{Ra^{\star}}{C^{\star}} \qquad\qquad (5)$$

where Ra and Ra* are the rates of infusion (appearance) of the unlabelled and labelled species of insulin respectively, C and C* are their concentrations. Equation[5] is easily solved for Ra:

$$Ra = \frac{Ra^{\star}C}{C^{\star}} \qquad\qquad (6)$$

so that it is obvious that if the tracer is appropriate, then the systemic rate of appearance of insulin in steady state can be calculated using equation.[6] The equivalence of the validity of the tracer with a MCR which is equal for both labelled and unlabelled insulin and with the correctness of the calculation of Ra is, therefore, evident.

One of the disadvantages of the insulin labelled with H^3 is its relatively low specific activity. Although iodinated insulins are theoretically of a higher specific activity, this becomes low as the number of iodine atoms per molecule is decreased in an effort to achieve a biologically more appropriate tracer.[58] It was possible to use the H^3-insulin at an infusion rate of about 5% or less of the basal endogenous secretion rate. From our calculations, this was found to still be a minor pertubation.[59]

2. THE DETECTION OF INSULIN TRACER IN PLASMA

Following the incubation of radioactive labelled insulin with isolated cells and chromatography of the labelled material by gel filtration, several peaks have been found by different investigators.[60-63] Three principal peaks have been identified – a large molecular weight peak, a peak eluting in the insulin position and an small molecular weight peak. That the labelled material which elutes in the insulin position may not be only intact insulin has been shown by studies where the binding activity of the peak eluting with the molecular size of insulin is decreased by up to 50%.[64-66] Reverse phase high performance liquid chromatography (RP-HPLC) had been used for some time to separate species of insulin[67, 68] and more recently iodinated insulin from incubation mixtures.[69] Because this method has a much higher resolving power for individual peptides,[70] it was chosen to separate insulin from any degradation products in plasma in our own work. We were also able to demonstrate[71] that the H^3-insulin counts recovered from plasma using RP-HPLC were 22% lower than the counts found using gel filtration (Sephadex G50) to separate insulin from the labelled substances. H^3-insulin standards mixed with plasma in vitro and run under ths same conditions showed only a 5% difference. These data show that in vivo it is also important to purify the H^3-insulin peak obtained by molecular sieve chromatography further and that this can be accomplished using RP-HPLC.

3. MATHEMATICAL MODELS FOR INSULIN KINETICS

The insulin system, particularly its secretory kinetics, has been a prime candidate for model development. An increased understanding of the large amount of data obtained was sought using a variety of mathematical descriptions to integrate it. For a

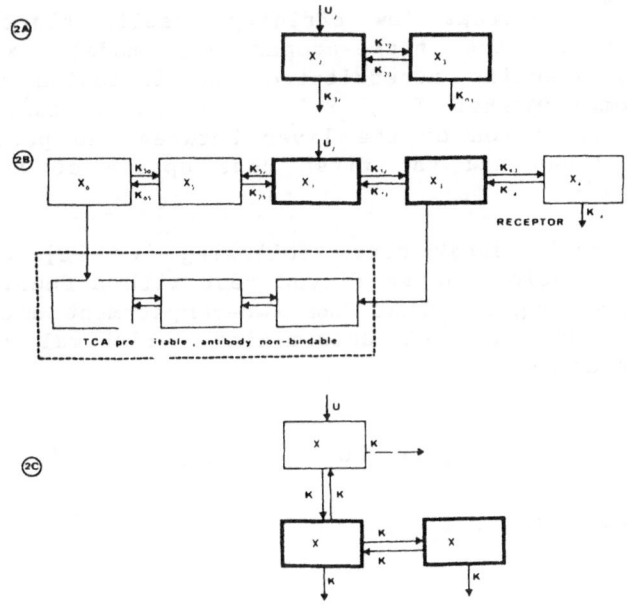

Fig. 3   A) A two-compartment model for insulin kinetics.

          B) A multiple-compartment model for kinetics of insulin
          and some of its degradation products according to Berman
          et al.[76] x_2, x^5 and x_6 represent insulin concen-
          trations in peripheral compartments. x_3 and x_4
          represent insulin bound to receptors. The part of the
          model enclosed by dashed lines represents TCA precipi-
          table, but antibody non-bindable insulin degradation
          products.

          C) A three-compartment model for insulin kinetics where
          x, represents the liver and insulin secretion (U_7)
          takes place in the portal vein. First-pass uptake of
          insulin by the liver is thus accounted for. Extraction
          of insulin by the liver on subsequent passes can be
          described if $K_{72}=0$.

review see, for example reference.[72]   The models which are
relevant to our discussion here can be placed in three categories
and are summarized in Figure 3.

     The first model (A) represents the model used most fre-
quently[73-75] to describe peripheral insulin kinetics.   In order to
account for the fact that insulin with high affinity for receptors
had higher effective volumes of distribution than low affinity
insulins, these were differentially labelled and their kinetics

analysed (b).[76] Whereas low affinity insulin kinetics could be accounted for by the three-compartment model (x_2, x_5, x_6), high affinity insulins necessitated the inclusion of additional "receptor" compartments: (x_3, x_4). The third model (C) represents the interposition of the liver between the portal and peripheral circulations and the first pass uptake of insulin by the liver (k_{07}).[77,78]

The H^3-insulin decay curve following its injection into the peripheral circulation can be fitted best with a double exponential function. This suggests that the two-compartment model is sufficient for the purposes of determining peripheral (post-hepatic) rates of appearance:

$$\dot{x}_2 = - (k_{02} + k_{32}) \ x_{23}x_3 + U_2 \qquad (7)$$

$$\dot{x}_3 = k_{32}x_2 - (k_{03} + k_{23})x_3 \qquad (8)$$

where

x_2 = insulin concentration in a central compartment (which includes plasma)

x_3 = insulin concentration in a more distal compartment (which most likely includes receptors)

k_{ij} = exchange and removal coefficients

Insulin is assumed to be removed from either the central compartment proportional to x_2,[74,75] or the second compartment proportional to x_3 [73] or both.[73] In our work the first of the above assumptions was used. In addition, the fractional removal rate k_{02} was assumed to contain all nonlinearities and time variations.

4. VALIDATION AND PHYSIOLOGY OF INSULIN DEGRADATION

a) <u>Steady state calculations - validation of tracer</u>

The most precise method of comparing the kinetics of a labelled insulin to native insulin <u>in vivo</u>, is to determine their rates of metabolic clearance. Early studies were done by Ooms and colleagues[15] to compare the catabolic rate of cristalline insulin with insulins labelled with 0.2-4 atoms of I^{125} or I^{131} per molecule. Stepwise infusions of a mixture of labelled and unlabelled insulins to give insulin levels from 100 µU/ml to 5000/µU/ml showed that MCR (labelled insulin) = 0.7 MCR (unlabelled insulin) even for the species labelled with only 0.2 atoms/ molecule.

A similar protocol to that of Ooms[15] was used in our studies: unlabelled insulin was infused in a stepwise fashion so that insulin levels in different studies varied from 20 to 1000/μU/ml. H^3-BI-insulin was infused at constant rates which, in terms of insulin mass, amounted to no more than 5-10% of basal secretion rates.

The results of a typical study are shown in Figure 4. The figure shows insulin measured in plasma and after purification on a C-18 column. Similarly H^3-insulin is measured after purification using gel filtration and the C-18 column. The values used in all calculations were those after reverse-phase chromatography. It was found that the rates of appearance at different infusion rates were 97.3 ± 1.8% of the rates of infusion. This means that the MCR of labelled insulin was also 97% of the MCR of the unlabelled species (see Equation #6).

At basal insulin concentrations (7.9 ± 1.8 μU/ml), the mean value of MCR (tracer determined) was 29.9 ± 3.4 ml/kg/min. These values are comparable to those found in man by Sonksen et al.[16,79]: 24.7 ml/kg/min at a mean concentration of 16 μU/ml. Iodinated insulins have in general, however, been metabolised differently from native insulin. For nonspecifically labelled insulins the rate of catabolism decreased as the degree of iodination increased.[46-48] As noted above even with 0.2 atoms of iodine per molecule the metabolic clearance was only 70% of the native molecule.[15] When 0.05 atoms iodine molecule of insulin were used[55] similar decay curves were obtained, but a non-tracer dose of insulin was introduced into the system. The development of specifically labelled tracers gave an improved correlation between the behaviour of labelled and unlabelled insulins. In particular BI-3,5-diiodotyrosine insulin and A-14-insulin have been used.[52-54] It was shown recently[80] that B1 tracers yielded values of MCR insulin in greyhounds which were 16.7 ± 0.7 ml/kg/min compared to A14-monoiodoinsulin (10.2 ± 0.7 ml/kg/min), A19-monoiodoinsulin (10.1 ± 1.0 ml/kg/min) and unfractionated tracer preparations (7-8.5 ml/kg/min). For the best available iodinated tracers the results are only approximately half of those obtained in our studies and similar to those found using a tracer labelled non-specifically, but to a low degree.[81] Similarly, in man, the metabolic clearance rate of iodinated insulin have been found in be between 2.6 and 10.7 ml/kg/min.[43,44,58]

The differences among the results might be explained by differences in the quality of the iodinated insulin used. The values are only one-tenth to one-half of those found in our studies[59] and of the measurements of Sonksen et al.[16] This may provide additional evidence for the difficulties in using radio-iodoinsulin as a tracer. The values for the MCR of unlabelled insulin published previously[43,73,83] are also small (11.5 to 14.8 ml/kg/min)

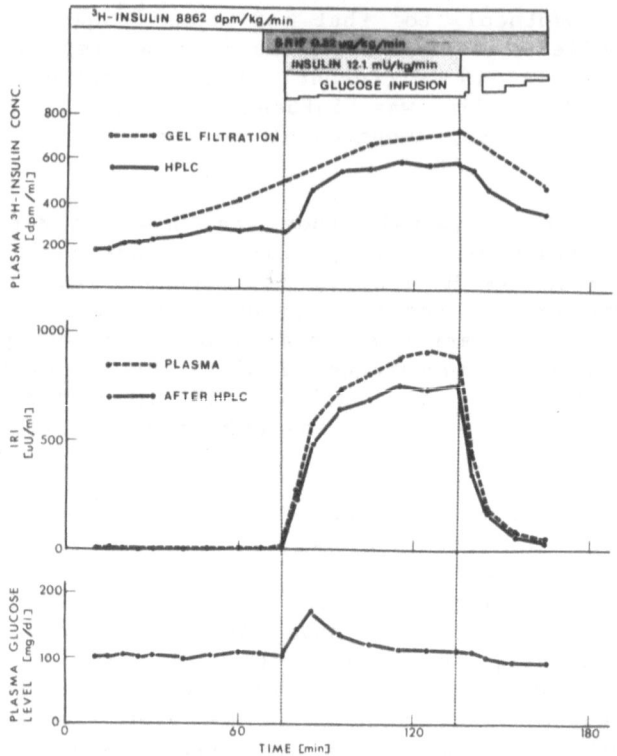

Fig. 4   Data from a representative study: Tritiated insulin was
           infused from time zero.   At 75 min. unlabelled porcine
           insulin infusion was started at a high rate along with
           somatostatin and glucose.   The upper panel shows the
           tritiated insulin concentrations assessed following HPLC
           (solid line) as well as some of the samples assayed after
           purification by Sephadex G-50 (dotted line).   The middle
           panel shows the immunoreactive insulin concentrations
           assayed both in unextracted plasma (dotted line) and in
           plasma extracted by HPLC (solid line).   The lower panel
           shows plasma glucose levels.

compared with the value reported in our studies. This discrepancy
may be because of species differences, but is most likely due to the
decrease in MCR caused by the elevation of plasma insulin concentrations following exogenous administration of unlabelled insulin.
What this discussion serves to emphasize is that the criteria for a
valid tracer must be established in vivo. To date, the comparison
of the metabolic clearance rate appears to be the most sensitive
indicator.

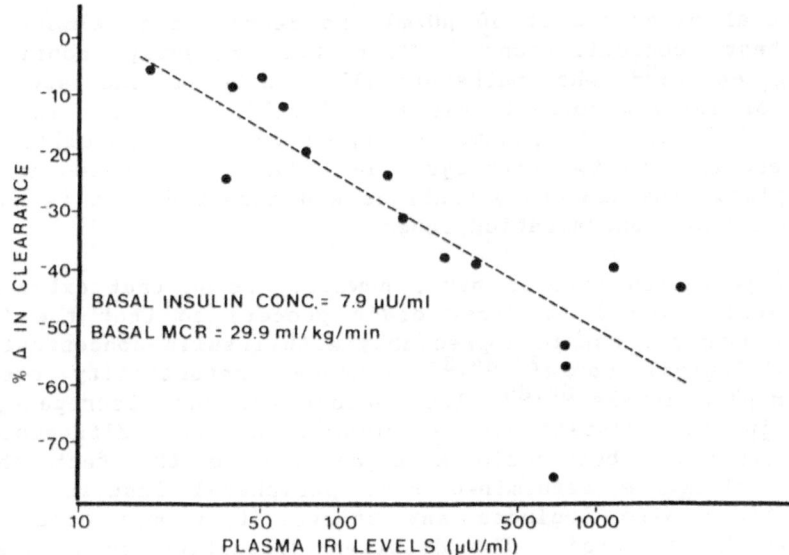

Fig. 5   Relationship   between   plasma   immunoreactive   insulin
concentrations and metabolic clearance rate of insulin in
steady state.   The linear regression line is y=-11.6 x +
30.6.   x = ln (plasma immunoreactive insulin concentration), y = percent difference in MCR from basal MCR.

b. The relationship of the metabolic clearance of insulin and its
    concentration

    In our studies we found that the MCR of insulin decreased as
the   concentration   of   insulin   increased.[59]   Figure   5   showed   a
negative correlation between the percent difference in MCR from
basal (y) and the logarithm of plasma insulin concentrations, ln
(IRI), (p < 0.001).

    y = 30.6 - 11.6 (IRI)   (9)

This relationship held for an insulin range of 20 µU/ml to
1000/µU/ml.   It is analogous to the decreasing MCR seen by Ooms et
al.[47] in dogs and Sonsken et al.[16] in man.   Our results also
show a tendency of the MCR to saturate near an insulin concentration
of 1000 µU/ml at a level about 60% below basal.   This is analogous
to the results of Franckson and Ooms[17] who found that the total
clearance of insulin (hepatic and renal catabolism as well as
urinary clearance) decreased from about 11 ml/kg/min at 50 µU/ml
to 4 ml/kg.min at 10^6 µU/ml.   Moreover it was demonstrated that
the renal metabolic clearance plus urinary clearance remained
virtually unchanged at all concentrations while liver catabolism was

65% of total clearance at 50 μU/ml and decreased to almost zero at the highest concentrations. This was recently confirmed by Fugleberg et al[83] who mathematically analysed the steady-state response of insulin concentrations to insulin infusions in man. It was concluded that the plasma disappearance of unlabelled insulin may be described by two pathways – one that is saturated at physiological plasma insulin concentrations and a second that is nonsaturable over a wide concentration range.

Most perfusion studies have, however, found that extraction by the isolated liver is a first order process so that the fraction extracted does not change appreciably with insulin concentrations in the physiological range[27,84,85] although saturability occurs at higher insulin levels.[84,86] The reasons for the discrepancy in _in vivo_ and _in vitro_ results may be primarily due to a difference in _in vitro_ metabolism, but could also be due to the fact that the metabolic clearance determined from peripheral insulin or tracer concentrations also includes any changes that may occur in the volume of distribution. The detailed dissection of removal from volume of distribution remains to be performed.

c. <u>Degradation products of insulin in plasma</u>

It was stated in Section 2, above, that H^3-insulin counts recovered from plasma using reverse phase HPLC were on average, 22% lower than the counts found using gel-filtration (sephadex G50) to separate insulin from labelled substances. When a C-18 SepPak alone was used to fractionate the labelled substances the results seen were analagous to those following purification by molecular sieve chromatography. Since a C-18 SepPak will not retain either large molecular weight proteins or amino acids and di-or tri-peptides (70), it effectively eliminates the large and small molecular weight peaks found on gel-filtration.[60-63] The two methods are, therefore, likely to give similar results in the present application and have used interchangeably in our preliminary investigations.

It was also found (Figure 6) that the fraction of the counts which are not insulin, but are in the molecular weight range of insulin, decreases with the plasma insulin concentration,[71] suggesting saturability of the process which alters the insulin molecule. This suggestion is strengthened by the fact that standards with both high and low contents insulin gave the same recoveries which were over 90%. A similar saturability occurs in the difference of immunoreactivity between plasma and the eluate from the C-18 column. The difference in immunoreactivity, however, remains lower suggesting a partial cross reactivity of the degradation products of insulin considered with the insulin antibody.

The development of these products in time was also investigated.[87] $B1-H^3$-insulin was infused at a constant rate

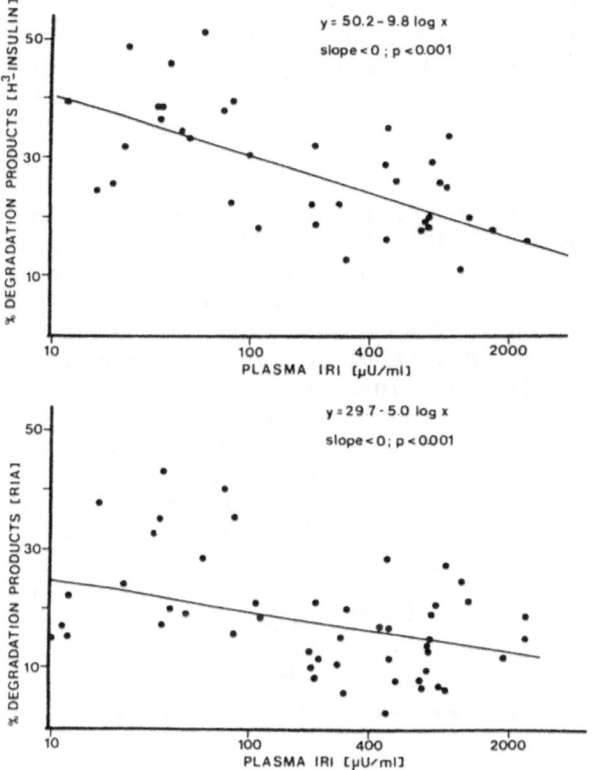

Fig. 6   Top: Regression line between the fraction of H³-insulin which is present as degradation product in plasma and different plasma insulin concentrations.

Lower: Regression line showing relationship between fractional increase in immunoreactivity in plasma between the insulin fraction on RP-HPLC and total immunoreactivity at different insulin concentrations.

and plasma samples were extracted for insulin using either reverse phase chromatography, C-18 SepPak alone or gel-filtration. Controls were obtained by incubating the labelled insulin with plasma _in vitro_ for the same length of time. It was found that, in the _in vivo_ studies, the HPLC extracted counts fall relative to either those determined by gel-filtration of SepPak, starting at about 3 min and equilibrating within 15 min at 15–20% below the value at time zero. In contrast to this, the counts obtained following _in vitro_ incubation, after purification by HPLC, remain at about 92% of those found by SepPak or gel-filtration, no matter what the incubation period.

All this evidence, although indirect strongly points to the existance of partial degradation products of insulin of intermediate size which are produced by a saturable process with a time course which is near that of the disappearance of insulin from plasma. Those products also appear to retain some cross reactivity with insulin antibody.

The existence of these products in vivo reflects the findings in vitro. Various studies[66,69,88-90] have pointed out inconsistencies in immunoprecipitability and biological activity, chromatographic separation and immunoreactivity of labelled "insulins" found in perfusing media. The number and structure of degradation products is unknown. A metabolite has been identified following the incubation of a [(^{125}I) iodotyrosine B1] insulin with isolated hepatocytes which corresponds to insulin with the B chain cleaved between the interchain disulfide bonds.[91] This is also an early product of the action of insulin protease on insulin.[92] The possibility of the presence of ß—chain secondary to cell surface glutathione[93] also exists. In studies on the biologically active centre of the insulin molecule and its mechanism of action, the biological activity of various degraded insulins and insulin fragments have been studied.[94-96] The potential interest of these fragments rests in that they may correspond to intra—cellular second messengers for insulin action,[97,98] or perhaps the partial degradation of the insulin may terminate the activity of the molecule on a cell.

d.   Validation of the calculation of nonsteady state rates of systemic insulin appearance.

From our work and that of others described above, it is evident that the insulin system cannot be linear under all circumstances — that is the metabolic clearance of insulin is dependent at least on the concentration of insulin. It has also been suggested that glycemia,[77] route of nutrient entry[18,22] and other factors may influence at least the hepatic uptake of insulin. Because of these observations, in the general case, it is essential to use tracers to estimate this changing MCR. In some cases, however, it may be permissible to forego the use of a tracer. For example, Turner et al.[99] infused insulin at low rates and using a deconvolution procedure based on the observed insulin concentrations, obtained satisfactory results for the calculated infusion rates. This, obviously, cannot always hold.

In our own studies[100] insulin was infused into dogs at time-varying rates concurrently with somatostatin to suppress endogenous secretion and B1—H^3—insulin at constant rates. The response to a preliminary tracer injection was obtained prior to the study. Plasma H^3—insulin and immunoreactive insulin were measured after extraction on a C—18 column. The mathematical model for insulin kinetics, described by equations[7, 8] was used for both insulin and tracer. k_{03} was set to zero and k_{02} was assumed to be the time varying quantity. The remainder of the constant parameters were obtained from the response to the tracer injection. The rate of insulin appearance was calculated continuously after fitting the insulin and tracer data with a set of polynomials. The results of a typical study are shown in Figure 7. The top panel gives the results obtained using the tracer. It can be seen that the two curves superimpose quite well. In contrast to this, the lower panel shows the results obtained by deconvolution - i.e, assuming that the system is linear or that k_{02} also is constant during the study. It is very clear that the calculated values seriously overestimate the rate of infusion since, in fact, the fractional disappearance rate of insulin had decreased during the insulin infusion. In some studies, there was little difference whether nonlinearity was assumed or not, in others the difference was greater. The overall conclusion that can be drawn is that without a prior knowledge as to the constancy of insulin clearance, tracers must be used to compensate for possible variations in the MCR.

III THE NONINVASIVE CALCULATION OF THE HEPATIC EXTRACTION OF INSULIN

As indicated above, it has been frequently suggested that, for example, the oral introduction of nutrients, especially glucose, will alter the hepatic extracion of insulin (as well as glucose).

The classical method of measuring insulin extraction in vivo is to determine its concentration in the portal, hepatic venous and arterial blood, the blood flow in the portal vein and hepatic artery and perform the appropriate calculation.[10,20,22] This method is, however, too invasive for use in man and, furthermore, may not always be accurate out of steady-state.

C-peptide yields a measure of insulin secretion which is equivalent to the prehepatic appearance of insulin. The post-hepatic appearance can be calculated using the tracer methods discussed above. The difference between these two quantities, therefore, gives the first-pass hepatic uptake of insulin. Dividing this by the insulin secretion rate finally gives its fractional extraction by the liver.(Figure 8)

This perception has been used by many authors in the quantitative estimation of changes in hepatic extraction of insulin (e.g., 6,40, 101, 102). The derivation of this can be seen as follows:

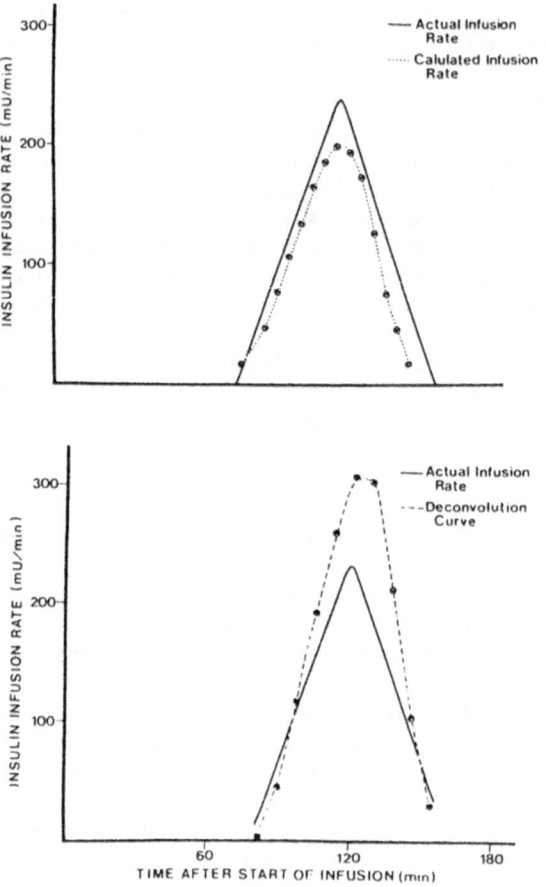

Fig. 7   Top: Actual infusion rate of insulin and that calculated using both tracer and insulin concentrations.
Lower: Actual infusion rate and that calculated using the tracer response to an injection and insulin infusions only, i.e., assuming insulin displays linear kinetics.

Rate of C–peptide appearance = MCR(C–peptide) x concentration (C–peptide).

Rate of insulin appearance = MCR (insulin) x concentration (insulin).

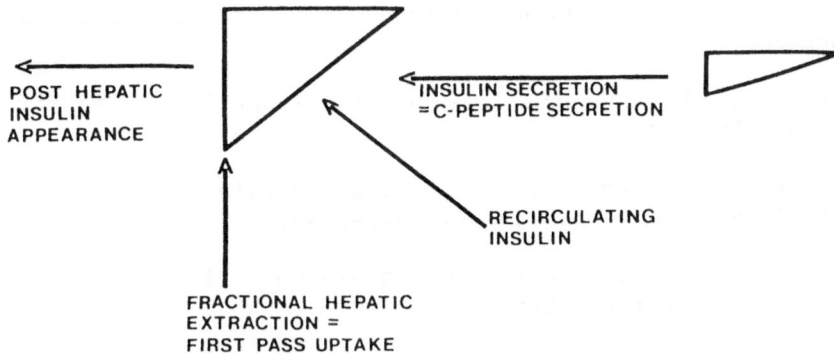

Fig. 8   Schematic representation of the determination of frac-
          tional hepatic extraction of insulin.

Now, the two rates of appearance are equal since we have an equimolar secretion of the two peptides. Therefore, the ratio of MCR's
is inversely proportional to the ratio of concentrations. If one
assumes that the MCR of C-peptide does not change, then changes in
the MCR of insulin will indeed be reflected in changes of the ration
of concentrations of insulin to C-peptide. If it is assumed that
the major clearance of the insulin which is secreted into the portal
vein occurs in the liver then changes in the concentration ratios
will, in fact, reflect changes in hepatic extraction. Under physiological conditions, the assumptions mentioned are probably quite
reasonable (e.g. 17), but some care must be taken in interpreting
the results. The parameters which determine the distribution of
both peptides and the removal rate of C-peptide must be similar if
two groups of subjects being compared. In addition two factors, for
example, both hyperinsulinemia and cirrhosis may decrease the
hepatic extraction of insulin simultaneously.

With the validations performed above   the following general
protocol is suggested for the measurement of hepatic extraction out
of steady-state;

Out of steady-state, various approaches are again possible.
Waldhausl et al.[21] measured arterial-hepatic venous difference of
both C-peptide and insulin, as well as liver blood flow, to calculate the rate of secretion and post-hepatic appearance of insulin
and, therefore, its hepatic extraction. Meistas[103] integrated
both insulin and C-peptide concentrations over a 24-hour period.

With the validations performed above   the following general
protocol is suggested for the measurement of hepatic extraction out
of steady-state;

i.   Injection of C-peptide and tracer insulin to determine their
      basal kinetic parameters.

ii.   During the perturbation studied – infause insulin tracer at a constant rate.

iii. Use C-peptide concentrations to calculate the pre-hepatic rate of insulin appearance.

iv.   Use the labelled and unlabelled insulin concentrations to calculate post-hepatic insulin appearance.

v.   Subtract (iv) from (iii) and divide by (iii) to obtain the fractional hepatic extraction.

     With this methodology, different groups and circumstances can be compared since the hepatic extraction is effectively dissected away from other considerations.

IV.   APPLICATIONS TO DIABETES AND OTHER PATHOLOGICAL CONDITIONS

     The secretion of insulin, its disappearance or clearance from the systemic circulation as well as its uptake by the liver have been investigated in a variety of metabolically abnormal condi- tions: diabetes, obesity, glucose intolerance, cirrhosis. It was shown by Faber et al.[34] that insulin secretion could be studied in normals and insulin-dependent diabetics using C-peptide concentra- tions. It was noted, however, that the clearance of C-peptide in the two cases was different emphasizing the importance of deter- mining individual responses to C-peptide injections. Meistas et al.[40] estimated insulin secretion rates in diabetics and obese patients with urinary C-peptide excretion. Using an I^{125} labelled insulin tracer Navalesi et al.[58], demonstrated an insulin deficiency as well as insulin resistance in non-insulin dependent diabetics. This was accompanied by a derangement of insulin distribution. Using only step-wise insulin infusions with a two-compartment model, Frost et al. also showed changes in insulin distribution and catabolism manifested by a larger distribution space and lower metabolic clearance rate in diabetics. Using more invasive arteriohepatic venous differences, both insulin and C-peptide in type 2 diabetics, Waldhausl et al.[21] showed an increased basal insulin secretion rate which, however, became exhausted during a large glucose challenge. Hepatic extraction of insulin remained as in normals. Using molar ratios of C-peptide to insulin Faber et al.[6] suggested a reduced insulin extraction by the liver. Bonora et al.[105] found by comparing both the C-peptide: insulin molar rations and areas under response cures, that both hypersecretion of insulin and its decreased hepatic uptake contribute to the hyperinsulinemia present in simple obese and mildly glucose intolerant patients. With severe glucose intoler- ance, decreased hepatic uptake appeared to be the major cause of the hyperinsulinemia.

It is evident that a large amount of work has been done which established a set of fundamental problems. The inconsistencies present in some of the results as well as more detailed mechanisms of, for example, the pathogenesis of hyperinsulinemia will be carried out in the future as a result of the careful application of validated methods.

ACKNOWLEGEMENTS

All the work reported from our laboratories has been funded by the Canadian Diabetes Association. We would like to express our gratitude to Professor R.E. Offord, G. Davies, C. Bradshaw, S. Pye and K. Kranz for their essential contributions to this work and to J. Blais for her careful typing of the manuscript.

REFERENCES

1. D.M. Kipnis, Insulin secretion in diabetes mellitus, Ann. Intern. Med. 69:891-901 (1969).
2. J.M. Olefsky, G.M. Reaven, Insulin binding in diabetes: relationships with plasma insulin levels and insulin sensitivity, Diabetes 26:680-688 (1977).
3. C.R. Kahn, Role of insulin receptors in insulin-resistant states, Metabolism 29:455-466 (1980)
4. H. Beck-Nielsen, The pathogenetic role of an insulin-receptor defect in diabetes mellitus of the obese, Diabetes 27:1175-1181 (1978).
5. O.G. Kolterman, R.S. Gray, J. Griffin, P. Burstein, J. Insel, J.A. Scarlett, and J.M. Olefsky, Receptor and post-receptor defects contribute to the insulin resistance in non-insulin dependent diabetes mellitus, J. Clin. Invest. 68:957-969 (1981).
6. O. Faber, K. Christensen, H. Kehlet, S. Madsbad, and C. Binder, Decreased insulin removal contributes to hyperinsulinemia in obesity, J. Clin. Endocrinol Metab. 53:618-621 (1981).
7. I. Mandelbaum, C.R. Morgan, Pancreatic blood flow and its relationship to insulin during extracorporeal circulation, Am. J. Surg. 170:755-758 (1969).
8. Y. Kanazawa, T. Kuzuya, T. Ide, Insulin output via the pancreatic vein and plasma insulin response to glucose in dogs, Am. J. Physiol. 215:620-626 (1968).
9. A.M. Rappaport, J.K. Davidson, T. Kawamura, B.J. Lin, S. Zelin, J. Henderson, and R.E. Haist, Quantitative determination of insulin output following an intravenous glucose tolerance test in the dog, Can. J. Physiol. Pharm. 46:373-381 (1968).
10. J.B. Field, Insulin extraction by the liver, in: "Endocrinology," vol. 1, Endocrine Pancreas, R.O Grey, E. B. Astwood, eds., Am Physiol Society, Washington, 505(1972).

11. L.L. Madison, and N. Kaplan, The hepatic binding of I^{131} labeled insulin in human subjects during a simple transhepatic circulation, J. Lab. Clin. Med. 52:927-932 (1958).

12. J.B. Field, Extraction of insulin by the liver, Ann. Rev. Med. 309-314 (1973).

13. C.E. Mondon, J.M. Olefsky, C.B. Doldas, and G.M. Reaven, Removal of insulin by perfused rat liver: effect of concentrations, Metab Clin. Exp. 51:912-921 (1975).

14. A.H. Rubenstein, A.H. Pottenger , M.E. Mako, G.S. Getz, and D.F. Steiner, The metabolism of proinsulin and insulin by the liver, J. Clin. Invest. 51:912-921 (1972).

15. A. Ooms, Y. Arnould, U. Rosa, G.F. Pennisi, and J.R.M. Franckson, Clearances metaboliques globales de l'insuline cristalline et d'insulines substituees au radioiode, Path Biol. 16:241-245 (1968).

16. P.H. Sonksen, C.V. Tompkin, C. Srivastava, and J.D.N. Nabarro, A comparative study on the metabolism of human insulin and porcine proinsulin in man, Clin. Sci. Mol. Med. 45:633-654 (1973).

17. J.R.M. Franckson, and H.A. Ooms, The catabolism of insulin in the dog: evidence for the existence of two pathways, Postgrad. Med. J. 49:931-939 (1973).

18. M. Kaden, P. Harding, and J.B. Field, Effect of intraduodenal glucose adminsitration on hepatic extraction of insulin in the anaesthetized dog, J. Clin. Invest. 52:2016-2028 (1973).

19. P.E. Harding, G. Bloom, and J.B. Field, Effect of infusion of insulin into portal vein on hepatic extraction of insulin in anaesthetized dogs, Am. J. Physiol. 228:1580-1588 (1975).

20. J. Jaspan, and K. Polonsky, Glucose ingestion in dogs alters the hepatic extraction of insulin: in vivo evidence for a relationship between biologic action and extraction of insulin, J. Clin. Invest. 69:516-525 (1982).

21. W. Waldhausl, P. Bratusch-Marrain, S. Gasic, A. Korn, and P. Nowotny, Insulin production rate, hepatic insulin retention and splanchnic carbohydrate metabolism after oral glucose ingestion in hyperinsulinemia Type 2 (non-insulin-dependent) diabetes mellitus, Diabetologia 23:6-15 (1982).

22. T. Ishida, Z. Chap, J. Chou, R. Lewis, C. Hartley, M. Entman, and J.B. Field, Differential effects of oral, peripheral intravenous, and intraportal glucose on hepatic glucose uptake and insulin and glucose extraction in conscious dogs, J. Clin. Invest. 72:590-601 (1983).

23. K. Polonsky, J. Jaspan, D. Emmanuouel, K. Holmes, and A.R. Moossa, Differences in hepatic and renal extraction of insulin and glucagon in the dog; evidence of saturability of insulin metabolism, Acta Endocrinol 102:420-427 (1983).

24. A.H. Rubenstein, J.L. Clark, F. Melani, and D.F. Steiner, Secretion of proinsulin C-peptide by pancreatic beta cells and its circulation in blood, Nature 224:697-699 (1969).

25. D.L. Horwitz, J.I. Starr, M.E. Mako, W.G. Blackard, and A.H. Rubenstein, Proinsulin, insulin, C-peptide concentrations in human portal and peripheral blood, J. Clin. Invest. 55:1278-1283 (1975).

26. K. Polonsky, J.B. Jaspan, W. Pugh, D. Cohen, M. A. Schneider, T. Schwartz, A.R. Moossa, H. Tager, and A.H. Rubenstein, Metabolism of C-peptide in the dog: in vivo demonstration of the absence of hepatic extraction, J. Clin. Invest. 72:1114-1123 (1983).

27. R.W. Stoll, J.L. Touber, L.A. Menahan, R.H. Williams, Clearance of porcine insulin, proinsulin and connecting peptide by the isolated rat liver, Proc. Soc. Exp. Biol. Med. 133:894-896 (1970).

28. C. Kulh, O.K. Faber, P. Hornes, and S.L. Jensen, C-peptide metabolism and the liver, Diabetes 27:197-200 (1978).

29. D.L. Horwitz, H. Kuzuya, and A.H. Rubenstein, Circulating serum C-peptide. A brief review of diagnostic implications, New Engl. J. Med. 295:207-209 (1976).

30. L.H. Heding, Insulin, C-peptide and proinsulin in nondiabetics and insulin treated diabetics. Characterization of the proinsulin in insulin-treated diabetics, Diabetes 27, Suppl. 1:178-183 (1978).

31. K.S. Polonsky, and A.H. Rubenstein, C-peptide as a measure of the secretion and hepatic extraction of insulin. Pitfalls and limitations. Diabetes 33:486-494 (1984).

32. W. Waldausl, P. Bratusch-Marrain, S. Gasic, A. Korn, and P. Nowotry, Insulin production rate following glucose ingestion estimated by splanchnic C-peptide output in normal man, Diabetologia 17:221-227 (1979).

33. P.R. Bratusch-Marrain, W.K. Waldhausl, S. Gasic, A. Hofer, Hepatic disposal of biosynthetic human insulin and porcine C-peptide in humans, Metabolism 33:151-157 (1984).

34. O.K. Faber, C. Hagen, C. Binder, J. Markussen, V.K. Naithani, P.M. Blix, H. Kuzuya, D.L. Horwitz, A.H. Rubenstein, and N. Rossing, Kinetics of human connecting peptide in normal and diabetic subjects, J. Clin. Invest. 62:197-203 (1978).

35. R.P. Eaton, R.C. Allen, D.S. Schade, K.M. Erickson, and J. Standefer, Prehepatic insulin production in man; kinetic analysis using peripheral connecting peptide behaviour, J. Clin. Endoc. Metab. 51:520-528 (1980).

36. J. Radziuk, The numerical solution from measurement data of linear integral equations of the first kind, Int. J. Num. Meth. Engng. 11:729-735 (1977).

37. T. Morishima, K. Polonsky, H. Tager, and J. Radziuk, The measurement and validation of nonsteady C-peptide secretion rate in dogs, Diabetologia (1985).

38. T. Kuzuya, and A. Matsuda, Disappearance rate of endogenous human C-peptide from blood, Diabetolgia 12:519-521 (1976).

39. O.K. Faber, S. Madsbad, H. Kehlet, and C. Binder, Pancreatic beta cell secretion during oral and intravenous glucose administration, Acta. Medica. Scand. Suppl. 624:61-64 (1979).

40. M.T. Meistas, M. Rendell, S. Margolis, and A.A. Kowarski, Estimation of the secretion rate of insulin from the urinary excretion rate of C-peptide: study in obese and diabetic subjects, Diabetes 31:449-453 (1982).

41. C.W. Sheppard, "Basic principles of the tracer method," John Wiley and Sons, Inc., New York (1962).

42. J. Radziuk, An integral equation approach to meaning turnover in nonsteady compartmental and distributed systems, Bull. Math. Biol. 38:679-693 (1976).

43. S.M. Genuth, Metabolic clearance of insulin in man, Diabetes 21:1003-10102 (1972).

44. M.P. Stern, J.W. Farquhar, A. Silvers, and G.M. Reaven, Insulin delivery rate into plasma in normal and diabetic subjects, J. Clin Invest. 47:1947-1957 (1968).

45. S.W.D. Shen, G.W. Reaven, J.W. Farquhar, Comparison of impedance to insulin-mediated glucose uptake in normal subjects and in subjects with latent diabetes, J. Clin. Invest. 49:2151-2160 (1970).

46. J.L. Izzo, A. Roncone, M.J. Izzo, and W.F. Bale, Relationship between degree of iodination of insulin and its biological, electrophorectic and immunochemical properties, J. Biol. Chem. 239:3749-3754 (1964).

47. H.A. Ooms, Y. Arnould, U. Rosa, G.F. Pennisi, J.R.M. Franckson, Clearance metabolique globale de l'insuline cristalline et d'insulines substitutees au radioiode, Path. Biol. 16:241-245 (1968).

48. E.R. Arquilla, H. Ooms, and K. Mercola, Immunological and biological properties of iodoinsulin labelled with one or less atoms of iodine per molecule, J. Clin. Invest. 47:474-487 (1968).

49. R.H. Jones, D.I. Doon, M.J. Ellis, Sonksen, and D. Brandenberg, Biological properties of chemically modifed insulin, 1. Biological activity of proinsulin and insulin modified at A_1-glycine and B_{29}-lysine. Diabetologia 12:601-608 (1976).

50. T. Blundell, G.G. Dodson, D. Hodgkin, and D. Mercola, Insulin: the structure in the crystal and its reflection in chemistry and biology, Adv. Protein Chem. 26:279-402 (1972).

51. R. Geiger, and D. Langner, Insulin-Analoga mit N-terminal ver- kurzter B-Kette, Selektiner Edmann-Abbau an der B-Kette des Insulins, Hoppe Selyer's Z, Physiol Chem. 354:1285-1290 (1973).

52. M.J. Ellis, R.H. Jones, J.H. Thomas, R. Geizer, V. Teetz, and P.H. Sonksen, B1-3, 5-diiodotyrosine insulin: a valid tracer for insulin, Diabetologia 13: 257-261 (1977).

53. J.L. Hamlin, E.R. Arquilla, Monoiodoinsulin, preparation, purification and characterization of a biologically active derivative substituted predominantly on tyrosine A14, J. Biol. Chem. 249:21-32 (1974).

54. S. Linde, B. Hansen, O. Sonne, J.J. Holst, and J. Gliemann, Tyrosine A14[^{125}I] monoiodoinsulin. Preparation, biologic properties and long term stability, Diabetes 30:1-8 (1981).

55. R. Navalesi, A. Pilo, and E. Ferranini, Kinetic analysis of plasma insulin disappearance in nonketotic diabetic patients and in normal subjects. A tracer study with ^{125}I-insulin, J. Clin. Invest. 61:197-208 (1978).

56. P. Halban, R.E. Offord, The preparation of a semisynthetic tritiated insulin with a specific radioactivity of up to 2 Curies per millimole, Biochem. J. 151:219-225 (1975).

57. P.A. Halban, C. Karakash, J.G. Davies, and R.E. Offord, The degradation of semisynthetic tritiated insulin by perfused mouse livers, Biochem J. 160:409-412 (1976).

58. R. Navalesi, A. Pilo, and E. Ferrannini, Kinetic analysis of plasma insulin disappearance in nonketotic diabetic patients and in normal subjects, J. Clin. Invest. 61:197-208 (1978).

59. T. Morishima, C. Bradshaw, and J. Radziuk, Measurement and validation of steady state turnover of insulin using tritiated insulin as tracer in dogs - relationship of insulin clearance to concentration, Am. J. Physiol. (in press).

60. S. Terris, and D.F. Steiner, Binding and degradation of ^{125}I-insulin by rat hepatocytes, J. Biol. Chem. 250:83-89 (1975).

61. J. Gliemann, and V. Sonne, Binding and receptor-mediated degradation of insulin in adipocytes, J. Biol. Chem. 253:7857 (1978).

62. M. Berger, P.A. Halban, W.A. Muller, R.E. Offord, A.E. Renold, M. Vranic, Mobilization of subcutaneously injected tritiated insulin in rats: effects of muscular excercise, Diabetologia 15:133-140 (1978).

63. W.C. Duckworth, Insulin degradation of liver cell membranes, Endocrinology 140:1758 (1979).

64. B.I. Posner, B. Patel, A.K. Verma and J.J.M. Bergeron, Uptake of insulin by plasmalemma and Golgi subcellular fractions of rat liver, J. Biol. Chem. 255:735 (1980).

65. C.R. Kahn, and K. Baird, The fate of insulin bound to adipocytes. Evidence for compartmentalization and processing, J. Biol. Chem 253:4900 (1978).

66. T.R.I. Misbin, J.G. Davies, R.E. Offord, P.A. Halban, and R.D. Mehl, Binding and degradation of semisynthetic tritiated insulin by IM-9 cultured human lymphocytes, Diabetes 29:730 (1980).

67. U. Damgaard, and J. Markussen, Analysis of insulins and related compounds by HPLC, Horm. Metab. Res. 11:580-581 (1979).

68. A. Dinner, and L. Lorenz, High perforamance liquid chromato-
     graphic determination of bovine insulin, Anal. Chem.
     51:1872-1873 (1979).
69. F.B. Stentz, H.L. Harris, A.E. Kitabchi, Early detection of
     degraded ^{125}I-insulin in human fibroblasts by the use of high
     performance liquid chromatography, Diabetes 32: 474-477 (1983).
70   H.P.J. Bennett, C.A. Browne, P.I. Brubaker, and S. Solomon, A
     comprehensive approach to the isolation and purification of
     peptide hormones using only reverse-phase liquid chromato-
     graphy, in: "Biological/Biomedical Applications of Liquid
     Chromatography III," G.L. Hawk, ed., Marcel Dekker, Inc., New
     York and Basel p.197-209 (1981).
71. J. Radziuk, T. Morishima, H.P.J. Bennett, P.A. Halban, and R.E.
     Offord, The presence of partially-degraded insulin in plasma of
     dogs. A method of measuring the plasma concentrations of
     tritiated insulin, Metabolism (in press).
72. J. Radziuk, and G. Hetenyi, Jr., Modelling and the use of
     tracers in the analysis and exogenous control of glucose
     homeostasis, in: "Modelling in Metabolism with Clinical
     Applications," D. Cramp, ed., J. Wiley and Sons, London, 1981,
     p.p. 73-142.
73. K.G. Tranberg, and H. Dencker, Modelling of fractional
     disappearance of unlabelled insulin in man, Am. J. Physiol.
     235:E577-E585 (1978).
74. P.A. Insel, J.E. Liljenquist, J.D. Tobin, R.S. Sherwin, P.
     Watkins, R. Andres, and M. Berman, Insulin control of glucose
     metabolism in man. A new kinetic analysis, J. Clin. Invest.
     55:1057-1066 (1975).
75. E.A. McGuire, J.D. Tobin, M. Berman, and T.R. Andres, Kinetic
     of native insulin in diabetic, obese and aged man, Diabetes
     28:110-120 (1979).
76. M. Berman, R.A. McGuire, J. Roth, and A.H.J. Zeleznik, Kinetic
     modelling of insulin binding to receptors and degradation in
     vivo in the rabbit, Diabetes 29:50-59 (1980).
77. K.G. Tranberg, Hepatic uptake of insulin in man, Am. J.
     Physiol. 237:E509-E518 (1979).
78. C. Cobelli, G. Felderspil, G. Pacini, W.A. Salvan, and C.
     Scandellari, Modelling and stimulation of the blood glucose
     regulation system, in: "Stimulation of Systems," L. Dekker, G.
     Savastano and G.C. Vansteenkisto, eds., North Holland,
     Amsterdam, pp. 675-687 (1979).
79. P.H. Sonksen, K.H. Jones, C.V. Tompkins, M.C. Srivastara, and
     J.D.N. Nabarro, The metabolism of insulin in vivo. Excerpta
     Medica. Int. Congress Series #413, 204-213 (1976).
80. C.S. Cockram, S. Bahrami, M.A. Bordujerdi, R.H. Jones, and D.
     Brandenburg, B1-monoiodoninsulin: a comparison with other
     tracers, Diabetologia 21:260 (1981).
81. R. Navalesi, A. Pilo, and E. Ferrannini, Insulin kinetics after
     portal and peripheral injection of ^{125}I insulin. II experi-
     ments in the intact dog, Am. J. Physiol. 230:1630-1636 (1976).

82. R.S. Sherwin, K.J. Kramer, J.F.D. Tobin, P.A. Insel, J.E. Liljenquist, M. Berman and R. Andres, A model of the kinetics of insulin in man, J. Clin. Invest. 53:1481-1492 (1974).

83. S. Fugleberg, K. Kolendorf, B. Thorsteinsson, H. Bliddal, B. Lund, and F. Bojsen, The relationship between plasma concentrations and plasma disappearance rate of immunoreactive insulin in normal subjects, Diabetologia 22:437-440 (1982).

84. J.S. Striffler, and D.L. Curry, Kinetics of insulin clearance by the liver in perfused liver-pancreas, Endoc. Res. Comm. 7:231-239 (1980).

85. S.S. Solomon, L.F. Fenster, J.W. Ensinck, and R.H. Williams, Clearance studies of insulin and non-suppressible insulin-like activity in the rat liver, Proc. Soc. Exp. Biol. Med. 126:116 (1967).

86. R.I. Misbin, T.J. Merimee, and J.M. Lowenstein, Insulin removal by isolated perfused rat liver, Am. J. Physiol. 230:171-177 (1976).

87. T. Morishima, R.E. Offord, and J. Radziuk, Time-course of the development of plasma partially-degraded insulin fragments in dog in vivo. Diabetologia (in press).

88. W.C. Duckworth, K.R. Runyan, R.K. Wright, P.A. Halban, and S.S. Solomon, Insulin degradation by hepatocytes in primary culture, Endocrinology 108:1142-1147 (1981).

89. W.C. Duckworth, and A.E. Kitabchi, Insulin metabolism and degradation, Endocrine Reviews 2:210-233 (1981).

90. R.I. Misbin, and E.C. Almira, The fate of insulin in rat hepatocytes. Evidence for the release of an immunologically active fragment, Diabetes 33:355-361 (1984).

91. R.K. Assoian, H.S. Tager, [(^{125}I) Iodotyrosyl[1]] insulin. Semisynthesis, receptor binding, and cell-mediated degradation of a B chain-labelled insulin, J. Biol. Chem. 256:4042-4049 (1981).

92. W.C. Duckworth, F. Stentz, M. Heinemann, and A.E. Kitabchi, Initial site of cleavage of insulin by insulin protease, Proc. Natl. Acad. Sci. USA 76:635(1979).

93. P.T. Varandani, and M.A. Nafz, Insulin degradation. XVI. Evidence for the sequential degradative pathway in isolated liver cells, Diabetes 25:173-179 (1976).

94. G. Weitzel, K. Eisele, V. Schulz, and W. Stock, Structure and activity of insulin. XII. Further studies on biologically active synthetic fragments of the B chain, Hoppe-Selyer Z., Physiol Chem. 354:321 (1973).

95. K. Kikuchi, J. Larner, R.J. Freer, A.R. Day, H. Morris, and A. Dell, Studies on the biological activity of degraded insulins and insulin fragments, J. Biol. Chem. 255:9281-9288 (1980).

96. K. Kikuchi, J. Larner, R.J. Freer, and A.R. Day, Effect of insulin fragments in biological activity of insulin and desoctapeptide insulin. 1. Potentiation of biological activities, J. Biol. Chem. 256:9445-9449 (1981).

97. J. Larner, G. Galasko, K. Cheng, A.A. DePaoli-Roach, L. Huang, P. Daggy, and J. Kellogg, Generation by insulin of a chemical mediator that controls protein phosphorylation and dephosphorylation, Science 205:1408 (1979).

98. J.R. Seals, and L. Jarett, Pyruvate dehydrogenase activation in adipocyte mitochondria by an insulin-generated mediator from muscle, Science 206:1407-1408 (1979).

99. R.C. Turner, J.A. Grayburn, G.B. Newman, and J.D.N. Nabarro, Measurement of insulin delivery rate in man, J. Clin. Endocrinol 33:279-286 (1971).

100. T. Morishima, C. Bradshaw, and J. Radziuk, Measurement and validation of the post-hepatic rate of insulin appearance under nonsteady state conditions, Am. J. Physiol. (in press).

101. D.G. Johnston, K.G. M.M. Alberti, O.K. Faber, C. Binder, and R. Wright, Hyperinsulinism of hepatic cirrhosis diminished degradation or hypersecretion? Lancet 1:10-12 (1977).

102. R. Rossell, R. Yomis, Casamitjana, R. Segura, E. Vilardell, and F. Rivers, Reduced hepatic insulin extraction in obesity: relationship with plasma insulin levels, J. Clin. Endocrinol. Metab 56:608-611 (1983).

103. M.T. Meistas, S. Margolis, and A.A. Kowarski, Hyperinsulinemia of obesity is due to decreased clearance of insulin, Am. J. Physiol. 245:E155-E159 (1983).

104. D.P. Frost, M.C. Srivastava, R.H. Jones, J.D.N. Nabarro, and P.H. Sonksen, The kinetic of insulin metabolism in diabetes mellitus, Postgrad. Med. J. 49:949-954 (1973).

105. E. Bonora, I. Zavaroni, C. Coscelli, and U. Butturini, Decreased hepatic insulin extraction in subjects with mild glucose intolerence, Metabolism 32:438-446 (1983).

ATHEROSCLEROSIS, THE MAJOR COMPLICATION OF DIABETES

George Steiner

Departments of Medicine and Physiology, University of Toronto, Division of Endocrinology and Metabolism, Toronto General Hospital

MAGNITUDE OF THE PROBLEM

Atherosclerosis accompanies diabetes so commonly that it is almost not considered when discussing the complications of diabetes mellitus. While approximately one-third of the general North American population will die of atherosclerosis, this or a related disorder will underlie the death of three-quarters of the diabetics in North America.[1] This picture is very different from that which was seen before the discovery of insulin, when only about one-fifth of diabetic deaths were due to vascular disease.[2] This change has often been attributed to the discovery of insulin and the consequent increase in the survival of diabetics. The problem with such a facile explanation is that approximately 80% of diabetics are type 2 (NIDDM) diabetics, most of whom would not have died of ketoacidosis even before the discovery of insulin and most of whom do not depend on insulin for their survival. Hence, if the change in mortality pattern were to be explained by prolonged survival due to the discovery of insulin, one would expect that almost all of the cardiovascular disease in diabetics should be found in type 1 (IDDM) and/or in insulin-treated type 2 diabetics. This is probably not the case. Therefore one must look to other explanations, such as changing diagnostic criteria, changing general disease patterns, changing treatment methods in general, etc.

The Framingham study is one of several pointing out the increased risk of mortality due to macrovascular disease in the diabetic, particularly in the diabetic woman.[3] This is most dramatic in those living in countries with a high rate of atherosclerotic disease. The situation is somewhat less clear in those countries where atherosclerosis is less prevalent. For example, in Uganda, only 4 of 156 diabetics over 40 years of age had ischemic changes on their ECGs.[4] However, in 384 hospitals surveyed in Japan between 1968 and 1970, 5.9% of the deaths in non-diabetics were due to ischemic heart disease. The comparable figure for diabetics was 9.7%, much less than that seen in North America but still almost double that seen in non-diabetics.[5]

This increase in mortality is not confined to heart attacks. For example, in an autopsy study Alex et al. found about the frequency of cerebrovascular accident in diabetics to be about 1.5 times that found in non-diabetics. This was entirely attributable to brain infarction and not to hemmorhage.[6]

The impact of diabetes on the third major vascular bed, that supplying the lower extremities, only becomes apparent from morbidity data. This is because peripheral vascular disease is more likely to cause intermittent claudication or gangrene, with consequent lower extremity amputation, than it is to cause death. The Framingham study has pointed out that the increase in morbidity attributable to peripheral vascular insufficiency is even greater than the increase seen in coronary or cerebrovascular insufficiency. Using non-invasive techniques both Janka et al.[7] and Beach et al.[8] demonstrated a very greatly increased incidence of peripheral vascular disease in diabetics. Beach et al. pointed out that this was particularly so if the diabetics were smokers.[8] Most and Sinnock[9] have pointed out that in six of the United States that they surveyed the likelihood of diabetics having a lower extremity amputation was fifteen times greater than that of non-diabetics. However, one must also realize that this could be influenced by the greater likelihood of diabetics having neuropathy and/or infections also affecting their lower extremities.

TYPE 1 vs TYPE 2 DIABETES

The figures given up to this point have related to diabetics as a whole. The differentiation of diabetics into those dependent on insulin (type 1) and those not dependent on insulin (type 2) has been fairly recent and therefore much less data have been amassed that can relate the epidemiology of macrovascular disease to each of these types of diabetes. However, some suggestions can be deduced by re-examining previously acquired data attempting to apply the new diagnostic criteria to it. This was done for macrovascular disease in a Rochester, Minnesota population.[10] Applying the new National Diabetes Data Group diagnostic criteria to the previously examined population, it was found necessary to delete 16.5% of the original diabetic cohort. However, even after this was done, the incidence of macrovascular disease was almost the same as that which had been determined for people diagnosed, by older criteria, as having diabetes.

Approximately 80% of diabetics have the type 2 form of diabetes, and both this and atherosclerosis are disorders that are much more common in older age populations. Hence, it is easy to understand why the problem of atherosclerosis in diabetics is greatest in the type 2 diabetic. However, postmortem studies have also shown a significant increase in coronary atherosclerosis in diabetics who had the onset of their diabetes before age 15, and hence were probably type 1 diabetics.[12] Furthermore, in examining the observed: expected deaths, Kessler[12] suggested that the maximum increase in risk was in those diabetics between ages 30-35 years. In older diabetics, although still being greater than that in non-diabetics, the increase in risk was not as great as in the 30-35 year old age group. In American diabetics, with onset before age 15, the number of deaths due to atherosclerosis between the ages of 20 and 39 was about double that seen in the nondiabetic population.[13] It has also been reported that Krolewski and his colleagues found that "by age 50 the cumulative prevalence of coronary heart disease in type 1 diabetics with proteinuria (60%) is three times greater than that of type 1 diabetics without proteinuria and twelve times greater than in the general population".[14] This information indicates that not only is the increased incidence of coronary artery disease a problem in the type 2 diabetic, it also is in the type 1 diabetic.

The information with respect to cerebrovascular accidents is somewhat more vague. In postmortem studies examining the circle of Willis in 107 diabetics, atherosclerosis was found in 84% of those individuals whose urine was positive for acetone in more than 30% of the samples tested and only in 50% of those whose urine had acetone in less than 30% of the samples tested. While this may suggest that the more ketosis-prone individual was more likely to have cerebrovascular atherosclerosis, the reverse conclusion is suggested when atherosclerosis was related to the type of treatment. Cerebrovascular atherosclerosis was found in 86% of diet-controlled diabetics and 75% of sulfonylurea-controlled diabetics, presumably both type 2 diabetics. By contrast approximately 60% of insulin-treated, possibly a mixture of type 1 and type 2, diabetics had cerebrovascular atherosclerosis.[15]

The only study that has examined atherosclerosis specifically in relation to the type of diabetes has examined peripheral vascular disease by noninvasive methods (Beach, 1980). In that study it was found that 20% of nondiabetics with a mean age of 56 had peripheral vascular disease. This figure compared to 19% for type 1 diabetics with a mean age of 34; 41% for diet-treated type 2 diabetics with a mean age of 59; 34% for sulfonylurea-treated type 2 diabetics with a mean age of 61; and 32% for insulin-treated type 2 diabetics with a mean age of 57. It is clear from these data that there is a great increase in peripheral vascular disease in type 2 diabetics. It

does not appear that the treatment modality influences the prevalence of vascular disease in the type 2 diabetic. The data with
respect to type 1 disease is harder to interpret in view of the great
age difference. At first inspection it appears that there is less
atherosclerosis in the type 1 diabetic than in the type 2 diabetic.
However, it was reported that, for the same age, the prevalence of
arterial disease was actually 6.5% greater in the type 1 diabetic.
The only other point of note is that duration of diabetes appeared
to be weakly related to the prevalence of arterial disease. However, it should be noted that it is extremely difficult to date the
onset of diabetes, particularly in those with type 2 disease.

Obviously much remains to be done in order to obtain accurate
data about the prevalence of atherosclerosis in type 1, as compared
to type 2 diabetes. The problems are compounded by the potential
impact of other factors such as age, onset and duration of diabetes,
and the presence of other risk factors. Hence, at this point one
must turn to an examination of those factors that are potentially
atherogenic and compare them in the type 1 and in the type 2 diabetic in order to try to gain further insight into the problem.

PATHOLOGY

In beginning to examine those factors that may be potentially
atherogenic in the diabetic it is reasonable to ask whether there
are any atherogenic factors that are unique to the diabetic, or
whether diabetes merely accentuates those atherogenic factors that
also operate in the non-diabetic. One may make an initial approach
to this question by asking whether there is anything distinctive
about the atherosclerotic lesion in the diabetic. The evidence to
date would suggest that there is not.[16,17] However, there is general agreement that the process is more rapid and extensive in the
diabetic. Although the plaque appears to be the same, there have
been some suggestions that the distribution of the lesions may be
different in the diabetic. Some suggest that there may be an
increase in the frequency of left main coronary artery involvement.[18] Also most agree that peripheral vascular disease in the
diabetic tends to be more distal, while that in the nondiabetic is
more proximal in location.[8,19]

Many studies of atherosclerosis in diabetics use ischemic manifestations of heart disease as the endpoint with which to assess
vascular disease. It may therefore be appropriate to insert a note
of caution to indicate the possibility that ischemia need not always
indicate atherosclerotic vascular narrowing. This is particularly
relevant in view of the recent suggestions that microvascular disease
may be found in the heart of the diabetic.[20,21,22] However, the
impact of this is still uncertain. For example, there is a high
frequency of microangiopathy in diabetics of both Hong Kong and Japan

and yet there is a low frequency of macrovascular disease.[23,24]

ATHEROGENIC FACTORS

The many atherogenic factors that can promote macrovascular disease, particularly in the diabetic, have been extensively reviewed.[1,14,17,25,26] This chapter will not attempt to be a general review in the way that those were. Rather, it will attempt to focus on those atherogenic factors that have been identified as being, or those that could reasonably be presumed to be different in type 1 and in type 2 diabetics.

Hyperglycemia

Type 2 diabetes, even that relatively mild asymptomatic form that is diet controllable, has been shown to be associated with an increased incidence of atherosclerosis. Because the plasma glucose cut point between hyperglycemia per se and type 2 diabetes is somewhat arbitrary many have asked whether asymptomatic hyperglycemia is a risk factor for diabetes. There have been a number of studies with data relating to this issue. Some have used fasting glucose values. Others have used post-load glucose values and still others, casual glucoses values. Most have shown by univariate analysis that there is an association of hyperglycemia with coronary artery disease. This has even persisted if the diabetics are excluded from the study populations. The Whitehall Study showed that in men given a 50 g oral glucose load there was no effect of increasing blood glucose except in the top 5% of the population. In them there was a doubling of coronary artery disease.[27] This suggested that although glucose may not be linearly related to the risk of atherosclerosis there may be a threshold effect. Others were unable to demonstrate this.[28,29] The fifteen different groups that had examined blood glucose and coronary artery disease came together to try to pool their data in order to reach a consensus on this question.[30] After considering the data of all groups, the conclusion was reached that at present it does not appear that there is an association between asymptomatic hyperglycemia and coronary artery disease.

The failure to establish a risk relationship between asymptomatic hyperglycemia and coronary artery disease should not, on the other hand, be taken to mean that hyperglycemia itself plays no role in atherogenesis in the diabetic. There is much pathophysiologic data to indicate how hyperglycemia could have an atherogenic role. One possible role may be through sorbitol accumulation in the artery wall of hyperglycemics.[31] However, it may be necessary to be cautious as it has recently been suggested that endothelial cells derived from human umbilical veins do not have the polyol pathway.[32] A different influence of hyperglycemia on the arterial wall has been suggested by the demonstration that glucose inhibits the replication of cultured human endothelial cells.[33] This might imply that hyperglycemia could impair the ability to repair injury to endothelial cells and thus, could aggravate a first step in atherogenesis.

Another potential role that might be played by hyperglycemia itself could be through the non-enzymatic glucosylation of proteins. This process, which is well known in the case of hemoglobin Alc, has also been shown to occur with lipoproteins and with some of the structural proteins of the artery wall. Low density lipoprotein (LDL) has been shown to be nonenzymatically glucosylated in diabetics. This glucosylation itself may influence LDL catabolism.[34] It may also render LDL antigenic and the combination of LDL with the autoantibody directed against it may also alter its biological behavior.[35] In addition glucosylated LDL is unable to bind normally to the LDL receptor.[34,36] As a consequence of these changes, a high proportion of glucosylated LDL may be removed by a receptor independent pathway. That pathway could involve macrophages and conceivably could result in an increase in the production of foam cells.

Another possible way in which hyperglycemia could be atherogenic is through non-enzymatic glucosylation of collagen, a major structural protein in the artery wall. This has been shown to occur in animals and in humans.[37,38,39] Such glucosylated collagen has been found to be antigenic. Hence, as with glucosylated LDL, the influence of hyperglycemia could be directly on the properties of collagen itself, or indirectly through an autoimmune process.

Hyperinsulinemia

Hyperinsulinemia has recently been identified as a factor that may increase the risk of atherosclerosis, even in nondiabetics. This may be even more important in diabetics because their plasma insulin levels are frequently abnormal. The original epidemiologic evidence of the risk impact of hyperinsulinemia came from retrospective studies of patients who had had coronary artery, peripheral vascular or cerebrovascular disease.[40,41,42,43] More recently, three prospective studies have supported the notion that the presence of hyperinsulinemia identifies an increased risk for coronary heart disease.[44,45,46] Furthermore, this increased risk appears to be independent of hypercholesterolemia, blood glucose or blood pressure. One of these studies was done in Finnish policemen. Another was conducted on male Parisian civil servants. Only the third, undertaken in Busselton Australia, was performed in a population that included both men and women. That third study only showed the increased risk of coronary heart disease in men. Thus the role of hyperinsulinemia in women still remains unresolved.

Hyperinsulinemia of endogenous (pancreatic) origin generally reflects the beta-cell's attempt to compensate for insulin resistance. The association of such insulin resistance with obesity is well known.[47] Furthermore, obesity often accounts for at least some of the insulin resistance that is seen in patients with type 2 diabetes and patients with hypertriglyceridemia. However, in both of these conditions, insulin resistance may also be seen in the absence of obesity.[48,49,50] In addition to the hyperinsulinemia described above, hyperinsulinemia may be seen in the insulin-treated type 1 or type 2 diabetic. In that situation it is exogenous (injected) in origin. As will be pointed out later, these two forms of hyperinsulinemia may have different metabolic consequences. These differences may stem from the fact that the major impact of the hyperinsulinemia, in endogenous hyperinsulinemia, may be on the liver. On the other hand in exogenous hyperinsulinemia, the impact may be both on the liver and on extra-hepatic tissues.

Hyperinsulinemia may have an atherogenic impact on the artery wall itself. This was suggested by Cruz et al. who infused insulin into one femoral artery of diabetic dogs and showed that there was lipid accumulation and medial proliferation in that artery, but not in the contralateral control artery.[51] Stout also demonstrated that if chickens were fed a normal diet and injected with insulin every day for 19 weeks lipid deposits appeared in their arteries. Control chickens did not show the same lipid deposits.[52]

Although it has been shown that insulin may exert an in vivo effect on arterial wall metabolism,[53,54] in vitro effects have been much more difficult to demonstrate. Capron et al. recently suggested that these difficulties may be due to the differences in the pressures to which cells of the arterial media are exposed in vivo and in vitro.[55] They found that insulin had no in vitro effect on the media of rat aortae perfused at 34 mm Hg. However, insulin stimulated the metabolism of glucose by the media, when the aortae were perfused at 70 mm Hg. It has also been found that insulin can induce an increase in sterol synthesis in arterial smooth muscle cells in culture, possibly by increasing the activity of HMG CoA reductase.[56]

In addition to these direct effects on metabolism, it appears that insulin can promote the proliferation of arterial cells. This has been shown for both the smooth muscle cells of primates and of rats.[57,58] Insulin also enhances the synthesis of DNA by rat aortic smooth muscle cells.[59] However, it does not appear to do so with endothelial cells.[59] It is important to recognize that the behavior of endothelial cells derived from different sites is different.[60] Thus, insulin increases the conversion of glucose to glycogen in calf retinal endothelium but not aortic endothelium. Insulin also stimulates 3 the incorporation of H-thymidine into DNA by these retinal endothelial cells, but not by calf aortic or human umbilical venous endothelial cells.

Hyperinsulinemia may also have played a role in two other atherogenic factors, blood pressure and lipoprotein metabolism. The impact of diabetes on blood pressure will be discussed later. However, at this point, it is appropriate to indicate that insulin can promote expansion of the plasma volume, probably by decreasing urinary sodium excretion.[61,62] With respect to lipoprotein metabolism, it will be pointed out that the production of VLDL and IDL are increased in both the hyperinsulinemic human and rat.[50,63,64,65] Furthermore hyperinsulinemia, particularly if it is extrahepatic, will increase the activity of lipoprotein lipase which can increase the degradation of the triglyceride rich lipoproteins.[66] This increase in the activity of lipoprotein lipase has also been suggested to have an effect on HDL.[67] In fact that may even account for the unexpected increase in HDL—cholesterol that has been observed in a number of diabetics, particularly those with type 1 diabetes. To date there has been no reported effect of insulin on the uptake of lipoproteins by the arterial cells. However, Chait et al. did find that insulin stimulated the binding of LDL to cultured human fibroblasts.[68] These insulin-induced changes may have an atherogenic effect that is additive to any independent risk effect of hyperinsulinemia.

Hypertension

The association of hypertension with atherosclerotic vascular disease, particularly cerebrovascular disease, has been well documented.[69] Although it is generally true that hypertension plays a causal role in atherosclerosis, it is worthwhile to remember that atherosclerosis, through its effect on aortic elasticity may also influence blood pressure particularly systolic blood pressure.[70] Furthermore, atherosclerosis, if it affects the renal arteries may lead to hypertension.

The pathophysiologic role of hypertension in atherogenesis has generally been attributed to the vessel injury that it may induce.[71] The possibility that blood pressure may directly influence the metabolism of the aorta has already been discussed.[55] In view of these observations, when considering atherosclerosis in the diabetic, it is important to examine the possibility that diabetes and hypertension are associated. If they are, it is then relevant to ask whether any such association is different in type 1 diabetes from that in type 2 diabetes.

Any examination of hypertension in diabetics must recognize the many spurious factors that may influence such a relationship. For example, the thiazide diuretics are frequently used to treat hypertension. They may also decrease an individual's glucose tolerance and create a picture much like type 2 diabetes. Other medications such as the oral contraceptives may cause both an increase in blood pressure and glucose intolerance. Certain endocrinopathies such as acromegaly, pheochromocytoma, primary aldosteronism and Cushing's syndrome may have both hypertension and carbohydrate intolerance, as a part of their manifestations. Finally, and most commonly, obesity is frequently associated with diabetes (especially type 2) and hypertension. The diabetes may result from, or be exacerbated by the obese person's resistance to insulin.[47] The mechanisms underlying hypertension in the obese have been recently reviewed.[72] Obesity can increase cardiac output. It can increase sodium retention as a consequence of the hyperinsulinemia that results from insulin resistance in the obese person. It can alter the relationships between renin and aldosterone, and it can produce neuroendocrine changes. Any, or all of these could lead to hypertension in the obese, be he diabetic or not.

Even if one corrects for obesity, there have been many epidemiologic suggestions that diabetes and hypertension are associated with each other. However, Keen et al. have pointed out the importance of matching diabetics and controls closely in order to avoid misinterpretations.[73] Bearing this in mind, it has been suggested by the Framingham study that hypertension is more common in diabetics, particularly diabetic women, than in non-diabetics.[74] The association of diabetes and hypertension is very much stronger in the elderly, raising the possibility that the problem is greatest in type 2 diabetics.[75] A similar inference may be made from the observations of Jarrett et al., that blood pressure correlated with blood glucose in men over 40 years of age, and that this was independent of obesity.[76] It has also been suggested that the blood pressure may be lower in those diabetics who require over 50 units of insulin per day than it is in those diabetics who require less insulin.[77] That would be consistent with hypertension being more of a problem in the type 2 diabetic. Drury has summarized those flimsy pieces of evidence that may be used to compare hypertension in type 1 to type 2 diabetics.[78] He suggests that diabetes is mainly a problem of the older population. Further, he suggests that any hypertension seen in young type 1 diabetics is likely to be systolic hypertension. Diastolic hypertension in type 1 diabetics appears to be an accompaniment of renal disease.

Lipoproteins

As in the other sections of this chapter, the aim here will be to review those aspects that may provide further insight into the comparison of types 1 and 2 diabetes. It will not be an attempt to provide an overall review of lipoproteins in diabetes. Furthermore, the emphasis will be placed on those abnormalities that are associated with hyperinsulinemia (endogenous or exogenous) rather than with those aspects that are associated with insulin deficiency. It is now known that insulin deficiency is accompanied by an increase in free fatty acids, the substrate for lipoprotein triglyceride, and with a deficiency of lipoprotein lipase, the enzyme responsible for triglyceride clearance.[79] However, gross insulin deficiency is rarely seen in diabetic humans today, and when it occurs, it is generally short lived. Therefore, this is unlikely to be a risk for atherosclerosis. By contrast, as noted earlier, diabetics today are more generally hyperinsulinemic.

Most agree that the most common lipid abnormality in the general diabetic population is hypertriglyceridemia. There is also some evidence, but less general agreement, to suggest that plasma choles- terol is also elevated.[1,80,81]

It is no longer sufficient to consider only the total plasma concentration of lipids. One must now consider the concentrations of specific lipoproteins and of their apolipoproteins. This neces- sitates a definition of the different lipoprotein classes. This task is made all the more difficult by the fact that the physical and chemical means used to separate the lipoprotein classes do not separate the lipoproteins into functionally homogeneous species. Most methods that are used to separate "LDL" yield the Sf 0-20 frac- tion of lipoproteins. The Sf 20-400 fraction was considered to be "VLDL". It is now recognized, from kinetic studies, that the rem- nants of VLDL catabolism are found in the Sf 12-60 fraction.[82,83] Hence, the fraction previously considered to be LDL, in fact, has a large portion of VLDL-remnants (also called IDL). This may explain the "triglyceride enrichment of LDL" reported in the diabetic.[84,85,86,87]

It is also important to consider possible changes in the com- position of other lipoproteins, as may be reflected in their apoli- proteins. Thus, it has been shown that in diabetics, animals and humans there is a reduction in the apo C-II/apo C-III ratio.[88,89] Such a change may make the triglyceride-rich lipoproteins a poorer substrate for lipoprotein lipase. It has also been suggested that there is a reduction in plasma apo A-I, but not in plasma apo A-II.[88] By contrast Eckel et al. have suggested that HDL apo A-I/apo A-II ratios are increased in diabetics.[90] Type 1 and type 2 diabetics probably can not be compared, when they have been studied in separate centers, because of the highly different patterns of lipoproteins seen between different centers. There are only a few studies in which the lipoproteins of type 1 and 2 diabetics have been compared as a part of the same study. In one such study no difference was found.[88] In another, diet treated type 2 diabetics had the highest serum triglycerides and the lowest HDL cholesterols. Sulfonylurea-treated type 2 diabetics were next in showing this pat- tern. Insulin-treated type 2 diabetics and type 1 diabetics had similar values and were not different from nondiabetic males.[87] In a very comprehensive review of HDL levels seen in diabetics Nikkila has indicated that most centers have found that the HDL levels in the type 2 diabetics who do not receive insulin is either low or normal. This contrasts with the various reports relating to insulin-treated diabetics, whose HDL cholesterols are normal or high.[67]

Most studies of lipoproteins in diabetics have examined their concentrations. However, it is probably at least as important to examine their turnover. The two do not necessarily parallel each other. As already indicated, today most diabetics are hyperinsulinemic rather than insulin deficient. Hence, this consideration of lipoprotein kinetics will be confined to the effect of hyperinsulinemia. Furthermore, it was noted that the main abnormality is in the triglyceride-rich lipoproteins.

The vicious cycle linking hyperinsulinemia and hypertriglyceridemia was described when discussing hyperinsulinemia. As noted there, hyperinsulinemia in humans and in rats is associated with an increase in the production of plasma triglyceride.[50,63,64] It should be noted that it was not possible to reproduce this increase in triglyceride production in cultured rat hepatocytes.[91,92] However, such an in vitro system is clearly very different from the in vivo models. The impact of changes in triglyceride production on the plasma concentration of triglyceride will depend on the balance between production and removal. Thus in the rat made hyperinsulinemic, either by injection or by infusion of insulin into subcutaneous tissues, the production of triglyceride is greatly accelerated but the plasma concentration of triglycerides declines.[63,93] This probably reflects an even greater increase in triglyceride removal due to an effect of insulin on lipoprotein lipase.[66] It is possible that similar changes account for the decline of triglycerides seen in patients with insulinomas. It is also interesting to note that the balance between production and removal of triglycerides appears to be different in rats that receive insulin by intraperitoneal infusion compared to rats that receive insulin by subcutaneous infusion.[93] Both receive the same amount of insulin. Both have a similar portal venous concentration of insulin. The subcutaneously infused rats have a higher concentration of insulin in the peripheral venous blood. Both groups have the same increase in triglyceride production. However, the serum triglycerides decline in subcutaneously infused rats and, by contrast, do not change in the intraperitoneally infused rats. This may reflect a greater stimulation of the extrahepatic enzyme, lipoprotein lipase, in the subcutaneously infused rat.

Whatever the impact of hyperinsulinemia on plasma triglyceride concentrations, there are circumstantial reasons to suggest that an increase in the turnover of triglyceride-rich lipoproteins may promote atherogenesis. If the turnover of these lipoproteins is accelerated, there will be an increase in the generation of their catabolic remnants. There is mounting evidence to suggest that these remnants, or IDL, may be atherogenic. Type III hyperlipoproteinemia, a disorder associated with a great accumulation of IDL, is associated with early atherosclerosis. Zilversmit has reviewed the data that suggests the triglyceride-rich lipoproteins may be degraded to smaller more atherogenic particles by lipoprotein lipase on the arterial wall.[94] Epidemiologic studies have shown that male myocardial infarct survivors have elevated levels of Sf 12-20 lipoproteins, and that the levels of these lipoproteins can predict the likelihood of reinfarction.[95] Although kinetic studies have indicated that the remnants of VLDL are in the Sf 12-60 fraction, we have found (unpublished observations) that 75% of the Sf 12-60 particles are in the Sf 12-20 fraction. Thus, the studies on infarct survivors probably do represent findings that can be translated to IDL. Furthermore, we have investigated, in a preliminary manner, the concentrations of Sf 12-60 lipoproteins in the plasma of men undergoing aorto-coronary bypass grafting. They were found to be higher than those in control men undergoing valve surgery and free of coronary arteriosclerosis.[1] Thus, it is possible to develop an argument that hyperinsulinemia promotes atherogenic changes in the lipoproteins, even without altering their concentrations. This would have obvious implications on the hyperinsulinemic type 2 diabetic and on the insulin treated type 1 or 2 diabetic. It also suggests that there may be a difference in the atherogenic impact of hyperinsulinemia depending on the route of insulin administration, from the pancreas into the portal vein, or from a subcutaneous depot.

Platelets and soluble clotting factors

It has become increasingly apparent that platelets play a very significant role in the early process of atherogenesis. Furthermore, they and the soluble clotting factors are extremely important in the occlusion of an artery by thrombus. The role of the platelets in atherogenesis was suggested by the observations of Moore that, in the presence of anti-platelet antiserum, arterial injury could no longer initiate experimental atherosclerosis.[96] More recently Ross has demonstrated that, among its many constituents, the platelet contains a factor that stimulates the growth of arterial smooth muscles. He and Glomset have reviewed the way in which the platelet may adhere to the wall of an injured artery, then release from it granules that lead to further platelet aggregation, to arterial contraction, to thrombus formation and to smooth muscle proliferation.[98] The reasons for platelets to adhere to the injured vessel wall may involve the elaboration of von Willebrand factor and the decreased production of prostacylcin by the artery. Prostacyclin appears to have many effects that oppose those of the thromboxane. Thomboxane is a prostaglandin derivative that is produced during the process of platelet aggregation. It has been suggested that there is a delicate balance between the opposing effects of prostacyclin and thromboxane which, if disturbed may initiate or aggravate atherogenesis. It has been this that has also led some to suggest that antiplatelet drugs such as aspirin may, in the proper dose, inhibit atherogenesis by blocking prostaglandin production by the platelets more than that by the artery wall. There have been many descriptions of platelet and clotting factor abnormalities in diabetics. Although many of these have been inconsistent, there appears to be general agreement that platelet adhesiveness and platelet aggregation increase in the diabetic and that this may be related to glycemic control. There may also be changes in the soluble clotting factors in a general pattern that would increase thrombogenesis. The problem with most of these studies is that there is a great deal of inconsistency between them. Furthermore, many of the changes may not underlie atherosclerois, but may be secondary to it.[98] Finally, there is no appropriately controlled comparison of platelet function and of the clotting factors in type 1 and type 2 diabetes. For more details, the reader is referred to recent reviews.[17,99,100]

Obesity

The association of obesity with type 2 diabetes is well recognized. It is also well known that obese individuals have an increased risk of coronary artery disease. However, as pointed out earlier, it is also known that obesity is accompanied by dyslipoproteinemias, hyperinsulinemia and hypertension. Each of these, by itself, may increase the risk of atherosclerosis. Hence, the real question is whether obesity confers a risk for atherosclerosis that is independent of other risk factors. The Framingham study has suggested that although obesity may be associated with an increase in the incidence of angina and of sudden death, it is not associated by itself with an increase in the incidence of myocardial infarction. Keen and his colleagues have recently reviewed the arguments suggesting that the effects of obesity are mediated through other risk factors.[101]

SOME OUTSTANDING PROBLEMS

The heterogeneity of both diabetes and atherosclerosis have made the analysis of their association extremely complex. Perhaps, with the increasing recognition of all the different forms of diabetes and the multitude of atherogenic factors, it will be possible to be more specific in future studies relating diabetes to atherosclerosis and its causative factors. Although there are a number of studies that indicate the increased association of diabetes with atherosclerosis or with some of its underlying causes, there are still very few studies in which types 1 and 2 diabetes have been differentiated. In those few where this has been done, factors such as differences in the age and duration of diabetes have complicated the comparisons of both populations. Without good epidemiologic data, it has been necessary to turn to such data as is available about the frequency and nature of atherogenic factors in types 1 and 2 diabetes. From this one may make indirect guesses about the macrovascular disease in both of these populations. These will have to be tested by direct study in future.

It is clear that there is an increased frequency of atherosclerosis in the diabetic population. However, our present knowledge does not permit us to account for all of this increase in macrovascular disease on the basis of currently known risk factors. This raises the possibility that there are other atherogenic factors about which we do not yet know. Such factors may or may not be unique to the diabetic. New potential candidates, such as some of the apoprotein abnormalities, are being identified and explored. There is, however, another challenging possibility. Jarrett has asked whether diabetes is in fact causally related to atherosclerosis, or whether this is just a casual association.[102] His questions arise from one perception of the epidemiologic data. However, they do direct attention to fascinating recent studies of the molecular genetics of diabetes and atherosclerosis.[103] Mandrup-Poulsen et al. have observed that the frequency of U alleles in the region flanking the 5' end of the human insulin gene, on the short arm of chromosome 11 is increased 2.5 times in patients with atherosclerosis. It does not appear to exert its effect through blood glucose, triglyceride or cholesterol levels. Furthermore, they feel that the previously observed association of this genetic abnormality with an increase in the risk of diabetes disappears when the data is corrected for the presence of atherosclerosis. This would support the notion of an association between both disorders that need not be entirely due to cause and effect. Clearly this will merit further examination. Even if it does hold, one should not conclude that the impact of diabetes on other risk factors is not important. It may mean that one will have to examine the influence of interacting risk factors on atherosclerosis. From a further knowledge of the atherogenic influences in diabetes one can anticipate suggestions about the most effective preventive treatment. What is the most appropriate diet for the diabetic in relation not only to his glycemic control, but also in relation to his risk of macrovascular disease? What is the influence of achieving normglycemic control? Would such control be accompanied by hyperinsulinemia and, if so, would this have a deleterious effect? Is there a different risk in relation to the route of insulin administration? In fact could one construct a rational argument to treat diabetes by those means that would supply the body's insulin from the pancreas, even if it meant giving an oral hypoglycemic agent?

REFERENCES

1. G. Steiner, Diabetes and atherosclerosis: An overview, Diabetes, 30 (suppl. 2):1-7, (1981).

2. S. Warren, P.M. LeCompte, and M.A. Legg, "The Pathology of Diabetes Mellitus," Lea and Febiger, Philadelphia, p. 186, 4th ed. (1966).

3. T. Gordon, W.P. Castelli, M.C. Hjortland et al., Diabetes, blood lipids, and the role of obesity in coronary heart disease risk for women, Ann. Int. Med. 87:393-403, (1977).

4. A.G. Shaper, K.T. Lee, R.F. Scott et al., Chemico-Anatomic studies in the geographic pathology of arteriosclerosis, Comparison of adipose tissue fatty acids in diabetics from East Africa and the United States with different frequencies of myocardial infarction, Am. J. Cardiol. 10:390-399, (1962).

5. Y. Hirata, and T. Mihara, Principal causes of death among Japanese from 1968 to 1970, in: "Diabetes Mellitus in Asia," S. Baba, Y. Goto, and I. Fukui, eds., Excerpta Medica, Amsterdam, p 91-97 (1976).

6. M. Alex, E.K. Goldenberg, and H.T. Blumenthal, An autopsy study of cerebrovascular accidents in diabetes mellitus, Circ. 25:663-673 (1962).

7. H.U. Janka, E. Standl, and H. Mehnert, Peripheral vascular disease in diabetes mellitus and its relation to cardiovascular risk factors: Screening with the Doppler ultrasonic technique, Diabetes Care 3:207-213 (1980).

8. K.W. Beach, J.D. Brunzell, and D.E. Strandness, Jr., Severe arteriosclerosis obliterans in patients with diabetes mellitus, Relation to smoking and form of therapy, Arteriosclerosis 2:275-280 (1982).

9. R.I. Most, and P. Sinnock, The epidemiology of lower extremity amputations in diabetic individuals, Diabetes Care 6:87-91 (1983).

10. L.J. Melton, P.J. Palumbo, M.S. Dwyer, and C.P. Chu, Impact of recent changes in diagnostic criteria on the apparent natural history of diabetes mellitus, Am. J. Epidemiol. 117:559-565 (1983).

11. F.V. Crall, and W.C. Roberts, The extramural and intramural coronary arteries in juvenile diabetes mellitus, Analysis of nine necropsy patients aged 19-38 years with onset of diabetes before age 15 years, Am. J. Med. 64:221-230 (1978).

12. I.I. Kessler, Mortality experience of diabetic patients, A 26 year follow-up study, Am. J. Med. 51:715-724 (1971).

13. G. Goodkin, Mortality factors in diabetes, J. Occupational Med. 17:716-721 (1975).

14. N.B. Ruderman, and C. Haudenshild, Diabetes as an atherogenic factor, Prog. in Cardiovasc. Dis. 26:373-412 (1984).

15. M.L. Grunnet, Cerebrovascular disease: diabetes and cerebral atherosclerosis, Neurol. 13:486-491 (1963).

16. H.C. McGill, Diabetes and its vascular lesions in Diabetes and Atherosclerosis Connection, J. Moskowitz, ed., The Juvenile Diabetes Foundation, New York, :45-52 (1981) .

17. R.J. Jarrett, H. Keen, and R. Chakrabarti, Diabetes, hyper-glycemia and arterial disease in Complications of Diabetes, 2nd Ed. H. Keen and R.J. Jarrett eds., Edward Arnold Publishers Ltd., London, :179-204 (1982).

18. B.F. Waller, P.J. Palumbo, J.T. Lie, and W.C. Roberts, Status of coronary arteries of necropsy in diabetes mellitus with onset after age 30 years, Am. J. Med. 69:498-507 (1980).

19. D.E. Strandness, R.E. Priest, and G.E. Gibbons, Combined clini-cal and pathologic study of diabetic and non-diabetic peripheral arterial disease, Diabetes 13:366-372 (1964).

20. V.W. Fischer, H.B. Barner, and M.L. Leskin, Capillary basal laminar thickness in diabetic human myocardium, Diabetes 28:713-719 (1979).

21. S.M. Factor, E.M. Okun, and T. Minase, Capillary microaneurysms in the human diabetic heart, N. Eng. J. Med. 302:384-388 (1980).

22. M.D. Silver, V.F. Huckell, and M. Lorber, Basement membranes of small cardiac vessels in patients with diabetes and myxedema; preliminary observations, Pathology 9:213-220 (1977).

23. H. Keen, and R.J. Jarrett, The WHO multinational study of vas-cular disease in diabetes: 2 Macrovascular disease prevalence, Diabetes Care 2:187-195 (1979).

24. R.J. Jarrett, and H. Keen, The WHO multinational study of vas-cular disease in diabetes: 3 Microvascular disease, Diabetes Care 2:196-201 (1979).

25. J.A. Colwell, M. Lopes-Virella, and P.V. Halushka. Patho-genesis of atherosclerosis in diabetes mellitus, Diabetes Care 4:121-133 (1981).

26. G.M. Reaven, and G. Steiner, Proceedings of a conference on diabetes and atherosclerosis, Diabetes 30(2):1-110 (1981).

27. J.H. Fuller, P. McCartney, R.J. Jarrett, H. Keen, G. Rose, M.J. Shipley, and P.J.S. Hamilton, Hyperglycemia and coronary heart disease: The Whitehall study, J. Chronic Dis. 32:721-728 (1979).

28. R. Stamler, J. Stamler, H.A. Lindberg, J. Marquardt, D.M. Berkson, O. Paul, M. Lepper, A. Dyer, and E. Stevens, Asympto-matic hyperglycemia and coronary heart disease in middle aged men in two employed populations in Chicago, J. Chronic. Dis. 32:805-815 (1979).

29. R. Stamler, J. Stamler, J.A. Schoenberger, R.B. Shekelle, P. Collette, S. Shekelle, A. Dyer, D. Garside, and J. Wannamaker, Relationship of glucose tolerance to prevalence of ECG abnor-malities and to 5-year mortality from cardiovascular disease: Findings of the Chicago Heart Association detection project in industry, J. Chronic Dis. 32:817-828 (1979).

30. R. Stamler, and J. Stamler, eds., Asymptomatic hyperglycemia and coronary heart disease, A series of papers by the Inter-national Collaborative Group, based on studies in fifteen pop-ulations, J. Chronic Dis. 32:683-837 (1979).

31. K.H. Gabbay, Hyperglycemia, polyol metabolism and complications of diabetes mellitus, Ann. Revs. Med. 26:521-536 (1975).

32. R.P. Boot-Hanford, and H. Heath, The absence of sorbitol pathway activity in primary cultures of human umbilical vein endothelial cells, IRCS Med. Sci. Biochem. 9:451(abs) (1978).

33. R.W. Stout, Glucose inhibits replication of cultured human endothelial cells, Diabetologia 23:436-439 (1982).

34. Y.A. Kesaniemi, J.L. Witztum, and U.P. Steinbrecher, Receptor-mediated catabolism of low sensity lipoprotein in man, J. Clin. Invest. 71:950-959 (1983).

35. J.L. Witztum, U.P. Steinbrecher, M. Fisher, and A. Kesaniemi, Non-enzymatic glucosylation of homologous low density lipoprotein and albumin renders them immunogenic in guinea pigs, Pro. Nat. Acad. Sci. (U.S.A.) 80:2757-2761, (1983).

36. M.F. Lopes-Virella, G.K. Sherer, A.M. Lees, H. Woltmann, R. Mayfield, J. Sagel, E.C. LeRoy, and J.A. Colwell, Surface binding, internalization and degradation by cultured human fibroblasts of low density lipoproteins isolated from type 1 (insulin-dependent) diabetic patients:changes with metabolic control, Diabetologia 22:430-436 (1982).

37. A.R. Bassiony, H. Rosenberg, and T.L. McDonald, Glucosylated collagen is antigenic, Diabetes 32:1182-1184 (1983).

38. H. Rosenberg, J.B. Modrak, J.M. Hassing, W.A. Al-Turk, and S. Stohs, Glucosylated collagen, Biochem. Byophys. Res. Comm. 91:498-501, (1982).

39. B.W. Vogt, E.D. Schleicher, and O.H. Wieland, E Aminolysine bound glucose in human tissue obtained at autopsy, Diabetes 31:1123-1129 (1982).

40. N. Peters, and C.N. Hales, Plasma insulin concentrations after myocardial infarction, Lancet 1:1144-1145 (1965).

41. E.A. Nikkila, T.A. Miettinen, M.R. Vessenne, and R. Pelkonen, Plasma insulin in cononary heart disease, Lancet 2:508-511 (1965).

42. F. Sorge, W. Schwartzkopff, and G.A. Neuhaus, Insulin response to oral glucose in patients with a previous myocardial infarction and in patients with peripheral vascular disease, Diabetes 25:586-594 (1976).

43. M.M. Gertler, H.E. Leetma, E. Saluste, D.A. Covalt, and J.L. Rosenberg, Covert diabetes mellitus, ischemic heart disease and cerebrovascular disease, Geriatrics 27:105-120 (1972).

44. T.A. Welborn, and K. Wearnw, Coronary heart disease incidence and cardiovascular mortality in Busselton with reference to glucose and insulin concentrations, Diabetes Care 2:154-160 (1979).

45. K. Pyorala, Relationship of glucose tolerance and plasma insulin to the incidence of coronary heart disease: results from two population studies in Finland, Diabetes Care 2:131-141 (1979).

46. P. Ducimitiere, L. Eschwege, P.L. Papoz, R.J.R. Claude, and G. Rosselin, Relationship of plasma insulin levels to the incidence of myocardial infarction and coronary heart disease mortality in a middle-aged population, Diabetologia 19:205-210 (1980).

47. M. Vranic, S. Morita, and G. Steiner, Insulin resistance in
     obesity as analyzed by the response of glucose kinetics to glu-
     cagon infusion, Diabetes 29:169-176 (1980).
48. G.M. Reaven, and J.M. Olefsky, Role of insulin resistance in
     the pathogenesis of hyperglycemia, in: "Diabetes, Obesity and
     Vascular Disease," H.M. Katz and R.J. Mahler eds., John Wiley
     and Sons, New York, :229-266 (1978).
49. G. Steiner, S. Morita, and M. Vranic, Resistance to insulin but
     not to glucagon in lean human hypertriglyceridemics, Diabetes
     29:899-905 (1980).
50. G. Steiner, and M. Vranic, Insulin and hypertriglyceridemia: A
     vicious cycle with atherogenic potential, Int. J. Obesity
     6(suppl. 1):117-124 (1982).
51. A.B. Cruz, D.S. Amatuzio, F. Grande, and L.J. Hay, Effect of
     intraarterial insulin on tissue cholesterol and fatty acids in
     alloxan-diabetic dogs, Circ. Res. 9:39-43 (1961).
52. R.W. Stout, Development of vascular lesions in insulin treated
     animals fed a normal diet, Brit. Med. J. 3:685-687 (1970).
53. A.V. Chobanian, G.C. Gerritsen, P.I. Brecher and L. McCombs,
     Aortic glucose metabolism in the diabetic Chinese hamster,
     Diabetologia 10:589-593 (1974).
54. H. Wallinsky, S. Goldfischer, L. Capron, F. Capron, B.B.
     Coltoff-Schiller, and L. Kasak, Hydrolase activities in the rat
     aorta, I Effects of diabetes mellitus and insulin treatment,
     Circ. Res. 42:821-831 (1978).
55. L. Capron, M. Phillipe, J.L. Guilmot, J.N. Feissinger, and E.
     Housset, Effect of insulin exposure upon the metabolism of rat
     aortic media: Influence of hydrostatic forces, Arterio-
     sclerosis 1:345-352 (1981).
56. R.W. Stout, Relative insensitivity to glucagon of sterol synthe-
     sis in cultured rat aortic smooth muscle cells, Atherosclerosis
     27:271-278 (1977).
57. B. Pfeifle and H. Ditschuneit, Effect of insulin on the growth
     of smooth muscle cells in vitro, Diabetologia 20:155-158 (1981).
58. R.W. Stout, E.L. Bierman, and R. Ross, Effect of insulin on the
     proliferation of cultured primate arterial smooth muscle cells,
     Circ. Res. 36:319-327 (1975).
59. H. Taggart, and R.W. Stout, Control of DNA synthesis in cultured
     vascular endothelial and smooth muscle cells, Atherosclerosis
     37:549-557 (1980).
60. G.L. King, S.M. Buzney, R.C. Kahn, N. Hetu, S. Buchwald, S.G.
     MacDonald, and R.I. Rand, Differential responsiveness to insulin
     of endothelial and support cells from microand macrovessels, J.
     Clin. Invest. 71:974-979 (1983).
61. J.H. Miller, and M.D. Bogdanoff, Antidiuresis associated with
     administration of insulin, J. Appl. Physiol. 6:509-512 (1954).
62. R.A. DeFronzo, C.R. Cooke, R. Andres, G.R. Faloona, and P.J.
     Davis, The effect of insulin on renal handling of sodium, potas-
     sium, calcium and phosphate in man. J. Clin. Invest. 55:845-855
     (1975).

63. G. Steiner, F. Haynes, G. Yoshino, and M. Vranic, Hyperinsulinemia and in vivo very-low-density lipoprotein tri-glyceride kinetics, Am. J. Physiol. 246:E187-E192 (1984).

64. D.A. Streja, E.B. Marliss, and G. Steiner, The effects of pro-longed fasting on plasma triglyceride kinetics in man, Metabolism 26:505-516 (1977).

65. D.C. Cattran, G. Steiner, D.R. Wilson, and S.S.A. Fenton, Hyper-lipidemia after renal transplantation: natural history and pathophysiology, Ann. Int. Med. 91:554-559 (1979).

66. C.N. Sadur, and R.H. Eckel, Insulin stimulation of adipose tissue lipoprotein lipase, Use of the euglycemic clamp tech-nique, J. Clin. Invest. 69:1119-1125 (1982).

67. E.A. Nikkila, High density lipoproteins in diabetes, Diabetes 30(suppl. 2):82-87 (1981).

68. A. Chait, E.L. Bierman, and J.J. Albers, Low density lipoprotein receptor activity in cultured human skin fibroblasts, Mechanism of insulin-induced stimulation, J. Clin. Invest. 64:1309-1319 (1979).

69. K. Asplund, E. Hagg, C. Helmers, F. Lithner, T. Strand, and P. Wester, The natural history of stroke in diabetic patients, Acta Med. Scand. 207:417-424 (1980).

70. C.J. Pepine, and W.W. Nichols, Aortic input impedance in cardio-vascular disease, Prog. Cardiovac. Dis. 24:307-318 (1982).

71. S. Glagov, Hemodynamic risk factors: Mechanical stress mural architecture, medial nutrition and vulnerability of arteries to atherosclerosis, in: "The Pathogenesis of Atherosclerosis," R.W. Wissler and C.J. Geer eds., Williams and Wilkins, Baltimore, :164-199 (1972).

72. H.P. Dustan, Mechanism of hypertension associated with obesity, Ann. Int. Med. 98:860-864, (1983).

73. H.Keen, N.S. Track, and G.S.C. Sowry, Arterial pressure in clinically apparent diabetics, Diabete et Metabolisme 1:159-178 (1975).

74. T.R. Dawber, "Diabetes and cardiovascular disease in The Framingham Study," Harvard University Press, Cambridge :190-201 (1980).

75. E. Barrett-Connor, M.H. Criqui, M.R. Klauber, and M. Holdbrook, Diabetes and hypertension in a community of older adults, Am. J. Epidemiol. 113:276-284 (1981).

76. R.J. Jarrett, H. Keen, M. McCartney, J.H. Fuller, P.J.S. Hamilton, D.D. Ried, and G. Rose, Glucose tolerance and blood pressure in two population samples: their relation to diabetes mellitus and hypertension, Int. J. Epidemiol. 7:15-24 (1978).

77. S. Pell, and C.A. D'Alonzo, Some aspects of hypertension in diabetes mellitus, Am. Med. Assoc. J. 202:104-110 (1967).

78. P.L. Drury, Diabetes and arterial hypertension, Diabetologia 24:1-9 (1983).

79. G. Steiner, M.A. Poapst, and J.K. Davidson, Production of chylomicron-like lipoproteins from endogenous lipid by intestine and liver of diabetic dogs, Diabetes 24:263-271 (1975).

80. J.D. Brunzell, Mechanisms of hyperlipidemia in diabetes mellitus in Diabetes and Atherosclerosis Connection, J. Moskowitz ed., Juvenile Diabetes Foundation, New York, (1981), p 181-192.

81. B.R. Zimmerman, P.J. Palumbo, W.A. O'Fallon, R.D. Ellofson, P.J. Osmundson, and F.J. Kazmier, A prospective study of peripheral occlusive arterial disease in diabetes, III. Initial lipid and lipoprotein findings, Mayo Clin. Proc. 56:223-242 (1981).

82. M.F. Reardon, N.H. Fidge, and P.J. Nestel, Catabolism of very low density lipoprotein B apoprotein in man, J. Clin. Invest. 61:850-860 (1978).

83. M.F. Reardon and G. Steiner. The use of kinetics in investigating the metabolism of very low and intermediate density lipoproteins, in: "Lipoprotein Kinetics and Modeling," M. Berman, S.M. Grundy and B. Howard eds., Acad. Press, New York (1982).

84. G. Schonfeld, C. Birge, J.P. Miller, G. Kessler, and J. Santiago, Apolipoprotein B levels and altered lipoprotein composition of diabetes, Diabetes 23:827-834 (1974).

85. M. Mancini, A. Rivellese, P. Rubba, and G. Riccardi, Plasma lipoproteins in maturity onset diabetes, Nutr. Metab. 24(suppl 1):65-73 (1980).

86. M.R. Taskinen, E.A. Nikkila, T. Kuusi, and K. Harno, Lipoprotein lipase in untreated type 2 (insulinindependent) diabetes associated with obesity, Diabetologia 22:44-50 (1982).

87. W. Beach, J.D. Brunzell, L.L. Conquest, and D.E. Strandness, The correlation of arteriosclerosis obliterans with lipoproteins in insulin-dependent and non-insulin-dependent diabetes, Diabetes 28:836-840 (1979).

88. E.R. Briones, S.J.T. Mao, P.J. Palumbo, W.M. O'Fallon, W. Chenoweth, and B.A. Kottke, Analysis of plasma lipids and apolipoproteins in insulin-dependent and non-insulin-dependent diabetics, Metabolism 33:42-49 (1984).

89. H. Bar-On, P.S. Roheim, and H. Eder, Serum lipoproteins and apolipoproteins in rats with streptozotocin-induced diabetes, J. Clin. Invest. 57:714-721 (1976).

90. R.H. Eckel, J.J. Albers, M.C. Chung, P.W. Wahl, F.T. Lindgren, and E.L. Bierman, High density lipoprotein composition in insulin-dependent diabetes mellitus, Diabetes 30:132-138 (1981).

91. P.N. Durrington, R.S. Newton, D.B. Weinstein, and D. Steinberg, Effects of insulin and glucose on very low density lipoprotein triglyceride secretion by cultured rat hepatocytes, J. Clin. Invest. 70:63-73 (1982).

92. W. Patsch, S. Franz, and G. Schonfeld, Role of insulin in lipoprotein secretion by cultured rat hepatocytes, J. Clin. Invest. 71:1161-1174 (1983).

93. T. Kazumi, M. Vranic, and G. Steiner, Comparison of portal vs peripheral hyperinsulinemia on VLDL-triglyceride kinetics, Proc. 7th Int. Endoc. Cong. (abst) (1984).

94. D.B. Zilversmit, Atherogenesis, a post-prandial phenomenon, Circulation 60-473-485 (1979).

95. H.B. Jones, J.W. Gofman, F.T. Lindgr, T.P. Lyon, D.M. Graham, B. Strisower, and A.V. Nichols, Lipoproteins in atherosclerosis, Am. J. Med. 11:358-380 (1951).
96. S. Moore, R.J. Friedman, D.P. Singal, J. Gauldie, M.A. Blajchman, and R.S. Roberts, Inhibition of injury induced thromboatherosclerotic lesions by anti-platelet serum in rabbits, Thromb. Haemostasis 35:70-81 (1976).
97. R. Ross, and J.A. Glomset, The pathogenesis of atherosclerosis, N. Eng. J. Med. 295:369-377 and 420-425 (1976).
98. J.F. Mustard, and M.A. Packham, Platelets and diabetes mellitus, N. Eng. J. Med. 297:1345-1347 (1977).
99. J.A. Colwell, P.D. Winocour, M. Lopes-Virella, and, P.V. Halushka, New concepts about the pathogenesis of atherosclerosis in diabetes mellitus, Am. J. Med. 67-80 (1983).
100. E. Standl, and H. Mehnert eds., Pathogenetic concepts of diabetic microangiopathy, Hormone Metb. Res. 11(suppl.):1-58 (1981).
101. H. Keen, B.J. Thomas, and R.J. Jarrett, Obesity and cardiovascular risk, Int. J. Obesity 6(suppl. 1):83-89 (1982).
102. R.J. Jarrett, Type 2 (non-insulin-dependent) diabetes mellitus and coronary heart disease - chicken, egg or neither? Diabetologia 26:99-102 (1984).
103. T. Mandrup-Poulsen, P. Owerbach, S.A. Mortensen, K. Johansen, H. Meinertz, H. Sorensen, and J. Nerup, DNA sequences flanking the insulin gene on chromosome 11 confer risk of atherosclerosis, Lancet 1:250-252 (1984).

A COMPARISON OF KIDNEY DISEASE IN

TYPE I AND TYPE II DIABETES

S. Michael Mauer and
Blanche M. Chavers

Department of Pediatrics
University of Minnosota Medical School
Minneapolis, Minnseota 55455

It should be self-evident that the manifestations of clinical diabetic nephropathy are dependent upon the development of serious lesions in the kidney.[1] Thus, a comparison of nephropathy in Type I and Type II diabetes might logically focus on a comparison of the natural history of these lesions in these two disorders of glucose metabolism. Unfortunately, there is insufficient information available to provide a very precise description of either of these progressive processes let alone a comparison of the two. Herein we will attempt to summarize what, in our view, are some of the central issues in this area.

INCIDENCE

Marks reported that uremia caused 42% of the deaths in Type I diabetes.[2] Uremia was considered the cause of death in approximately 2.5% of Type II diabetic patients aged 40 to 59 at onset of disease and 0.8% of patients beyond age 60 at the onset of disease.[3] Among 702 patients presenting with ESRD in Brooklyn 24.6% were diabetic and approximately one-half had each type of diabetes.[4] Thus, diabetes represents the most important cause of renal insufficiency. One-third of the diabetic patients with end-stage renal disease (ESRD) receiving hemodialysis treatment at the Regional Kidney Disease Center in Minneapolis, Minnesota, between 1966 and 1981 were Type II diabetics.[5] Uremia, resulting from discontinuation of dialysis, caused 16% of the total deaths in this group.

IS DIABETES REQUIRED FOR THE DEVELOPMENT OF DIABETIC NEPHROPATHY?

It has been argued that the secondary microvascular complications of diabetes may represent an inherited tendency which,
although genetically linked to diabetes, is separate from the
diabetic dysmetabolism.[6] However, Osterby has shown that the
kidney is structurally normal at the onset of Type I diabetes and
develops progressive lesions only with time.[7] Further, we have
evidence that non-diabetic individuals who have identical twins with
Type I diabetes have completely normal kidney structure despite
discordance for diabetes for as long as three decades (unpublished
data). Although there are individual case studies proporting to
illustrate that the lesions of diabetic nephropathy can develop in
patients with Type II diabetes prior to manifestation of glucose
intolerance, a careful review of these reports failed to substan-
tiate these claims.[8] Thus, it appears that in both Type I and
Type II diabetes glucose dysmetabolism is a necessary prerequisite
for renal lesions. We feel, however, that hyperglycemia is not, per
se, a sufficient cause.[9] Patients with many years of either type
of diabetes may escape the development of significant renal
lesions. Thus, there appears to be a spectrum of susceptibility to
renal disease in diabetes.

THE LESIONS OF DIABETIC NEPHROPATHY

The pathology of the kidney has been more thoroughly studied in
Type I compared to Type II diabetes. The most sensitive indicator
of diabetes is glomerular basement membrane (GBM) thickening while
the most specific, widening of the glomerular mesangium, especially
the Kimmelsteil-Wilson nodule, and afferent and efferent arteriolar
hyalinosis, are found in uremic patients with both Types I and II
diabetes.[1,10] Recent studies, using quantitative electron micro-
scopic morphometric analysis in Type I patients have indicated that
the functional abnormalities of diabetic nephropathy (proteinuria,
hypertension and decreased glomerular filtration rate) are correlated with mesangial expansion and not with GBM thickening.[11]
Mesangial expansion appears to adversely influence glomerular
function through its effects on constricting glomerular capillary
lumenal space and peripheral capillary wall filtration surface.[11]
Progressive interstitial fibrosis may also be an important component
of the renal pathology.[12] Although much less well studied, the
pathology of Type II diabetic nephropathy appears to be essentially
similar to that of Type I.[10,13]

THE ROLE OF GLYCEMIC CONTROL IN THE TREATMENT AND PREVENTION OF
CLINICAL DIABETIC NEPHROPATHY

Once clinical proteinuria is well established in Type I

diabetes, the subsequent course is almost always characterized by an inexorable progression to end-stage renal failure. Institution of strict glycemic control in Type I diabetes does not alter this outcome.[14] Structural studies suggest that this may be because the lesions of diabetic nephropathy are already very far advanced.[11] The effect of improved treatment of the diabetic state on earlier stages of the evolution of nephropathy in Type I diabetes is not directly known, although some studies do suggest that the incidence of this complication can be positively influenced by this aproach.[15] Recent evidence strongly suggests that persisting blood glucose levels between 150 to 200 mg/dl for 8 to 10 years constitutes a major risk factor for the development of pathology of nephropathy in Type II diabetes while lower levels of hyperglycemia either achieved spontaneously or through treatment with insulin or oral hypoglycemic agents were associated with much lower risks of the development of obvious glomerular changes of diabetes.[10] Thus, although strict proof is lacking, current evidence suggests that efforts to maximize glycemic control in both types of diabetes could be rewarded with a decreased incidence or a delay in presentation of overt diabetic nephropathy. The problem of selecting the patient at risk for renal complications for more intensive glycemic treatment is not completely solved. Renal biopsy is a useful tool.[11] More indirect renal assessment may also be important. Mogensen has found the urinary albumin excretion (UAE) rates may predict subsequent nephropathy in Type I[16] and II patients.[17] This microalbuminuria is reversible by strict glycemic control in Type I patients[16] (unstudied in Type II). It remains to be seen whether UAE, as measured under strict glycemic control, will indicate a better renal outcome for patients manifesting improvement in this parameter.

SUMMARY

Diabetes is the most important cause of ESRD in the Western world. Type I and II diabetes appear to contribute importantly to ESRD although, obviously, the prevalence of ESRD is higher in Type I. Microalbuminuria may predict later development of overt clinical nephropathy in both Type I and Type II patients. In both diabetes subtypes current evidence favours the dysmetabolism of diabetes as causative. There are clinical observations in Type I and renal morphologic evidence in Type II indicating that risk of nephropathy is, in part, related to the magnitude of hyperglycemia. Institution of strict glycemic control fails to reverse established clinical nephropathy in Type I diabetes. Efforts to determine if precise regulation of blood sugar can prevent nephropathy in patients with Type I and Type II diabetes are currently incomplete.

REFERENCES

1. S.M. Mauer, M. W. Stefes, D.M. Brown, The kidney in diabetes,
    Am J Med. 70:603 (1981).
2. H.H. Marks, Longevity and mortality of diabetics, Am J Public
    Health 55:416 (1965).
3. M.C. Balodimus, Diabetic nephropathy, in: "Joslin's Diabetes
    Mellitus," 11th edition, A. Marble, P. White, R.F. Bradley,
    L.P. Krall, ed., Lea and Febiger, Philadelphia 526-561 (1971).
4. T.K.S. Rao, E.A. Friedman, Diabetic nephropathy in Brooklyn,
    in: "Diabetic Renal-Retinal Syndrome," E.A. Friedman, F.A.
    L'Esperance Jr. eds., Grune and Stratton, New York, 3-8 (1982).
5. F.L. Shapiro, C.M. Comty, Hemodialysis in diabetics--1981
    update, in: "Diabetic Renal-Retinal Syndrome," vol 2, E.A.
    Friedman, F.A. L'Esperance Jr., eds., Grune and Stratton, New
    York 309-320 (1982).
6. M.D. Siperstein, R.H. Unger, L.L. Madison, Studies of muscle
    capillary basement membrances in normal subjects, diabetic and
    pre-diabetic patients, J Clin Invest 47:1973 (1968).
7. R. Osterby, Early phases in the development of diabetic
    glomerulopathy, Acta Med. Scand. 574 (Suppl):1 (1975).
8. G. Tchobroutsky, Prevention and treatment of diabetic
    nehrophathy, in: "Advances in Nephrology," vol. 9, J.
    Hamberger, J. Crosnier, J.P. Grunfeld, M.H. Maxwell, eds., Year
    Book Medical Publishers, Chicago, 663-86 (1979).
9. S.M. Mauer, M.W. Steffes, F.C. Goetz, D.E.R. Sutherland, D.M.
    Brown, Diabetic nephropathy: A prespective, Diabetes, 32:52
    (1983).
10. A.M. Carpenter, F. Goetz, P. LeCompte, J. Williamson, Glomerulo-
    sclerosis in non-ketotic (Type II) diabetes: Autopsied cases
    from the University Study Group, submitted.
11. S.M. Mauer, M.W. Steffes, E.N. Ellis, D.E.R. Sutherland, D.M.
    Brown, F.C. Goetz, Structural-functional relationships in
    diabetic nephropathy, J. Clin Invest. 74:1143 (1984).
12. R. Bader, K.E. Grund, S. Machensen-Haen, H. Christ, A. Bohle,
    Structure and function of the kidney in diabetic glomerulo-
    sclerosis. Correlations between morphologic and functional
    parameters, Path Res. Pract. 167:204 (1980).
13. J. Fabre, L. Balant, P.G. Dayer, H.M. Fox, A.T. Vernet, The
    kidney in maturity onset diabetes mellitus: A clinical study
    of 510 patients, Kidney Int. 21:730 (1982).
14. G.C. Viberti, R.P. Hall, R.J. Jarrett, A. Angyropoulos, M.
    Nahmud, H. Keen, Microalbuminuria as a predictor of clinical
    nephropathy in insulin dependent diabetes mellitus, Lancet
    1:1430 (1982).
15. E. Takazakura, Y. Nakamota, H. Hayakawa, et al., Onset and
    progression of diabetic glomerulopathy, Diabetes 24:1 (1975).
16. C.E. Mogensen, C.K. Christensen, Pedicting diabetic nephropathy
    in insulin-dependent patients, New Engl J. Med. 311:89 (1984).

17. C.E. Mogensen, Microalbuminuria predicts clinical proteinuria
     and early mortality in maturity-onset diabetes, New Engl J.
     Med. 310:356 (1984).
18. G.C. Viberti, J.C. Pickup, R.J. Jarrett, H. Keen, Effect of
     control of blood glucose on urinary excretion of albumin and
     B2-microglobulin in insulin-dependent diabetes, New Engl J.
     Med. 300:638 (1979).

DIABETIC NEUROPATHY

Peter James Dyck, Anthony Windebank, Hitoshi Yasuda,
F. John Service, Robert Rizza, and Bruce Zimmerman

Peripheral Nerve Laboratory
Department of Neurology
Mayo Clinic
Rochester, MN

ABSTRACT

The incidence and prevalence of diabetic neuropathies in
Insulin Dependent (IDDM) and Non-Insulin Dependent (NIDDM) Diabetes
Mellitus is not known because in previous studies the heterogeneity
of diabetes and of the neuropathies was not taken into account,
criteria for diagnosis and surveillance for neuropathy were
variable, and studies were not prospective or population based. We
have begun such prospective epidemiologic studies using a uniform
algorithm for the classification of the diabetic disorders and
uniform and validated approaches for the assessment of symptoms,
neurologic deficits and various quantitative end-points of neural
dysfunction. As regards cause, a key question which we are trying
to answer is whether hyperglycemia and associated metabolic alterations affect neural tissue directly or whether there is an intervening tissue alteration between metabolic derangement and tissue
change. Improved control of hyperglycemia does not appear to be
associated with rapid neurologic improvement, possibly arguing for
an intervening tissue alteration. The recently observed decrease in
nerve oxygen tension and blood flow in streptozotocin diabetes
suggests that an alteration of the nerve microenvironment may relate
importantly to the cause of diabetic neuropathy.

I. INTRODUCTION

Are the complications of diabetes, such as neuropathy, different among various disorders? Specifically, is the frequency of

neuropathy, underlying mechanisms, and treatment different between insulin dependent (IDDM) and non-insulin dependent (NIDDM) diabetes? These are the questions posed by the organizers. Although neuropathy, of various types, is known to occur in both IDDM and NIDDM, we do not yet know the answers to these questions because in previous reports: 1) operational definitions for IDDM and NIDDM were not used; 2) criteria for the diagnosis, staged severity and type of neuropathy were not applied; 3) tests used to detect and characterize neuropathy were often insensitive and unreliable, and 4) patient selection was not population based.

In this report, we define peripheral neuropathy, discuss minimal criteria, indicate tests suitable for diagnosis and characterization, list some key questions related to pathogenetic mechanisms, describe the variability of neuropathic expression and address the question of whether improved hyperglycemia control ameliorates or at least stops the progression of worsening nerve function in diabetic neuropathy.

II. HETEROGENEITY OF DIABETES MELLITUS

As discussed elsewhere, we now know that the syndrome of diabetes mellitus is composed of several different disorders. Although it was generally assumed, and still is, that chronic hyperglycemia is a major factor in the development of complications, it probably has not been sufficiently appreciated that risk factors might be different for the various types of neuropathic manifestations and diabetic disorders. Below we show the algorithm we use in designating IDDM from NIDDM. (Fig. 1).

III. CRITERIA FOR DIAGNOSIS, SEVERITY AND TYPE OF DIABETIC NEUROPATHY

In a recent review of the subject of Diabetic Neuropathy, Thomas and Eliasson[43] state that the incidence of diabetic neuropathy differs considerably among the reported series, ranging from less than 5% to nearly 60%.[43] This variability presumably reflects differences in: 1) patient selection; 2) criteria for the diagnosis of diabetes, and for the presence and type of neuropathy; 3) types of evaluation for the complication of neuropathy, and 4) lack of exclusion of neuropathies of other cause. Some series represent patients from a physicians practice, a city clinic, and electromyographic laboratory, or from a specialized laboratory. Although useful information has come from such studies, they may not be representative of the frequency and severity of events in an unselected community based diabetic population. Possibly the best reports of diabetic complications have come from hospital practices of a geographic region[34] or from population based studies.[31]

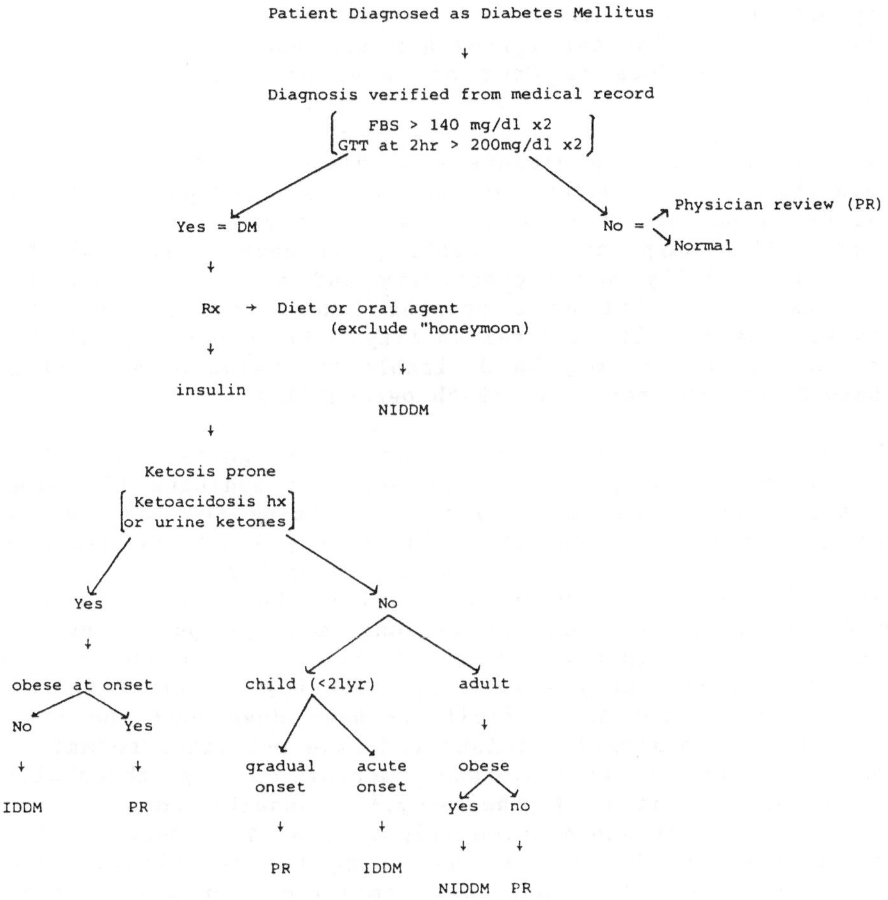

Patient Diagnosed as Diabetes Mellitus

↓

Diagnosis verified from medical record

$$\left[\begin{array}{l} \text{FBS} > 140 \text{ mg/dl x2} \\ \text{GTT at 2hr} > 200\text{mg/dl x2} \end{array} \right]$$

Yes = DM   No =   ⟋ Physician review (PR)
                                                             ⟍ Normal
↓

Rx   →   Diet or oral agent
            (exclude "honeymoon)
↓   ↓

insulin   NIDDM

↓

Ketosis prone

$$\left[\begin{array}{l} \text{Ketoacidosis hx} \\ \text{or urine ketones} \end{array} \right]$$

        Yes   No

        ↓   ⟋   ⟍

   obese at onset   child (<21yr)   adult

   No   Yes   ↓

   ↓   ↓   gradual   acute   obese

  IDDM   PR   onset   onset   yes   no

                           ↓   ↓   ↓   ↓

                           PR   IDDM   NIDDM PR

Fig. 1   The algorithm we use in our prospective or retrospective
            studies of diabetic neuropathy.

To date there is no prospective study of the incidence or prevalence
of diabetic neuropathy which: 1) is population based; 2) is
prospective; 3) employs defined criteria for the detection and
characterization of diabetic and neuropathic disorders; and 4) uses
a battery of sensitive and reliable tests.

The lack of accepted criteria for the diagnosis of neuropathy
is an important reason for variability in the reported frequency of
neuropathy among diabetes. Several approaches to setting the minimal criteria for the diagnosis of neuropathy may be considered. The
first is recognition of a clinical pattern of symptoms and signs
typical of neuropathy. A somewhat different criteria is whether the
patient has symptoms of neuropathy. A third criteria is based on
finding an abnormality of nerve conduction and EMG. A fourth, is

finding pathologic abnormalities. Unless specific criteria, testing procedures and statistical approaches are used the decision about whether a patient does or does not have neuropathy will be quite variable.

We suggest that the diagnosis of diabetic neuropathy be based on quantitative evaluation of neuropathic end-points by using percentile responses derived from a healthy control population. This approach presupposes that testing procedures are available to measure hyperactivity and hypoactivity and absence of function of motor, sensory, and autonomic neurons (axons) and classes of such neurons with sensitivity and reliability. In an operational definition of neuropathy, it may be desirable to insist on more than one attribute being abnormal (e.g. >95th percentile).

The approaches that we are using to recognize abnormality of sensory neurons (axons) will be listed. To evaluate the symptoms (pain, paresthesia, and other symptoms) arising from hyperactivity, presumably from ectopic generators in sensory axons, we use a questionnaire of symptoms associated with neuropathy. This battery of questions is being validated by having the same questionnaire answered by groups of healthy persons and groups of neuropathy patients. This Neuropathy Symptom Profile (NSP) undoubtedly will find a use in assessing the type and severity of neuropathic symptoms. To measure sensory deficit we have developed the Computer Assisted Sensory Examination (CASE) and have published normal values of touch-pressure, vibration, and thermal cooling thresholds at various cutaneous sites of the body.[10] Results for a group of diabetic patients are shown below (Figs. 2, 3, 4). Nerve conduction parameters are most helpful in assessing the function of sensory nerves. The nerve action potential amplitude, or more correctly, the area beneath the compound action potential provides an approximate measure of the number of afferent nerve fibers in the nerve. Graded severity can be clinically scored by summing selected items of the neurologic examination. The Neurologic Disability Score (NDS) which we employ is shown in Fig. 5. We have found the NDS to be helpful in studies of inflammatory-demyelinating, uremic and diabetic neuropathy.[7]

Definition and criteria for types of diabetic neuropathy need also be set. Eichhorst[11] originally described paralytic, hyperalgesic and ataxic forms of neuropathy. Others have added autonomic, cranial nerve, compression, ischemic neuropathy, mononeuropathy (e.g. femoral neuropathy or lumbosacral plexus neuropathy), or multiple mononeuropathy to the list.[43] Operational definitions, criteria, and limits to these neuropathies need to be set.

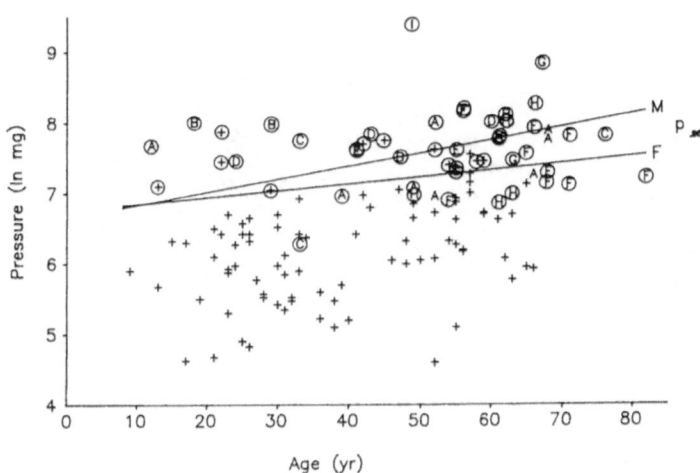

Fig. 2   Thresholds of touch-pressure plotted against age for
          patients with diabetes mellitus as described in text.
          The ninety-fifth percentile (P95) lines for males (M)
          and females (F) are shown.   The circle values are
          abnormal (>P95) by criteria of raised threshold of
          sensitive points or by too many insensitive points (A=1,
          B=2, etc.).   (With permission from: Dyck P.J. et al.:
          Computer assisted sensory examination to detect and
          quantitate sensory deficit in diabetic neuropathy.
          Neurobehav. Toxicol. Tetrat. 5:697-704, 1983).

IV OBSERVATIONS WHICH MIGHT BEAR ON THE CAUSE(s) OF DIABETIC
    NEUROPATHIES

    The mechanisms underlying diabetic neuropathies are not known.
At first ischemia, due to arteriosclerosis of vasa nervorum, was
thought to be responsible.   Increasingly, however, metabolic
derangement is blamed.   Recent alterations of capillary and of the
nerve microenvironment has again raised the question of the role of
ischemia in the development of diabetic neuropathy.   The simple
scheme below reflects the important differences in the two
hypotheses.

    1.   Hyperglycemia → metabolic alterations → intervening
         tissue alteration e.g. vessel abnormality → nerve
         dysfunction.

    2.   Hyperglycemia   →   metabolic   alteration   →   nerve
         dysfunction.

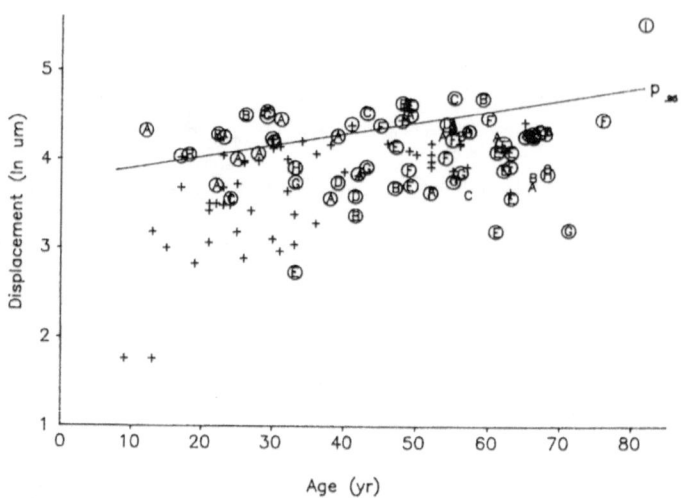

Fig. 3   Thresholds of vibration plotted against age for patients
          with diabetes mellitus as described in text. (With
          permission from: Dyck P.J. et al.: Computer assisted
          sensory examination to detect and quantitate sensory
          deficit in diabetic neuropathy. Neurobehav. Toxicol.
          Tetrat. 5:697-704, 1983).

     In the following paragraphs we will list without comment,
observations that will need to be taken into account in formulating
a view regarding the mechanism underlying the development of
neuropathy. For references see the recent review by Thomas and
Eliasson (1984).

1.   Diabetes mellitus is not one but several disorders.

2.   Diabetic neuropathy is not one but several types. This
      variability implies different mechanisms or different
      factors involved in common mechanisms.

3.   Since neuropathy is associated with types of diabetes,
      one assumes that hyperglycemia and associated metabolic
      derangements play a role in the development of neuropathy.

4.   Various metabolic abnormalities are characteristic of
      diabetes and could be involved in neuropathy: a) tissue
      decrease of myo-inositol;   b) tissue decrease of
      Na^+K^+ ATPase activity;   c) increased sorbitol and
      fructose in tissue; d) altered lipid composition and
      metabolism; and e) altered non-enzymatic glycosylation.

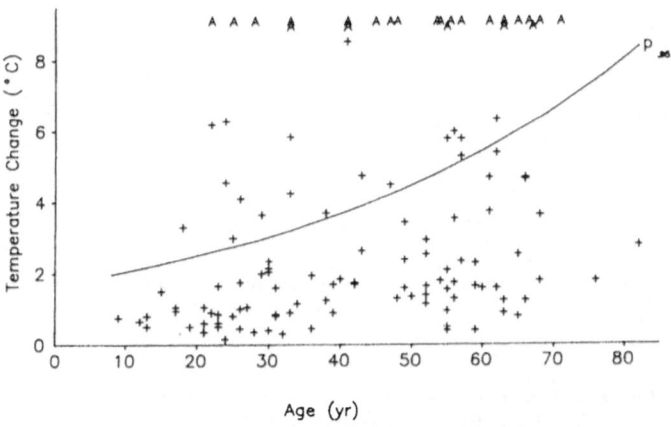

Fig. 4   Thresholds of thermal cooling plotted against age for
          patients with diabetes mellitus studies in our labora-
          tory. The letter A indicates that a threshold was not
          obtained when the maximal intensity of stimulus was used.
          (With permission from: Dyck P.J. et al.: Computer
          assisted sensory examination to detect and quantitate
          sensory deficit in diabetic neuropathy. Neurobehav.
          Toxicol. Tetrat. 5:697-704, 1983).

5.   Retinopathy, nephropathy and neuropathy are associated in
     the same patient thus suggesting common mechanisms for the
     three complications.

6.   There is both clinical and pathologic evidence of premature
     atherosclerosis, arteriosclerosis and capillary disease.
     The prominent basement membrane thickening which
     characterized diabetic endoneurial capillaries is shown in
     Fig. 6.

7.   Euglycemia does not reverse abnormal nerve conduction or
     clinical end-points of neuropathy as rapidly as expected or
     not at all (Service et al., in preparation).

8.   Axonal attenuation (either a failure of development,
     shrinkage or atrophy) has been observed in experimental
     diabetes.

9.   An abnormality of axonal flow has been reported in both
     experimental and human diabetic neuropathy.

DIABETIC NEUROPATHY NEUROLOGIC DISABILITY SCORE (NDS 2)

Name_____   Pt# _____

Age_____   Sex _____   Date_____

Scoring by examiner's standards of normal considering site tested, age
and sex, and of strength of unaffected muscles:

Muscle strength: 0=no weakness; 1=mild weakness; 2=moderate weakness;
3=severe weakness (minimal resistance to examiner's force); 3.25=
just able to move part against gravity; 3.5=not able to move part
against gravity, but can move it in horizontal plane; 3.75=flicker
of the muscle, but joint movement does not occur; 4=no observed
muscle contraction.

Tendon reflexes: 0=normal, 1=decreased, 2=absent.

Sensation (dorsal index finger and great toe): 0=normal, 1=decreased,
2=absent (using tapered cotton wool wisp, hat pin, 250 hz tuning fork).

		Right	Left
Cranial Nerves			
1	3rd nerve		
2	6th nerve		
3	facial weakness		
4	palate weakness		
5	tongue weakness		
Muscle Weakness			
6	respiratory		
7	neck flexion		
8	shoulder abduction		
9	elbow flexion		
10	brachioradialis		
11	elbow extension		
12	wrist flexion		
13	wrist extension		
14	finger flexion		
15	finger spread		
16	thumb abduction		
17	hip flexion		
18	hip extension		
19	knee flexion		
20	knee extension		
21	ankle dorsiflexors		
22	ankle plantar flexors		
23	toe extensors		
24	toe flexors		
Reflexes			
25	biceps brachii		
26	triceps brachii		
27	brachioradialis		
28	quadriceps femoris		
29	triceps surae		
Sensation			
I.Finger: 30 (terminal 31 phalanx) 32 33	Touch-pressure / Pricking pain / Vibration / JP		
G.Toe: 34 (terminal 35 phalanx) 36 37	Touch-pressure / Pricking pain / Vibration / JP		
	SUM		

TOTAL:_____

Fig. 5   Neurologic Disability Score (With permission from Dyck
            P.J. et al.: Human diabetic endoneurial sorbitol,
            fructose, and myo-inositol related to sural nerve
            morphometry. Ann. Neurol. 8:590-596, 1980).

10. The pathologic alteration of experimental diabetic nerves has not closely mirrored the pathologic changes in the human disease, perhaps suggesting:

   a. that long-term experimental studies of hyperglycemia are needed.

   b. that study of human disease and tissue be emphasized.

11. Marked alterations of the microenvironment of experimental diabetic nerves are being discovered possibly emphasizing that:

   a. there are mechanistic steps interposed between metabolic alterations and nerve fiber damage.

   b. that this may be a fruitful area for further study.

12. The results of clinical trials in diabetic neuropathy show that:

   a. supplementation of the diet with myo-inositol has been disappointing in correcting diabetic neuropathy.

   b. the use of aldose reductase inhibitors awaits completion but some pilot studies appear to be promising.

   c. the use of tight blood glucose control with insulin pumps or by frequent insulin injections has not thus far shown a prompt unequivocal reversal of diabetic neuropathy.

V. HETEROGENEITY OF DIABETIC NEUROPATHY

The diversity of presentation was recognized in earliest accounts of diabetic neuropathy. Pain, paresthesia, lumbago and sciatica were described. Absent knee reflexes[2] were attributed to diabetic neuritis.[5] Pryce[35] commented on the special vulnerability of sensory nerve fibers. A chronic progressive atrophic weakness associated with diabetes mellitus was reported[30] but some of the patients had features of amyotrophic lateral sclerosis. Leyden[26] described hyperesthetic or neuralgic, motor or paralytic and ataxic or pseudotabetic forms of diabetic neuropathy, an indication that diabetic neuropathy presented in diverse forms. Bruns[4] diabetic patient developed severe pain, weakness and atrophy of one anterior thigh muscle soon followed by similar involvement of the other thigh. This condition, also called femoral neuropathy, was shown to occur occasionally also in

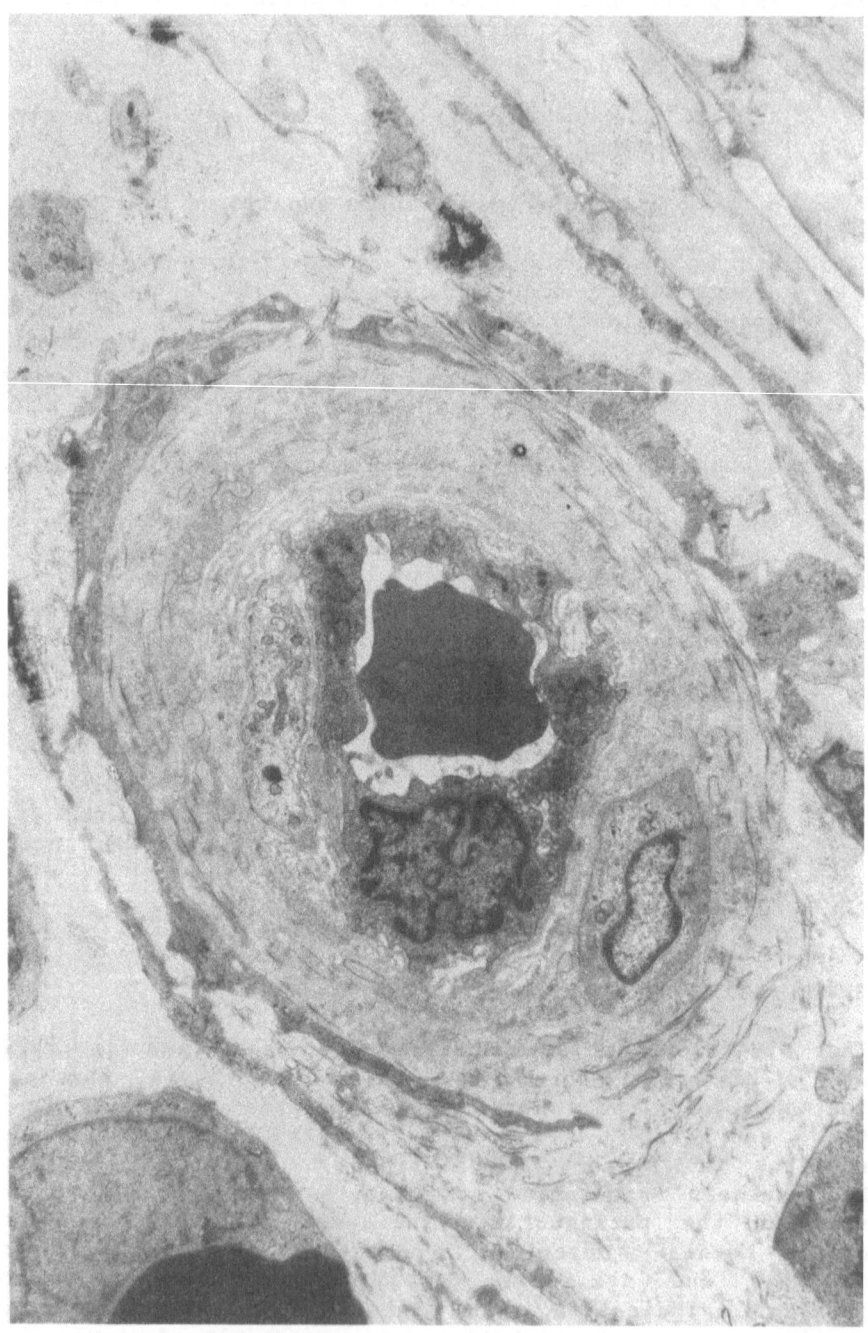

Fig. 6   An endoneurial capillary for a patient with diabetic
neuropathy showing prominent reduplication and thickening
of the basement membrane (X8400).

non-diabetics and to follow a monophasic course to improvement. Others used the term diabetic amyotrophy[15,16,17,23] for a similar syndrome to describe patients with proximal muscle weakness, pain and raised CSF protein. There appears to be considerable overlap between their patients and the other motor neuropathies referred to earlier. A recent study suggests that segmental radicular involvement is not uncommon among diabetics.[1] Some investigators associated ischemic gangrene with nerve damage.[32,36] By 1922, Kraus listed the diabetic neuropathic complications as cranial palsies, mononeuritis, polyneuritis, motor polyneuropathies and sensory polyneuropathies. Autonomic nerve involvement increasingly is recognized as causing an abnormality of pupillary reaction,[14] of esophageal[27] and gastric[47] and of bladder[13] and sexual dysfunction and of sudomotor function. An abnormality of nerve conduction may be present even when the patient does not have symptoms or neurologic signs of neuropathy. Patients may have neuropathic signs and pathologic abnormalities of biopsied nerves with symptoms and still others may have neuropathic symptoms without neuropathic signs.

VI. HYPERGLYCEMIA AND DIABETIC NEUROPATHY

The present state of knowledge concerning the relationship between blood sugar control and the prevention or cure of diabetic neuropathy remains unsatisfactory. This question remains unanswered for several reasons: the pathogenesis of diabetic neuropathy is unknown; there is not a good animal model of human diabetic neuropathy; and there is relatively little information from controlled trials of the effect or degree of control on symptomatic neuropathy.

The pathogenesis of the neuropathy is necessarily complex because it is unlikely that identical pathways produce the different end-points of diffuse distal small fiber disease (hyperalgesic-autonomic form), diffuse large fiber disease (ataxic form), polyradiculoneuropathy and mononeuritis multi-plex (cranial nerve palsies, diabetic amyotrophy). The former diffuse diseases may relate to a metabolic abnormality of nerve or Schwann cells while the latter focal disease may reflect small vessel pathology. Alternatively, all forms may represent abnormalities in vessels of different sizes or in the microenvironment of nerve. These questions will not even begin to be answered until detailed, three-dimensional, quantitative, pathologic studies of the nerves and their blood vessels are carried out among diabetic patients and linked to the clinical condition of the patient before death. Such studies are at present underway in this laboratory.

The lack of a good animal model of the neuropathic process continues to hamper the search for underlying mechanisms. The commonly used models of insulin deficiency are the alloxan induced and streptozotocin induced diabetic rats and spontaneously diabetic strains of mutant rats and mice. In all of these models there is a consistent reduction in motor nerve conduction velocity occurring soon after the appearance of hyperglycemia[12,22,24,39,41,42] which may be prevented by institution of insulin therapy.[19,24] This abnormality of nerve conduction velocity is not necessarily reversed by insulin once it has been established.[12,19] These conduction abnormalities are accompanied by axonal shrinkage;[21,42] however, it is still a matter of dispute whether they lead to actual fiber pathology in the form of axonal degeneration or demyelination.[3,28,41] Interpretation is further complicated by the observation that axonal shrinkage and reduction in conduction velocity may be induced in a few hours in the cat during intravenous infusion of glucose. This suggests that these acute changes may be a consequence of interstitial hyperosmolarity rather than due to a metabolic or fixed structural abnormality.[7,9,42]

The difficulty in interpreting the significance of conduction changes with treatment is equally apparent in the human disease. There is much evidence to suggest that, at the time of first diagnosis, and certainly before onset of symptomatic neuropathy, many diabetics show abnormalities of nerve conduction[6,20,29] and there is some evidence that these changes may be improved by the institution of blood sugar control.[6,18,21,33,45] However, there is little information directly implicating these electrophysiologic abnormalities as the forerunners or predictors of the later development of symptomatic neuropathy. They may merely reflect acute metabolic or osmolar abnormalities accompanying the uncontrolled hyperglycemic state. A single study relates the early presymptomatic electrophysiological changes to nerve fiber pathology.[7,8] Unfortunately, there is no information to tell us that reversal of the nerve conduction abnormalities is associated with the prevention or repair of symptomatic, clinically overt neuropathy. At this time, we stand with a variety of observations, which are either retrospective or uncontrolled. In 1968 Gregersen,[21] showed a small improvement in motor nerve conduction velocity in newly diagnosed diabetics after the institution of insulin therapy. A similar observation was made by Ward et al.[45] This was a heterogeneous group of diabetics who were initially controlled by diet therapy, sulphonylureas, phenformin or insulin, and it is of note that the greatest degree of improvement occurred in patients treated with sulphonylureas. More recent observations have concerned improvement in control of conventionally treated diabetics. Again, the majority of studies are uncontrolled. White et al.[46] reported two cases of improvement in severe neuropathy associated with the institution of improved control using either home glucose monitoring and multiple insulin injections or a continuous insulin infusion pump. A similar case report described a dramatic improvement in the neuropathy of a 16-year-old girl after control was improved using an insulin infusion pump.[44] In another uncontrolled study, Graf et al.[18] demonstrated that non-insulin dependent diabetics also showed an improvement in motor, but not sensory, nerve conduction velocity in the 12 months after institution of control with either oral agents or insulin. The improvement in nerve conduction velocity was small (3 meters per second or less) and this study did not address the question of any relationship of the electrophysiological changes to symptomatic neuropathy or neurologic impairment.

A single controlled trial was reported by Pietri et al.[33] who compared the nerve conduction velocities of type I diabetics treated with conventional or rigorous infusion pump insulin therapy over a six week period. Motor nerve conduction velocity in the median and peroneal nerves increased significantly while there was no change in the ulnar motor conduction velocity or in sensory conductions in general. Again, this study did not look at any relationship to the changes to symptomatic neuropathy.

In general, there has been a lack of rigorous quantitation of either symptomatology or neurologic deficit; very little attempt to measure changes in these variables; and a lack of distinction between changes induced by therapeutic maneuvers and the natural history of the disease. There are only two prospective, controlled trials relating the degree of control to the course of symptomatic neuropathy and changes in nerve conduction velocity.[37,38] Both studies were performed in this center, both were short term and both were negative. Although negative, however, they are of importance for two reasons. They represent the first attempts to perform controlled trials addressing the relationship of degree of glycemic control to function of peripheral nerves in terms of electro-physiology and symptomatic neuropathy in groups of carefully defined diabetics. Secondly, they used a quantitative multifactoral approach to evaluate the electrophysiologic parameters, measures of sensation and functional status of the patient. The only additional requirement in this armamentarium is a standardized and quantitative measure of patient symptoms. This has been developed in the Neuropathy Symptom Profile (NSP). Such trials are difficult to design and to perform; they are expensive and require a very cooperative and well defined patient population. In the long run, however, they have the potential to save a great deal of time, money and effort for both the patient and his physician. There is no point in embarking on the widespread use of costly infusion pumps if they offer no advantage over conventional treatment. Careful definition of the natural history of diabetic neuropathy in the whole population is an essential step in the evaluation of treatment.

REFERENCES

1. Bastron, J. A., and Thomas J. E., Diabetic polyneuropathy, Mayo Clin. Proc., 56:725-732 (1981).
2. Bouchard, M., Loss of the knee-phenomenon in diabetes, Br. Med. J., 237 (1884).
3. Brown, M. J., Sumner, A. J., Greene, D. A., Diamond, S. M., and Asbury, A. K., Distal neuropathy in experimental diabetes mellitus, Ann. Neurol., 8:168-178 (1980).
4. Bruns, L., Ueber neuritische Lahmungen beim diabetes mellitus, Berlin Klin. Wchnscht, 27:509-515 (1890).
5. Buzzärd, F., Illustrations of some less known forms of peripheral neuritis, especially alcoholic monoplegia and diabetic neuritis, Br. Med. J., 1:419 (1890).
6. Downie, A. W., and Newell, D. J., Sensory nerve conduction in patients with diabetes mellitus and controls, Neurol., 11:876-882 (1961).
7. Dyck, P. J., Low, P. A., Sparks, M. Hexum, L., and Karnes, J., Effect of serum hyperosmolarity on morphometry of healthy human sural nerve, J. Neuropath. Exp. Neurol, 39:285-295 (1980).
8. Dyck, P. J., Sherman, W. R., Hallcher, L. M., Service, F. J., O'Brien, P. C., Grina, L. A., Palumbo, P. J., and Swanson, C. J., Human diabetic endoneurial sorbitol, fructose, and myoinositol related to sural nerve morphometry, Ann. Neurol, 8:590-596 (1980).
9. Dyck, P. J., Lambert, E. H., Windebank, A. J., Lais, A. A., Sparks, M. F., Karnes, J., Sherman, W. R., Hallcher, L. M., Low, P. A., and Service, F. J., Acute hyperosmolar hyperglycemia causes axonal shrinkage and reduced nerve conduction velocity, Exp. Neurol, 71:507-514 (1981).
10. Dyck, P. J., Karnes, J. O'Brien, P. C., and Zimmerman, I. R., Detection thresholds of cutaneous sensation in humans, in: "Peripheral Neuropathy", Dyck P. J., Thomas P. K., Lambert E. H., Bunge R., eds., W.B. Saunders, Philadephia, 49:1103-1138 (1984).
11. Eichhorst H, Beitrage zur Pathologie der Nerven und Muskein. 3. Neuritis diabetica und ihre Bezie hungen zum fehlenden Patellarsehnenreflex, Virchows Arch. Pathol. Anat. Physiol., 127:1 (1892).
12. Eliasson, S. G., Nerve conduction changes in experimental diabetes, J. Clin. Invest. 43:2353-2358 (1964).
13. Fagerberg, S. E., Kock, N. G., Petersen, I., and Stener, I., Urinary bladder disturbances in diabetics. I. A comparitive study of male diabetics and controls aged between 20 and 50 years, Scand. J. Urol, Nephrol, 1:19-27 (1967).
14. Friedman, S.A., Feinberg, R., Podolak, E., and Bedell R. H. W., Pupillary abnormalities in diabetic neuropathy. A preliminary study, Ann. Int. Med., 67:977-983 (1967).
15. Garland, H., Diabetic amyotrophy, Br. Med. J. 2:1287 (1955).

16. Garland, H., Neurological complications of diabetes mellitus: clinical aspects, Proc. R. Soc. Med., 53:137 (1960).

17. Garland, H. and Taverner, D., Diabetic myelopathy, Br. Med. J., 1:1045 (1953).

18. Graf, R. J., Halter, J. B., Pfeifer, M. A., Halar, E., Brozovich, F., and Porte, D., Glycemic control and nerve conduction abnormalities in non-insulin dependent diabetic subjects, Ann. Int. Med., 94:307-311 (1981).

19. Greene, D. A., DeJesus, P. V., and Winegrad, A. I., Effects of insulin and dietary myo-inositol on impaired peripheral motor nerve conduction velocity in acute streptozotocin diabetes, J. Clin. Invest., 55:1326-1336 (1975).

20. Gregersen, G., Diabetic neuropathy: influence of age, sex, metabolic control and duration of diabetes on motor conduction velocity, Neurol, 17:972-980 (1967).

21. Gregersen, G., Variations in motor conduction velocity produced by acute changes of the metabolic state in diabetic patients, Diabetologia, 4:273-277 (1968).

22. Hildebrand, J., Joffroy, A., Graff, G., and Coers, C., Neuromuscular changes with alloxan hyperglycemia, Arch. Neurol, 18:633-641 (1968).

23. Isaacs, H., Gilchrist, G., Diabetic amyotrophy, S. Afr. Med. J., 34:501-505 (1960).

24. Jakobsen, J., Early and preventable changes of peripheral nerve structure and function in insulin deficient diabetic rats, J. Neurol. Neurosurg. Psych., 42:409-518 (1979).

25. Kraus, W.M., Involvement of the peripheral neurons in diabetes mellitus, Arch. Neurol. Psych., 7:202-209 (1922).

26. Leyden, E., Beitrag zur Klinik des Diabetes mellitus, Wien. Med. Wochenscher., 43:926 (1893).

27. Mandelstam, P., Esophageal dysfunction in clinical and roentgenological mainfestations, JAMA, 201:581-586 (1967).

28. Mendell, J. R., Sahenk, Z., and Warmolts, J. R., The spontaneously diabetic BB-wistar rat, Abstracts of the Peripheral Nerve Study Group, 4-1 (1981).

29. Mulder, D. W., Lambert, E. H., Bastron, J. A., and Sprague, R. G., The neuropathies associated with diabetes mellitus: A clinical and electromyographic study of 103 unselected diabetic patients, Neurol, 11:275-283 (1961).

30. Nonne, M., Berliner Klinische Wschr, 33:207-212 (1896).

31. Palumbo, P. J., Elveback, L. R., and Whinant, J.P., Neurologic complications of diabetes mellitus: transient ischemic attack, stroke and peripheral neuropathy, in: "Advances in Neurology", Schoenberg BS, ed., Raven Press, NY, 19:593 (1978).

32. Pavy, F. W., On diabetic neuritis, Lance, 2:71 (1904).

33. Pietri, A., Ehle, A. L., and Raskin, P., Changes in nerve conduction velocity after six weeks of glucoregulation with portable insulin infusion pumps, Diabetes, 29:668-671 (1980).

34. Pirart, J., Diabetes mellitus and its degenerative
     complications: a prospective study of 4,400 patients observed
     between 1947 and 1973, Diabetes Care, 1:168,252 (1978).
35. Pryce, T. D., On diabetic neuritis with a clinical and
     pathological description of three cases of diabetic
     pseudo-tabes, Brain, 16:416 (1893).
36. Rundles, R. W., Diabetic neuropathy, Bull, N.Y. Acad. Med.,
     26:598 (1950).
37. Service, F. J., Daube, J. R., O'Brien, P. C., and Dyck, P. J.,
     Effect of artificial pancreas treatment on peripheral nerve
     function in diabetes, Neurology, 31:1375-1380 (1981).
38. Service, F. J., Daube, J. R., O'Brien, P. C., Zimmerman, B. R.,
     Swanson, C. J., Brennan, M. D., and Dyck, P. J, Effect of blood
     glucose control on peripheral nerve function in diabetic
     patients, Mayo Clin. Proc., 58:283-289 (1983).
39. Sharma, A.K., and Thomas, P.K., Peripheral nerve structure and
     function in experimental diabetes, J. Neurol. Sci., 1-15 (1974).
40. Sima, A. A. F., Peripheral neuroapthy in spotaneously diabetic
     BB-wistar rat, Abstracts of the Peripheral Nerve Study Group,
     4-2 (1981).
41. Sima, A. A. F., and Robertson, D. M., Peripheral neuropathy in
     mutant diabetic mouse, Acta Neuropath, 41:85-89 (1978).
42. Sugimura, K., Windbank, A. J., Natarajan, V., Lambert, E. H.,
     Schmid, H., and Dyck, P. J., Interstitial hyperosomolarity may
     cause axis cylinder shrinkage in streptozotocin diabetic nerve,
     J. Neuropath. Exp. Neurol, 39:710-721 (1980).
43. Thomas, P. K., and Eliasson, S. G., Diabetic Neuropathy, in:
     "Peripheral Neuropathy", P. J. Dyck, P. K. Thomas, E. H.
     Lambert, R. Bunge, eds., W.B. Saunders, Philadelphia,
     76:1773:1810 (1984).
44. Tolamat, A., Roque, J. L., and Russo, L. S., Improvement of
     diabetic peripheral neuropathy with the portable insulin
     infusion pump, Southern Medical Journal, 75:185-189 (1982).
45. Ward, J. D., Barnes, C. G., Fisher, D. J., Jessop, J. D., and
     Baker, R. W. R., Improvement in nerve conduction following
     treatment in newly diagnosed diabetics, Lancet, 1:428-431
     (1971).
46. White, N. H., Waltman, S. R., Krupin, T., and Santiago, J. V.,
     Reversal of neuropathic and gastrointestinal complications
     related to diabetes mellitus in adolescents with improved
     metabolic control, J. Pediatrics, 99:41-45 (1981).
47. Zitomer, B. R., Gramm, H. F., and Kozak, G. P., Gastric
     neuropathy in diabetes mellitus: Clinical and radiologic
     observations, Metabolism, 17:199-211 (1968).

THE WISCONSIN EPIDEMIOLOGIC STUDY OF DIABETIC RETINOPATHY

A COMPARISON OF RETINOPATHY IN YOUNGER AND

OLDER ONSET DIABETIC PERSONS

Ronald Klein, Matthew D. Davis, Scot E. Moss,
Barbara E.K. Klein, and David L. DeMets

From the Departments of Ophthalmology and Statistics
University of Wisconsin Medical School
Madison, Wisconsin U.S.A.

ABSTRACT

In a population-based survey of diabetic persons, retinopathy was detected by stereoscopic color fundus photography in 70% of persons under 30 years of age at diagnosis and taking insulin (Group YO), in 62% of persons 30 years of age or older at diagnosis and taking insulin (Group OO-I) and in 36 % of persons 30 years of age or older at diagnosis not taking insulin (Group OO-N). The mean duration of known diabetes was 14.6 years in Group YO, 11.0 years in Group OO-I and 6.9 years in Group OO-N. After 20 years of diabetes, proliferative retinopathy was present in about 50% of Group YO, about 25% of Group OO-I and about 5% of Group OO-N. After 15 years of diabetes, macular edema was present in about 18% of Group YO, about 20% of Group OO-I and about 12% of Group OO-N.

When present, macular edema tended to be associated with more hard exudate in Group OO-N.

INTRODUCTION

Suprisingly little information is available to document similarities and differences in retinopathy characteristics of Type I and Type II diabetes. Such comparisons are limited by the difficulty of classifying patients objectively and accurately by diabetes type, by the lack of population-based studies and by the paucity of reports in which patients with both types of diabetes have been assessed concurrently with standardized methods such as masked grading of stereoscopic fundus photographs.

Nevertheless, certain concepts have become generally accepted. In Type I diabetes, retinopathy is rarely present sooner than two years after diagnosis[3,11,14] and is rarely a threat to vision until after ten years of known diabetes,[10] whereas in Type II diabetes, retinopathy may be present, even severe, at the time of diagnosis.[3] Proliferative diabetic retinopathy (PDR) is the most important ocular problem faced by individuals with Type I diabetes, while diabetic maculopathy has been considered the more important problem in Type II diabetes.[3,10,11,13,14]

The Wisconsin Epidemiologic Study of Diabetic Retinopathy (WESDR), in which a population-based sample of diabetic individuals was evaluated using stereoscopic fundus photography, provides a unique opportunity to evaluate these generally accepted concepts and look for other similarities and differences. Because it was not feasible to measure C-peptide or serum insulin levels in this study, patients are classified by age at diagnosis of diabetes and insulin use.

PATIENTS AND METHODS

The Population

The methods of identification and description of the population have appeared in detail in previous reports.[11,12] In brief, 452 of the 457 physicians who provided primary care to diabetic patients in an 11-county area in Southern Wisconsin (Health Service Area 1 [HSA-1]) participated in the study. Participation involved keeping lists of all diabetic patients for whom primary care was provided from July 1, 1979 to June 30, 1980. During this one-year period, 10,135 diabetic patients were identified by the physicians. Charts of 9,841 of these patients were reviewed. Three hundred thirty-eight patients were confined to nursing homes; 157 had died before July 1, 1979, forty-five did not have diabetes (incorrect computer coding), and 18 had moved before July 1, 1979 or had gestational diabetes. The charts of these 558 patients were reviewed for sociodemographic data only. Among the remaining 9,283 patients, the diagnosis of diabetes had been made in 1,396 before 30 years of age, and in 7,887 at 30 years of age or older.

Of the 1,396 younger-onset group, 1,210 were taking insulin and, of them 1,092 lived within HSA-1. All of these individuals were invited to participate in the examination phase of the study; 902 (82.6%) were examined, 122 (11.2%) had moved out of the area, could not be located or had died, and 68 (6.2%) refused.

For the older-onset group, eligibility criteria for inclusion in the examination phase of the study included a diagnosis of diabetes by the primary care physician, confirmed by random or post-

prandial serum glucose level of at least 200 mg/dl or a fasting serum
glucose level of at least 140 mg/dl on at least two occasions, and
residence in HSA-1 at the time the examination phase was to begin in
September 1980 (n=5,431). Of these 5,431 individuals, duration of
known diabetes was less than five years in 2,341, five to 14 years
in 2,465 and 15 or more years in 625. Random samples of 576 persons
from the first group, 579 persons from the second group, and all 625
persons from the third duration group were selected for examination
(a total of 1,780 persons). Of these three groups, 451, 452, and
467, respectively, were examined; 178 (10.0%) had died, moved out of
the area or could not be located, and 232 (13.0%) refused.

Because of the sampling procedure used, weighting was employed
when estimating rates in the population. To derive the weighting
factors, the number of persons eligible for selection in each diabetes duration group at the start of the study was divided by the
number examined. Thus, weighting factors of 1.2 (1,092/902), 5.2
(2,341/451), 5.5 (2,465/452), and 1.3 (625/467) were computed for
the younger-onset persons, and for the short-, intermediate-, and
long-duration subgroups of the older-onset persons, respectively.

Procedures

Letters were sent by the local physicians informing their
selected patients of the survey and offering them an opportunity to
participate. Participants were contacted by the project coordi-
nator, who arranged their appointment dates. The examinations were
performed in a mobile examination van in or near the cities where
the participants lived.

Examinations consisted of measuring the height, weight, blood
pressure (using a random-zero sphygmomanometer [Hawksley] following
the Hypertension Detection and Follow-up Program protocol,[16] and
best corrected visual acuity (using the Early Treatment Diabetic
Retinopathy Study [ETDRS] protocol;[6] performing a slit-lamp examination for chamber depth and the presence of iris neovascularization;
dilating the pupils; administering a questionnaire; examining the
lens with a slit-lamp; taking stereoscopic color fundus photographs
of seven standard fields and a nonstereoscopic red reflex (lens)
photograph for each eye; performing a semiquantitative determination
of glucose, ketone, and protein levels in the urine using a reagent
strip (Labstix); and determinining blood glucose and glycosylated
hemoglobin levels from a fingerprick capillary blood sample.

Grading Protocol

Two levels of grading were carried out on the fundus photographs. First a preliminary grading was performed by one of two
senior graders. After examining all of the photographic fields for
the entire eye, the grader recorded a determination of the overall

retinopathy level and the presence of macular edema (thickening of the retina with or without partial loss of transparency within one disc diameter from the center of the macula). Second, a detailed grading was performed by one of several graders. This assessment consisted of a field-by-field, lesion-by-lesion evaluation of each photograph set for each eye utilizing the ETDRS adaptation of the modified Airlie House Classification of Diabetic Retinopathy.[4,7] Results were recorded on the Detailed Color Grading Form (ETDRS Form 76). Macular edema was judged to be present if any area of the retina within one disc diameter of the center of the macula was thickened.

An algorithm was used to compare the presence of macular edema and severity of retinopathy for each eye as found in detailed grading with the findings from the preliminary grading. When the two determinations disagreed, the eye was regraded for presence of macular edema and severity of retinopathy by another grader. If that grader agreed with either of the first two determinations, that result was accepted. However, if discrepancies remained, the eye was referred to the most senior grader at the Fundus Photography Reading Center for adjudication.

Photograph sets were examined in random order for the detailed grading to avoid possible bias relating to particular physicians, clinics, localities or temporal trends. Both levels of grading involved concurrent examination of right and left eyes.

Definitions

For each eye, the maximum grade in any of the seven standard photographic fields was determined for each of the lesions used in defining "retinopathy level," modifying a previous scheme[9] as outlined below.

Retinopathy   Definition

Level

1   No retinopathy.

1.5 Retinal hemorrhages only, no microaneurysms.

2   Microaneurysms and one or more of the following: retinal hemorrhages, but total of hemorrhages and microaneurysms (H/MA) less than standard photograph (STD) #2A (4); hard exudates (HE) less than STD #3; soft exudates (SE) questionably present; intraretinal microvascular abnormalities (IRMA) questionably present; venous beading (VB) questionably present; or small venous loops definitely present.

4   Microaneurysms and one or more of the following, but definitions
        of level 5 not met: H/MA equaling or exceeding STD #2A; HE
        equaling or exceeding STD #3; SE definitely present; IRMA
        definitely present; VB definitely present; larger venous loops
        or reduplication definitely present.

5   In fields 4 through 7 only, either (a) any three of the follow-
        ing: H/MA equaling or exceeding STD #2A in at least one field,
        SE definitely present in at least two fields, IRMA definitely
        present in at least two fields, VB definitely present in at
        least two fields, or (b) IRMA definitely present in at least
        four fields and equaling or exceeding STD #8A in at least two
        fields.

6.0   Fibrous proliferations only.

6.1   No evidence of 6.0 or 6.5, but scars of photocoagulation either
        in "scatter" or confluent patches, presumably directed at new
        vessels.

6.5   New vessels on or within one disc diameter (DD) of the disc
        graded less than STD #10A; new vessels elsewhere of any extent,
        or preretinal or vitreous hemorrhage, but level 7 definition
        not met.

7   Diabetic Retinopathy Study (DRS) high-risk characteristics
        (HRC),[5] i.e. one or more of the following: new vessels else-
        where equaling or exceeding one-half disc area in any single
        photographic field and preretinal hemorrhage or vitreous hemor-
        rhage in any field; new vessels on or within one DD of the disc
        less than STD #10A with preretinal or vitreous hemorrhage; new
        vessels on or within one DD of disc equaling or exceeding STD
        #10A with or without preretinal or vitreous hemorrhage.

8   Eyes that could not be graded for retinopathy level because of
        vitreous hemorrhage obscuring the retina, phthisis bulbi, or
        enucleation secondary to a complication of diabetic retinopathy.

        Eyes that could not be graded for retinopathy level because of
opacities in the media or enucleation not related to diabetic retinopathy were classified as "cannot grade."

        Patients were classified by retinopathy level in the worse eye.

Macular Edema

        In all persons with previous photocoagulation treatment who had
no or questionable macular edema at the time of examination, previous presence of macular edema was determined from past history as
recorded and documented in clinic records and from examination of

old clinic fundus photographs.   Eyes were classified by macular
edema status as specified below.

0   Absent at examination, no prior photocoagulation treatment.

1   Questionable at examination, no prior photocoagulation treat-
     ment.

2   Present (regardless of prior photocoagulation treatment).

3   Absent at examination, prior history of macular edema, prior
     photocoagulation treatment.

4   Absent at examination, no prior history of macular edema, prior
     photocoagulation treatment.

5   Present but due to other nondiabetic condition (e.g. macular
     degeneration, central retinal vein occlusion, aphakic cystoid
     macular edema, etc. in the absence of diabetic retinopathy).

8   Cannot grade.

     The presence or absence of macular edema was determined for
each eye of every individual.   Macular edema was defined as being
present in an eye if macular edema status was classified as 2 or 3.
Patients were considered to have macular edema if it was present in
either eye.   If it was present in both eyes, findings in the right
eye were used to categorize the patient.

Hard Exudate

     The severity of hard exudates with one disc diameter of the
center of the macula was based on the area of retina involved and
was defined as follows:

0   no evidence of hard exudate;

1   questionable hard exudate present;

2   hard exudate present, but less than STD #3;

3   hard exudate equaling or exceeding STD #3 but less than in STD
     #5;

4   hard exudate equaling or exceeding STD #5.

Cataract

     Nuclear sclerosis was considered to be present if an increase
in the optical density of the lens nucleus with or without a color

change was found on slit lamp biomicroscopy through a dilated pupil. Severity was judged against a standard slit lamp camera photograph. One of three levels could be assigned: absent or questionable; definitely present but less than the standard photograph; or equal to or greater than the standard photograph. Posterior subcapsular cataract was defined as a granular-appearing opacity of the posterior subcapsular area found on slit lamp examination. It was judged as absent or questionable; present but less than the area of such a cataract in a standard photograph or present and equal to or greater than the standard photograph. For the analyses reported here, presence of cataract was defined as the most severe level of either type of lens opacity.

Current age was defined as the age at the time of examination. Age at diagnosis of diabetes was defined as age at the time the diagnosis was first recorded by a physician in the patient's office chart or hospital record. Duration of diabetes was that time period between age at diagnosis and current age.

Wisconsin Storage and Retrieval, and information processing software system, was used for processing all subject files and for calculating the X^2 statistic.[8]

RESULTS

Table 1 presents the distribution of retinopathy severity in each of the three groups, together with mean duration of diabetes and age at examination. In the younger onset group 29.6% were free of retinopathy (Level 1) and 22.2% had PDR (Levels 6-8). In the older-onset, insulin-taking group 38.3% were free of retinopathy and 10.4% had PDR. Among noninsulin-taking patients 64.0% were free of retinopathy and 2.5% had PDR.

Figure 1 displays the percent of each group with any degree of retinopathy by duration of diabetes. In the 0-4 years duration interval 13% of the younger-onset group had retinopathy, as did 40% of the older-onset insulin-taking group and 24% of the noninsulin-taking group. In the latter two groups prevalence of retinopathy increased with duration at similar rates, reaching 53% and 84%, respectively, in persons with 15-19 years of diabetes. In the younger-onset group prevalence rose rapidly, to 55% in persons with 5-9 years of diabetes and to 95% in those with 15-19 years.

Figure 2 presents prevalence of proliferative diabetic retinopathy (PDR) by duration of diabetes in each group. In the younger-onset group prevalence was zero when duration was less than five years, 2% in the 5-10 year duration interval and then rose rapidly to more than 50% in persons with 25 or more years of diabetes. In the older-onset insulin-taking group prevalence rose fairly steadily from 2% in persons with less than five years of diabetes to more

Table 1.   Percent of persons with specified retinopathy level by
           age at diagnosis of diabetes and insulin use (weighted*)

Retinopathy Level	Diagnosis before age 30 years %	Diagnosis at or after age 30 years Insulin %	No Insulin %	Total %
1	29.6	38.3	64.0	49.3
1.5	1.0	4.0	5.6	4.3
2	17.0	13.0	12.1	13.2
3	12.6	13.4	8.1	10.7
4	17.3	19.7	6.9	13.1
5	0.3	1.1	0.2	0.5
6.0	0.8	0.7	0.2	0.4
6.1	0.9	1.2	0.3	0.7
6.5	11.2	5.2	0.9	4.1
7	5.0	2.4	1.0	2.2
8	4.3	0.9	0.1	1.1
CG	0.0	0.0	0.5	0.3
Total 100.0	100.0	100.0	100.0	
(# examined)	(902)	(674)	(696)	(2272)
Mean duration of diabetes (years) 14.6	11.0	6.9	9.6	
Mean age at examination (years)	29.4	63.6	67.1	59.6

*See methods section for weighting procedure

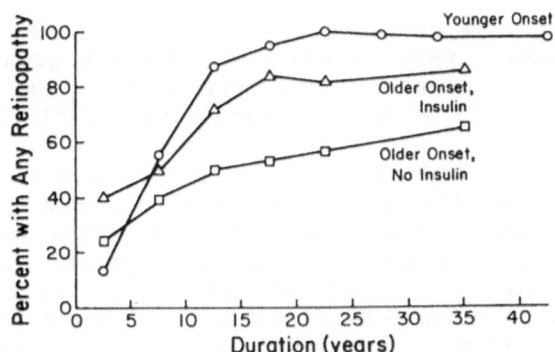

Fig. 1   Percent of persons with diabetic retinopathy by duration
          of diabetes in each of the three age-at-diagnosis,
          insulin-use groups. The number of persons in each dura-
          tion interval in each group was at least 70, with the
          following exceptions: younger-onset group, 30-34 year
          interval, 43; younger-onset group, 35 or more year inter-
          val, 44; noninsulin-taking group, 20-24 year interval,
          41; noninsulin-taking group, 25 or more year interval, 15.

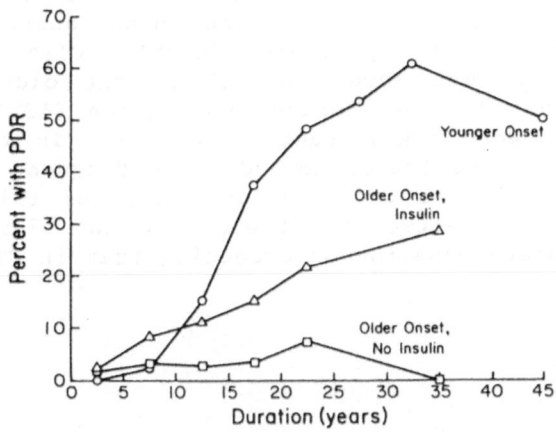

Fig. 2   Percent of persons with PDR by duration of diabetes in
          each of the three groups.

than 25% in those with 25 or more years of diabetes. In the noninsulin-taking group prevalence remained about 2-5% regardless of
duration.

     Figure 3 presents prevalence of macular edema in one or both
eyes by duration of diabetes. In the older-onset insulin-taking
group prevalence rose steadily from 5% in persons with less than five
years of diabetes to 21% in those with 20 or more years of diabetes.

In the other two groups prevalence was low during the first 10 years
of diabetes (virtually zero in the younger-onset group and about 2%
in the noninsulin-taking group) and then rose to about 18% and 11%,
respectively, in persons with 20 or more years of diabetes.

        Table 2 considers only patients with PDR (Levels 6.0 through 8)
who were examined, giving the distribution of PDR severity in the
worse eye and percent with macular edema in either eye in each age-
at-diagnosis, insulin-use group. Patients entered in this table as
having macular edema had either retinal thickening observed in the
photographs (macular edema status 2) or had scars of focal photocoagulation and a history of previous macular edema (status 3).
Macular edema occurred less frequently in the younger-onset group
than in the older-onset insulin-taking group (29.5% versus 47.4%,
X^2_1 = 8.24, p<.005).
        Table 3 considers only patients with macular edema who were
examined. Patients classified as having macular edema on the basis
of scars of focal photocoagulation and past history are included in
part A of the table and excluded in part B. Only the index eye of
each patient is considered (the right eye, if macular edema was present in it, otherwise the left). PDR was present in 65.4 % of the
younger-onset group, compared to 35.9% of older-onset insulin-taking
patients and 19.4% of the noninsulin-taking group. Visual acuity
less than 20/20 was more common in the older-onset groups (about
90%) than in younger-onset patients (70.4%). Clinically important
cataract or aphakia was more frequent in the older-onset groups
(about 35-40%) than in the younger-onset group (12%). All of the
above differences were significant (p <.001). In the noninsulin-
taking group there were trends towards more frequent involvement of
the center of the macula and a greater area of thickening within
disc-diameter of the center, but these were not significant. Presence of hard exudate equaling or exceeding that in STD #5 was least

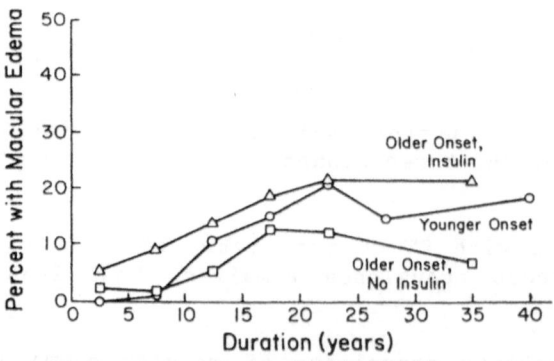

Figure 3   Percent of persons with macular edema (status 2 or 3, see
             methods) by duration of diabetes in each of the three
             groups.

Table 2.   Among persons with PDR examined, percent distribution of
           PDR severity in the worse eye and percent with macular
           edema in either eye, by age at diagnosis of diabetes and
           insulin use.

	Diagnosis before age 30 years	Diagnosis at or after age 30 years	
		Insulin	No Insulin
PDR without HRC (Levels 6.0–6.5)	58.0	66.3	50.0
HRC (Level 7)	22.5	21.1	35.0
Level 8	19.5	12.6	15.0
Total	100.0	100.0	100.0
Macular edema	29.5	47.4	35.0
(Number)	(200)	(95)	(20)

Table 3.   Among persons with macular edema (ME) examined, percent
           with specified characteristic in the index eye, by age at
           diagnosis of diabetes and insulin use.

	Diagnosis before age 30 years	Diagnosis at or after age 30 years	
		Insulin	No Insulin
A. ME present at examination or by history*			
PDR present	65.4	35.9	19.4
VA < 20/20	70.4	90.3	93.6
Cateract	7.4	27.2	32.3
Aphakia	4.9	5.8	9.7
(Number)	(81)	(103)	(31)
B. ME present*			
Extent ≥ 1 disc area	20.3	24.7	42.9
Center involved	54.2	58.0	67.9
HE ≥ STD. #5	1.7	8.6	17.9
(Number)	(59)	(81)	(28)

*See methods section for definitions

frequent in the younger-onset group (1.7%) and most frequent in the noninsulin-taking group (17.9%, Bartholomew's test[2] for linear trend = 7.18, p <.01).

   Table 4 presents the distribution of patients with PDR (Part A) and with macular edema in one or both eyes (Part B) between the three groups. When rates are weighted for the population from which the sample of patients examined was drawn, we estimate that 43.1% of persons with PDR belong to the younger-onset group, 42.3 % to the older-onset insulin-taking group and 14.6% to the noninsulin-taking group. Although PDR was present in 22.2% of the younger-onset group, as compared with 10.5% of the older-onset insulin-taking group, the latter group was twice as large, so that each contributed about equally to the total number with PDR. The non-insulin-taking group was about three times as large as the younger-onset group, so that its contribution to the total was about one-third as great, rather than one-ninth. The older-onset insulin-taking group contributed 59% of the total patients with macular edema, each of the other groups about 20%. Macular edema was about three times more common in the younger-onset group than in non-insulin-taking patients (9.0% versus 3.2%), but because the latter group was three times as numerous, the contribution of each to the total was about the same.

DISCUSSION

   The most striking difference observed in the study was in the prevalence of PDR, which rose rapidly with duration to reach 50%

Table 4.   Percentage distribution of persons with PDR (Part A) and with macular edema (Part B) by age at diagnosis of diabetes and insulin use (weighted*)

| | Diagnosis before age 30 years | Diagnosis at or after age 30 years | | Total |
		Insulin	No Insulin	
A. PDR	43.1	42.3	14.6	100.0
(% of group)	(22.2)	(10.5)	(2.6)	
B. Macular edema	20.1	59.0	20.9	100.0
(% of group)	(9.0)	(12.7)	(3.2)	
(# examined)	(902)	(674)	(696)	(2272)

*See methods section for weighting procedure

after 20 years of diabetes in the younger-onset group, rose at about one-half this rate in the older-onset insulin-taking group and remained at a constant level of about 2-5% with little or no relationship to duration in the noninsulin-taking group (Fig. 2). Given the presence of PDR, however, its severity did not appear to differ between these three groups (Table 2). Although only 2.6% of the noninsulin-taking group had PDR, this group was the largest and contributed 14.6% of the total number with PDR (Table 4).

Prevalence of macular edema was quite similar in the younger-onset and noninsulin-taking groups, although slightly greater in the former after 10 or more years of diabetes (Fig.3). But these groups did appear to differ in regard to certain retinopathy features (Tables 3). In the younger-onset group macular edema was accompanied by PDR in 65% of cases, as compared to 19% in the noninsulin-taking group. In only 2% of the younger-onset group was there a substantial amount of hard exudate within one disc diameter of the center of the macula, as compared to 18% of noninsulin-taking patients. The high frequency of PDR observed in younger-onset patients with macular edema is similar to the findings of others.[1,15] Macular edema was slightly more prevalent in the older-onset insulin-taking group at all diabetes durations, suggesting that both older age and greater severity of diabetes may be risk factors for its occurrence. Current age was not found to be related to macular edema in a multi-variate analysis of these data, but that analysis included only the older-onset groups.[12]

Several reports from ophthalmic clinics have found a substantial majority of patients with macular edema to be 20 years of age or older at diagnosis of diabetes (Kohner, 75% of an unspecified number of patients;[13] Aiello et al., 92 of 111 (83%) patients;[1] Sigelman, 57 of 95 (70%) patients 40 years of age or older at diagnosis.[15] If our patients 30 years of age or older at diagnosis are pooled without regard to insulin use, a comparable proportion of patients with macular edema is found here (80%, Table 4). From Table 4 it is clear that macular edema is seen more frequently in patients with older-onset diabetes largely because this type of diabetes is more common.

Our study, as most before it, relies on age at diagnosis of diabetes and insulin use to classify patients by diabetes type. Presumably nearly all of our younger-onset patients have Type I diabetes and nearly all of our noninsulin-taking group Type II. Comparisons between these groups have the advantage of reducing misclassification of diabetes type. But the more severe cases of Type II diabetes are (presumably) excluded by such a strategy. In this regard it is of interest that among older-onset patients, 27% of those with diabetes of 0-4 years duration were taking insulin, compared with 71% of those with 15 or more years of diabetes. Some of the patients who were started on insulin several years after diagnosis may have developed insulin-dependence, but presumably others have Type II diabetes for which insulin treatment was considered desirable. In some cases insulin treatment may have been started because retinopathy or other complications were observed. If we could identify accurately those older-onset patients who have Type II diabetes, presumably data from them would fall somewhere between those given here for the older-onset insulin-taking and noninsulin-taking groups. If we assume this to be the case, then our findings may be summarized as follows.

In Type I diabetes PDR is more common and is closely related to duration. Macular edema is seen mainly in eyes with PDR, and is rarely associated with more than a small amount of hard exudate.

In Type II diabetes PDR is less common, particularly in non-insulin-taking patients even after many years of diabetes. But because Type II diabetes is more common, it accounts for a substantial proportion of all patients with PDR. When present, PDR is not less severe in Type II than in Type I diabetes. In Type II diabetes macular edema occurs most frequently in the absence of PDR and is more often accompanied by hard exudate. Macular edema is most common in older-onset insulin-taking patients.

ACKNOWLEDGEMENTS

Supported by grant EY03083 (Dr. R. Klein) from the National Eye Institute, and by an unrestricted grant to the Department of Ophthalmology from Research to Prevent Blindness, Inc.

The authors are grateful to the 452 Wisconsin physicians and their staffs who participated and supported this study; to Moneen M. Meuer, BA for project coordination; to Stacy E. Meuer, BA for data management; to Steven D. Kessler, OD and Karen A. Richie, BA who examined participants; to Yvonne Magli, MA, Rose Brothers, BS, Magnus Harding, BS, Cheryl Hiner, BS, Mary Peckham, BA, and Anita Temple, BS for detailed grading of the fundus photographs; to Anik Ganguly, BE, MBA and Larry Hubbard, MA for programming and data management advice; and to the state of Wisconsin division of Health which donated the van.

REFERENCES

1. L.M. Aiello, L.I. Rand, and J.C. Briones, Diabetic retinopathy in Joslin Clinic patients with adult-onset diabetes, Opthalmology, 88:619-23 (1981).
2. D.J. Bartholomew, A test of homogeniety for ordered alternatives, Biometrika, 46:328, p. 36-48 (1959).

3. F.L. Caird, A. Pirie, and T.G. Ramsell, Diabetes and the Eye, Blackwell Scientific Publications, Oxford, England, Chap.6 (1969).

4. Diabetic Retinopathy Study Research Group, Report 7, A modification of the Airlie House classification of diabetic retinopathy, Invest. Ophthalmol. Vis. Sci. 21:210-226 (1981).

5. Diabetic Retinopathy Study Research Group, Photocoagulation treatment of proliferative diabetic retinopathy: Clinical application of Diabetic Retinopathy Study (DRS) findings, DRS report number 8, Ophthalmology, 88:583-600 (1981).

6. Early Treatment Diabetic Retinopathy Study Coordinating Center, Manual of Operations, Baltimore, Diabetic Retinopathy Coordinating Center, Chap. 11 (1980).

7. Early Treatment Diabetic Retinopathy Study Coordinating Center, Manual of Operations, Baltimore, Diabetic Retinopathy Coordinating Center, Chap. 5 and 18 (1980).

8. J. Harberg, D. Holladay, and S. Entine, WISAR: Wisconsin Storage and Retrieval System, Wisconsin Clinical Cancer Center, Madison, Wis., (1979).

9. B.E.K. Klein, M.D. Davis, and P. Segal, et al., Diabetic retinopathy, Assessment of severity and progression. Ophthalmology, 91(1):10-17 (1984).

10. R. Klein, B.E.K. Klein, and S.E. Moss, Visual impairment in diabetes, Ophthalmology. 91:1-8 (1984).

11. R. Klein, B.E.K. Klein, and S. Moss, et al., The Wisconsin Epidemiologic Study of Diabetic Retinopathy. 2. Prevalence and risk of diabetic retinopathy when age at diagnosis is less than 30 years, Arch. Ophthalmol. 102: 520-526 (1984).

12. R. Klein, B.E.K. Klein, and S.E. Moss, et al, The Wisconsin Epidemiologic Study of Diabetic Retinopathy, 4. Diabetic macular edema, Ophthalmology, in press.

13. E.M. Kohner, The evolution and natural history of diabetic retinopathy, Int. Opthalmol. Clin. 18:1-16 (1978).

14. P. Plamberg, M. Smith, and S. Waltman, et al., The natural history of retinopathy in insulin-dependent juvenile-onset diabetes, Ophthalmology, 88:613-618 (1981).

15 J. Sigelman, Diabetic macular edema in juvenile and adult-onset diabetes, Am. J. Ophthalmol. 90.287-96 (1980).

16. Writing Committe on Behalf of the HDFP Cooperative Group, The Hypertension Detection and Follow-up Program, Prev. Med. 5:207-315 (1976).

SOME SUMMARIZING THOUGHTS

George F. Cahill, Jr.

Howard Hughes Medical Institute
398 Brookline Avenue
Boston, MA 02215 USA

For the past ten to fifteen years diabetologists have emphasized the numerous differences separating that type of diabetes
mainly affecting children, associated with an autoimmune destruction
of the beta cells (Type I or IDDM, Insulin-Dependent Diabetes
Mellitus) and that type affecting primarily individuals in later
life and closely associated with aging, overnutrition and diminished
exercise (Type II or NIDDM, Non-Insulin-Dependent Diabetes
Mellitus). As a result of this trend in differentiating these two
broad categories, the National Diabetes Data Group published in 1979
an official classification which was subsequently accepted by the
World Health Organization and which demarcates the two disease
entities from each other (see chapter by Bennett). It is now
interesting that this apparently clear differentiation is becoming
less precise as more data accumulate. In fact, the ecumenical
exuberance of the late 1970s to segregate all diabetics into either
Type I or Type II was perhaps a little too unsophisticated in that
some individuals, such as those with maturity-onset diabetes occurring in youth, or those in whom a kind of insulin-dependent type
diabetes develops late in life after many years of what is clearly
Type II diabetes obviously can't be classified in either of the two
broad categories. The nomenclature itself is even confusing since
it is now obvious that there is a prodromal phase to Type I diabetes
when the patient is not dependent on insulin and, likewise, many in
the remission or "honeymoon" phase can go off insulin for variable
periods of time. Thus these subjects are strictly not
"insulin-dependent".

Conversely, as just mentioned above, there are elderly subjects
who have had a long history of progressively deteriorating beta cell

function, and who are absolutely dependent on at least one, and
frequently two, injections of insulin daily to remain out of ketoacidosis and in acceptable control. Thus operationally these
patients are physiologically insulin-dependent, but in a few
subjects who have been studied most are islet cell antibody
negative, and therefore are simply a result of a progressively
age-deteriorating demise of their beta cells. It is encouraging to
know that the National Institute of Arthritis, Digestive, Diabetes
and Kidney Disease (NIADDK) is now assembling a work group to
reconsider the entire classification, and particularly to make
subdivisions relative to the recent data of the past two to three
years. Thus the chapters in this volume by Bennett and Keen have
emphasized this need for new nomenclature in order to deal more
rationally with classification, both from a pathophysiological as
well as a therapeutic viewpoint.

     Dr. Permutt of St. Louis and Dr. Lernmark of Copenhagen, in
their respective chapters, have underscored the tremendous impact
that the new technology of molecular biology has brought to the
etiologic pathophysiology of some of the common diseases, particularly diabetes. All investigators now accept that the predisposition to Type I diabetes is inherited on chromosome #6 in close
linkage to the D locus. Thus approximately two-thirds of siblings
both with Type I diabetes are haplo-identical and over 90% of the
time they share at least one chromosome #6. Of more importance, the
risk for diabetics of being haploidentical to a known Type I
diabetic equals that of being a discordant identical twin, and this
therefore leaves little room for other inherited factors. Thus, not
only is the predisposition inherited on chromosome #6, but certain
markers, particularly DR-3 and DR-4 appear to be closely associated
with the disease. In the United States, just under half of the
total population bear a DR-3 or a DR-4, but of Type I diabetes 95%
have one or the other of these, and more interestingly, approximately half of all Type I diabetics have both DR-3 and DR-4, namely,
the mixed heterozygote. This mixed heterozygote in the general
population is only 1/2% meaning a 50-fold increase in prevalence as
compared to the general population.

     Turning it the other way around, one can state that of all of
the children in the United States who are the mixed heterozygote
DR-3/DR-4, about one in ten of these will be taking insulin by age
eighteen in comparison to about one in 300 in the general population. Thus we are at the point where we can almost predict which
child is at risk, and if one adds to the risk profile islet cell
antibody positivity as determined by one of several different
methods, as discussed by Lernmark and Permutt, then one is getting
to the point of not only giving an actuarial risk but essentially in
being able to single out which child will almost certainly come down
with the overt disease within the next few years. Thus, if one
assembles a number of factors, one can separate the high risk from

the low risk child, but the question then arises what does one do with this information? I'm not sure, were I a parent, would I want to know, as long as I was aware of the signs and symptoms should they appear and if so, would then begin to initiate appropriate therapy.

Thus, the paradigm for the peak risk child would be a twelve-year-old Finnish male who is the mixed DR-3/DR-4 heterozygote who is either an identical twin, and thus obviously shares the DR-3/DR-4 with his diabetic twin, or else is a haplo-identical sibling of a documented Type I diabetic. Finally, if one wants to add a final touch to the predisposition, one can state that this twelve-year-old Finnish lad has recently turned islet cell antibody positive and, although the definitive data have not yet been collected, were he to be islet cell antibody positive, both by the cytoplasmic technique and by the cell surface and by the complement fixing methodologies, this would probably all the more increase the degree of certainty that he is certainly getting the disease and is presently gradually destroying his beta cells as time passes. Also, if one could demonstrate cell-mediated cytotoxicity using his lymphocytes, as well as alterations in ratios of helper and suppressor cells and an increase in Ia bearing lymphocytes, these all would support that he is undergoing a progressive immuno-destruction of his insulin-producing tissues (see chapter by Lernmark).

Under the current nomenclature, what would you call this child if he still had normal glucose tolerance including a normal first-phase insulin release? By the old criteria, being haplo-identical or an identical twin to a known diabetic, he would fall in the "potential" category, but if he had all of the various components listed above, he really has classical Type I diabetes, but still not enough beta cell destruction to have any evidence of metabolic disturbance. Thus, reclassification is mandatory as this Symposium has emphasized.

Continuing along on the above hypothetical patient, a number of workers, particularly the Ganda, Soeldner, Eisenbarth group at the Joslin Clinic (see Lernmark chapter) have demonstrated that the first metabolic evidence of progressive beta cell destruction is the loss of first-phase insulin release to intravenous glucose stimulation. Insulin release to a number of other stimuli, such as sulfonylurea, glucagon, isoproterenol are all indistinguishable from normal. It is apparently the rapid insulin response to a glucose load given intravenously which is deficient. It is interesting that the insulin response to oral glucose may still persist, and this is very reminiscent of what happens in Type II diabetes where, again, the earliest and minimal lesion is the loss of first-phase insulin release to glucose stimulation with persisting maintenance of insulin release to a number of other secretogogues as reviewed by Porte in this volume. Thus, there is a commonality between Type I and Type II diabetes and the recent work of Gordon Weir and his colleagues in Virginia in experimental animals (see Porte chapter) have likewise shown that as time progresses in the rat after subtotal pancreatectomy, the earliest detectable lesion is loss of first-phase insulin release to glucose stimulation.

The molecular probes discussed by both Drs. Permutt and Lernmark (particularly the latter) have demonstrated that one can be much more precise in mapping genetic differences between individuals than simply by using serological antibody-determined polymorphisms. Thus the molecular probes for the Class II histocompatibility antigens have shown an even greater association of certain polymorphisms with Type I diabetes than have the immunological segregation into DR-3 and DR-4 categories. One has to keep in mind, however, that this may simply still be a closely-linked association of two genes without any pathophysiological meaning, one being the diabetes gene and the other the histocompatibility gene. Since, however, Type I diabetes appears to be due to an autoimmune destruction of the beta cells, it is not surprising (and, in fact, it might be expected) that the inheritance would be related to the inheritance of the immune response of Class II genes. Thus the molecular probe may be getting right to the specific target, which does or does not initiate the progressive autoimmune destruction of the beta cells and therefore separates the Type I diabetes-prone population from the rest.

However, the correlations on chromosome #11 5[1] to the insulin gene are not as clear. These may still represent a kind of founder effect in which certain gene groupings in a given population might be passed along to descendents of the population along with a gene causing some disease entity - the two not having any physiological or pathological correlation, except having both arisen in the same starting population. I always like to point out a rather ludicrous example of this, namely that dark skin by statistical association makes red cells sickle or, turning it around the other way, sickling red cells make the skin turn dark - both of these being obviously highly significant statistically, but with obviously no known pathophysiological connection! Thus the polymorphisms associated with Type I diabetes on chromosome #11 may simply be reflections of polymorphisms in Northern European populations in which one finds a higher incidence of Type I diabetes.

Next, a few words are in order concerning insulin resistance and beta cell secretion as discussed in the chapters by Porte and Olefsky. So much has been said over the past decade about insulin receptors and peripheral insulin resistance in Type II diabetes and other associated states, such as obesity, that one tends to lose the basic concept that in the fasting state it is the liver that sets the level of blood glucose. This is easily supported by the fact if one looks at an overnight fasted individual; glucose uptake is primarily by brain, red cells, white cells and other tissues such as peripheral nerve and renal medulla, and as far as we know, all of these are not acutely insulin-sensitive, as evidenced by glucose uptake. Thus very little glucose is removed by insulin-sensitive tissues in the fasted state, and what therefore sets the ambient level of glucose in the body is the interrelationship between insulin, blood glucose concentration and the liver.

Dr. Vranic in his introductory chapter has presented some very fascinating information that in the diabetic there appears to be a greater degree of hexose phosphate recycling in the liver, particularly after glucose loading, but it is still possible that a component of this may play a role in the fasted state. It is my guess that the major breakthrough in the therapy of the non-insulin-dependent or Type II diabetic will not relate to peripheral sensitivity or insensitivity to insulin, but rather to some mechanism in trying to reset the liver to an ambient glucose concentration of 80 or 90 mg/dl rather than 125 or greater.

Another point which deserves emphasis is that there are literally millions of Northern Americans walking around with a typical life style of physical inactivity, overnutrition and various degrees of obesity who do not have diabetes, and they do this because their beta cells are able to muster up the high levels of insulin needed to overcome their insulin resistance. Thus they may end secreting 200 or even 300 units of insulin per day and achieve perfectly normal glucose homeostasis, including first-phase insulin release. Likewise, Dr. Freinkel in his chapter on gestational diabetes has shown that normal (in fact, even super-normal) glucose homeostasis is achieved in the non-diabetic pregnant female, thanks mainly to augmented beta cell function. For years pathologists have pointed out the beta cell hyperplasia, both in non-diabetic pregnancy and in uncomplicated obesity. Thus there is in most normal individuals a capacity for the insulin-producing machinery to hypertrophy when challenged by counter-insulin processes. An inability to do this obviously leads to Type II diabetes and, for that matter, also to Type I diabetes after sufficient beta cell destruction has occurred in the latter, the commonality being perhaps loss of first phase insulin release. Thus it is this author's hypothesis that there is a spectrum in Type II diabetes in which there may be only a minimal senescence and depletion of beta cells but, because of sufficent insulin resistance, diabetes occurs. Conversely, there are on the other end of the spectrum others (and this is the thin, active, long-standing diabetic) with little if any peripheral insulin resistance who primarily have a progressive age-related beta cell demise, but still are Type II or non-insulin-dependent diabetics by classification, however may yet require insulin to avoid ketoacidosis.

Finally we come to the complications of both types of diabetes and the fact that every complication be it retinal maculopathy or proliferating diabetic retinopathy or peripheral neuropathy or classical nodular glomerulosclerosis - all of these appear in both the Type I and Type II diabetic (chapters by Mauer, Dyck and Davis). Generally speaking, it is true that the Type I is more at risk to develop proliferating retinopathy and the Type II diabetic the maculopathy, but there obviously are other effects contributing to both, namely, duration of diabetes as well as the age of the patient himself or herself.

It is interesting to point out, however, how much more aware the diabetologist is today of both types of diabetics developing precisely the same lesions. These observations really emphasize that the complications are probably secondary to the abnormal metabolic milieu and not due to a primary genetic disorder in which the complication is an expression of the inherited process. Instead the metabolic process results from relative or absolute insulin deficiency. More and more, it looks like the specific lesions - namely the retinopathy, nephropathy and neuropathy are secondary to the "hyperglycemia-years", but with the recent evidence that aldose reductase inhibition can improve neuropathy, the precise pathogenic sequence continues unclear. In other words, glycosylation of protein alone, due to the hyperglycemia, cannot be the sole offender if diminution of sorbitol production using aldose reductase inhibitors can provide symptomatic relief. In any case, the question is still up in the air and much research has yet to be done.

In conclusion, we are faced with many challenges. One is why inheritance of a factor on chromosome #6 leads to autoimmune destruction of beta cells, probably provoked by some environment signal such as a virus, as borne out by the fact that identical twins are concordant for Type I diabetes between one-quarter and one-half the time. In Type II diabetes there appears to be some age-related deficiency in beta cells function, and this appears to be unmasked by various degrees of ineffectiveness of insulin and thus Type II diabetes is a more heterogeneous disorder.

Finally, the increasing clarification of the pathological process in both Type I and Type II diabetes necessitates further diagnostic definitions, particularly as interventions are being initiated in the former. In both types the natural history continues to be elucidated in epidemiologic studies, particularly in relation to therapy, and again more definitive reclassifications are and will be developed.

INDEX